Making Research Relevant

Making Research Relevant is the ideal core textbook for master's-level introduction to research methods courses in any mental health field.

Accessible and user friendly, it is designed to help trainees and practitioners understand, connect, and apply research to clinical practice and day-to-day work with students and clients. The text covers foundational concepts, such as research ethics, the consumption of research, and how to analyze data, as well as an additional 11 applied, evaluative, and outcome-based research methods that can be applied in practice.

Easy to read, conversational chapters are infused with case examples from diverse settings, paired with brief video lectures and a practice-based application section which provide vignettes and practice to guide application and visual components that demonstrate how research methods can benefit mental health practitioners in real-world scenarios.

Kelly L. Wester, PhD, is a professor of counselor education at the University of North Carolina at Greensboro. She has taught graduate courses in research and provided workshops on research methodology.

Carrie A. Wachter Morris, PhD, is a professor of counselor education at the University of North Carolina at Greensboro and past president of the Association of Assessment and Research in Counseling.

"*Making Research Relevant* is true to its name. Wester and Wachter Morris have developed a textbook that contextualizes research within counseling practices. This is the exact textbook I needed for my research courses, and using it has transformed students' experiences: they better grasp research concepts and methods, take more ownership of their researcher identity, and feel inspired to integrate data gathering into their clinical work. What an essential resource for counseling students and practitioners, especially with the need to increasingly measure impact and conduct outcome-based research."

Maribeth F. Jorgensen, *PhD, LPC (TX/SD), LMHC (WA), LIMHP (NE),*
NCC, associate professor, Department of Counselor Education,
Sam Houston State University

"Reading this textbook felt like having conversations with the authors. The content is so accessible. Through the use of case examples, the authors demystify research methods by applying them to relevant counseling scenarios. I turned every page with a sense of connection as I was invited to consider my own identity as a researcher, the larger picture of our work with clients, and how research paves the way for greater efficacy and new possibilities."

Christina Jelinek, *master's counseling student*

"I never considered assuming a researcher identity before reading *Making Research Relevant*. I now see research as an integral part of becoming an effective counselor. I appreciated how the authors included case examples as that brought the material to life. Reading this book as a counseling student has inspired me to collect data from my future clients to ensure they are receiving effective counseling."

Brooke Angonia, *master's counseling student*

"*Making Research Relevant* is a practical guide for counselors in training to learn how to apply research methods to their future work, whether on a small scale like checking in-session effectiveness or on a large scale like a program evaluation. This book helped me to grow more confident in my counselor-researcher identity by showing me how research is intertwined with my responsibilities as a practitioner. Its straightforward nature and use of light humor kept me engaged from beginning to end. This book is a tool I plan to use during the remainder of my training and when I'm in the field."

Sydnee Jaynes, *master's counseling student*

"*Making Research Relevant* makes research accessible to students and practitioners. With these skills, counselors can evaluate their own effectiveness and collect evidence to inform their own practice. More importantly, the authors have considered the tools and resources counselors in the field will have access to so they can continue to use research to practice. Teaching with this text has brought students' practice to life so that they not only validate the client's experience but validate their development as counselors."

Jennifer D. Deaton, *PhD, LCMHC, assistant professor,*
University of North Carolina at Greensboro

Making Research Relevant

Applied Research Designs for the Mental Health Practitioner

Second Edition

Edited by Kelly L. Wester and Carrie A. Wachter Morris

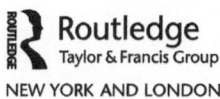
Routledge
Taylor & Francis Group

NEW YORK AND LONDON

Designed cover image: © Getty Images

Second edition published 2025
by Routledge
605 Third Avenue, New York, NY 10158

and by Routledge
4 Park Square, Milton Park, Abingdon, Oxon, OX14 4RN

Routledge is an imprint of the Taylor & Francis Group, an informa business

First edition published by Routledge 2018

ISBN: 978-1-032-69843-4 (hbk)
ISBN: 978-1-032-69008-7 (pbk)
ISBN: 978-1-032-70613-9 (ebk)

DOI: 10.4324/9781032706139

Access the Support Material: www.routledge.com/9781032690087

Typeset in Galliard
by SPi Technologies India Pvt Ltd (Straive)

Contents

Editors

Kelly L. Wester, PhD, NCC, LCMHC (NC) is a professor in the Department of Counseling and Educational Development at the University of North Carolina at Greensboro. She has worked in clinical practice with preadolescents through adults in juvenile correctional facilities, residential treatment facilities, college counseling centers, and outpatient mental health agencies. Her research focuses on non-suicidal self-injury and suicidal behavior among adolescents, young adults, and adults.

Carrie A. Wachter Morris, PhD, NCC, ACS is a professor in the Department of Counseling and Ed.ucational Development at the University of North Carolina at Greensboro. Her clinical focus is on school counseling. She is a past president of the Association for Assessment and Research in Counseling. Her research interests include school counselor education, crisis prevention and intervention, and innovation in pedagogy.

Contributors

Amy Allison, MRC, CRC has co-authored a previous text chapter on program evaluation and is currently doing clinical work with clients experiencing eating disorders, substance use disorders, and co-occurring disorders. Amy has a strong background in group work and spent a number of years doing group work with people experiencing eating disorders. Amy focuses on blending strong clinical counseling skills with movement-based therapeutic techniques. Amy is a certified yoga instructor and often blends her expertise into wellness-based programming aimed at helping at-risk populations through the recovery and rehabilitation process. Amy's strong group and clinical skills allow her a unique perspective in applying program evaluation principles to her work.

Arianna Alverio is a second year in her M.S. Clinical Mental Health Counseling program at Jacksonville University. She received a bachelor's degree in psychology from CUNY, Queens College. She is interested in substance use, marriage and family, and youth risk populations. She currently interns at SMA Project WARM, an all-women's inpatient treatment facility.

Jordan L. Austin is an assistant professor of Counseling in the School of Counseling and Human Services at Lenior-Rhyne University. Her research interests include counseling trainee development, clinical supervision, and emotional complexity and emotion regulation. In addition, she provides clinical services using a trauma- and attachment-informed lens to adults, couples, and families.

Yuliya Cannon, PhD is an organizational design and transformation consultant, specializing in supporting organizations through their digital transformation journeys. She holds a PhD in counselor education from the University of Texas at San Antonio (UTSA) and brings a deep understanding of behavioral science into the corporate world. With a unique blend of expertise in counseling, behavioral economics, and human-centered design, Dr. Cannon empowers organizational leaders and teams to consider the psychological impact of organizational change on individuals. She assists in developing the necessary skills and competencies to successfully navigate the human side of change.

Heather Delgado, PhD, LCMHCA, NCC is an assistant professor in the Department of Special Education, Rehabilitation, and Counseling at Auburn University. In this role, she teaches both masters and doctoral students and serves as the doctoral program coordinator. Her background is in clinical mental health counseling and she is a Licensed Clinical Mental Health Counselor Associate. Her research interests include issues of grief and loss in counseling, suicide prevention and intervention, and professional identify development of counselors.

Holly Downs is the director of the Propel Next project (a leadership and evaluation virtual learning journey for nonprofits) at the Center for Creative Leadership (CCL). Her research and evaluation work investigates the implementation and impact of programs delivered via traditional and virtual learning environments. She holds a Ph.D. in educational psychology from the University of Illinois at Urbana-Champaign.

Amanda L. Giordano, PhD, LPC (GA) is an associate professor in the Department of Counseling and Human Development Services at the University of Georgia. She specializes in addictions counseling and is the sole author of a clinical reference book titled *A Clinical Guide to Treating Behavioral Addictions* and co-author of a textbook titled *Addiction Counseling: A Practical Approach.* Dr. Giordano works to advance the counseling field with rigorous research and has published over 60 peer-reviewed articles and book chapters. She regularly offers community trainings and workshops related to addictions counseling, has been a guest on podcasts and keynote speaker, and writes a blog for *Psychology Today* called, "Understanding Addiction."

Ye He, is a professor in the Teacher Education and Higher Education Department at the University of North Carolina at Greensboro. She works with educators to engage students and families from diverse cultural and linguistic backgrounds. She teaches a doctoral-level course on mixed methods research, and her research focuses on the promotion of strength-based and community-engaged practices in education.

Maribeth F. Jorgensen, PhD, LPC (TX/SD), LMHC (WA), LIMHP (NE), NCC is an associate professor in the Department of Counselor Education at Sam Houston State University (SHSU). She also serves as the director of the College of Education Research Center at SHSU. Her primary area of scholarship is researcher identity development, with the goal of further integrating research and clinical practice. Maribeth primarily teaches research and clinical courses. In addition to her work as a counselor educator, she has been a licensed professional counselor since 2006 and sees individuals experiencing death and nondeath losses.

A. Stephen Lenz is a professor of counselor education at Texas A&M University-San Antonio. He is a licensed professional counselor who holds degrees in counselor education, clinical psychology, and health promotion. Dr. Lenz is interested in approaches to mental health prevention and intervention at the individual and community levels that support well-being and development across the lifespan. His research interests include holistic approaches to student development, assessment development and evaluation, and outcome research and evaluation.

W. Bradley McKibben, PhD, NCC, BC-TMH is an associate professor in the Department of Clinical Mental Health Counseling at Jacksonville University and editor for *Teaching and Supervision in Counseling*, the official journal of the Southern Association for Counselor Education and Supervision. His research interests include the supervisory relationship, influences of attachment strategies, counselor development, and multicultural considerations in clinical supervision, as well as clinical outcomes in emotionally focused therapy. He employs a variety of quantitative, qualitative, and mixed method research approaches, and he regularly publishes about research methodologies, including "how to" journal articles and book chapters on various research paradigms.

Casey A. Barrio Minton, PhD, NCC is a professor of counselor education at the University of Tennessee, Knoxville. Her scholarly work focuses on crisis intervention, clinical mental health issues, and professionalization through teaching and leadership. Casey is a past-president of Chi Sigma Iota International, the Association for Assessment and Research in Counseling, and the Association for Counselor Education and Supervision. She is founding editor of *Journal for Counselor Leadership and Advocacy* and editor of *Counselor Education & Supervision*. Casey is a Fellow of the American Counseling Association.

Dee C. Ray, PhD, LPC-S, NCC, RPT-S is Regents Professor and Elaine Millikan Mathes Professor in early childhood education in the counseling program and co-director of the Center for Play Therapy at the University of North Texas. Dr. Ray's scholarly research has focused on both quantitative and qualitative methods, with particular focus on the exploration of counseling interventions through randomized controlled trials. Dr. Ray additionally operates the counseling practice, EmpathyWell, in Highland Village, TX where she facilitates play therapy, training, and supervision.

Kathleen Brown-Rice, PhD, LPC-S (TX), LPC (SD), LCMHC (NC), ACS, NCC is a professor of counselor education in the College of Education at Sam Houston State University. She has worked as a professional counselor in various clinical settings and currently operates a private practice assisting clients with mental health, trauma, and substance abuse issues. Dr. Rice's scholarly research activity focuses on counselor supervision and training with an emphasis in ethical considerations, the implications of historical/generational trauma, and the impact of substance abuse on individuals, families, and the community. She also incorporates the use of biomarkers in her research to understand emotional regulation, risky behaviors, and resiliency.

Deborah L. Smith is a Licensed Professional Counselor, certified trauma-focused equine-assisted psychotherapist, and clinical professional counselor supervisor. She earned a bachelor's degree in psychology in 1992 from the University of Florida, a master's degree in clinical psychology from Wheaton College in 1994, and has worked as a clinician in residential, college, and private practice settings. She is currently a PhD student in the Counselor Education and Supervision program at the University of Georgia. Her research interests include trauma, equine therapy and its effectiveness, and the experiences of refugees and providers who serve the refugee population.

Heather Trepal, PhD, LPC-S (TX) is a professor of counseling and associate dean for Academic Programs and Student Success in the College of Education and Human Development at the University of Texas at San Antonio. She is the co-author of *Non-Suicidal Self-Injury: Wellness Perspectives on Behaviors, Symptoms, and Diagnosis*.

Lindsey K. Umstead, PhD, LCMHC, NCC, CEDS is a Licensed Clinical Mental Health Counselor, National Certified Counselor, and Certified Eating Disorders Specialist based in Raleigh, North Carolina. Dr. Umstead works in private practice with teens, adults, and families recovering from eating and feeding disorders, trauma, and anxiety and mood concerns. She remains active in teaching and research within counselor Eeducation in addition to serving as education chair for the North Carolina chapter of the International Association of Eating Disorders Professionals.

Shreya Vaishnav, PhD is an assistant professor in the Counseling Department at Palo Alto University. Her research focuses on the impact of microaggressions on students from marginalized identities and she has facilitated workshops on navigating and responding to microaggressions in academia. She has also led research projects on effective mentoring practices for students and faculty, strengths-based approaches in working with students from marginalized backgrounds, and social justice advocacy. Her clinical expertise lies in working with immigrant populations on cross-cultural issues, specifically South Asian immigrants and first-generation Asian Americans.

Edward Wahesh, PhD, ACS, NCC is an associate professor in the Department of Education and Counseling at Villanova University in Villanova, Pennsylvania. He has counseling experience in drug and alcohol, mental health, secondary, and collegiate settings. Dr. Wahesh actively researches, publishes, and presents on topics related to counselor training as well as the prevention and treatment of substance misuse and co-occurring disorders. He is also the co-author of *Motivational Interviewing in Clinical Mental Health Counseling.*

Michael Walsh, PhD, LPC (SC), CRC, CPRP is a clinical associate professor in the Counseling and Rehabilitation program at the University of South Carolina School of Medicine. Mike has served the field as an executive director for a psychiatric rehabilitation-based nonprofit organization, while also filling the clinical director role for the same organization. This allowed Mike to develop program evaluation skills in both organizational and clinical settings. A key part of much of Mike's experience with the nonprofit sector was grant writing and the inclusion of program evaluation tools as quality markers. Mike currently has a private practice assisting clients with mental health and wellness, as well as optimization of performance. Mike's scholarly research activity ranges from assessing and evaluating learning community–based counselor education programs to the utilization of innovative approaches such as virtual technologies in both clinical and educational settings.

1 Introduction

Carrie A. Wachter Morris, Kelly L. Wester, Shreya Vaishnav, and Jordan L. Austin

Research. Some may agree that it is necessary and required, thus engaging in it in their daily practice. Others may view research as a swear word, something that is done begrudgingly when it is **required**. Still others may even see it as something to be avoided at all costs. Yet, regardless of what your perspective is on research, all practitioners need to understand how to consume, apply, and conduct research. You might find yourself asking, "why?" That is a great question, and we have a lot of different answers to it, many of which we will explain in this text.

You'll notice that throughout this chapter—and indeed, throughout the book—we use the word "practitioner" to describe an individual who might work with clients or students in a variety of mental health and educational settings. This is done purposefully, as a variety of individuals can learn from the research generated not only within their own field, but also from sister professions with a similar goal of helping people. Thus, we hope that whatever your primary professional identity, whether it be that of counselor, school counselor, social worker, school social worker, marriage and family therapist, college counselor, student affairs specialist, psychologist, human development specialist, teacher, or one of the myriad of practitioners that we have not directly named, that you can see yourself and your work represented within this text when we say "practitioner." Working together, we can increase what we all know about how to help our clients and students be successful. Before we dive into research, we want you to take a moment and think about the work that you do, or the work that you hope to do in the future.

Picture yourself practicing—working with your clients or students. How do you want to impact them? How would you know whether you're effective as you help them navigate the challenges that they face? A practitioner's role is ultimately to help people find what they need to better function in their daily lives. This may be by helping them reduce psychological symptoms and maladaptive behaviors, by working with them to increase overall wellness, or by teaching them ways to cultivate healthier relationships. In working with others – whether you work with them in outpatient mental health, inpatient behavioral health, a K-12 school, a college or university, an integrated care setting, a private practice, or something else altogether – the fundamental outcome you are probably hoping for is to be effective in meeting your and your clients' or students' goals. This will mean that you want to be able to tell that what you are doing is, in fact, working.

And while your work with clients or students may be the primary reason that you want to be effective, it will not be the only reason. For example, in your work as a practitioner you will often be working *for* somebody else. We know that some of you may be your own boss in a private practice or an agency that you own (which we will get to shortly), but many others of

DOI: 10.4324/9781032706139-1

you will have bosses including principals, superintendents, directors, senior clinicians, department chairs, supervisors, or any number of other possible titles or roles. As your boss, *they* want to know that what you are doing is working. Otherwise, they may choose to replace you with another practitioner, or if budgets decrease, they may need to lay off individuals from their current jobs. If that is the case, they are more than likely going to select the individuals in their organization that are either (a) not necessary, or (b) not able to show that they are effective at what they do. For example, we have seen school counselors save positions that were scheduled to be cut in lean financial times because they were able to demonstrate to their superintendents and school boards what they did in their schools makes a difference through not just anecdotal evidence, but also through effectiveness data. When we are effective, we are more likely to be retained, receive pay increases or bonuses, and be promoted within an organization.

But, for argument's sake, let's say that you are your own boss. Though this may be true, your salary or payment may still come from third-party payers including insurance companies, grants, Medicare or Medicaid, or other outside payment agencies. More frequently, these agencies and organizations are asking for evidence that they are providing payment to practitioners who are effective. For some, this may mean that practitioners are solely utilizing empirically based treatments, such as cognitive behavior therapy. But other organizations and, we suspect, most third-party payers and insurance companies in the future, will require data and evidence that what you are doing is working – not only to allow you to have additional sessions with clients, but also to pay you for individual sessions. As a society, we have moved toward outcome-based evidence – and it may not be too far in the future that practitioners will have to provide evidence of their effectiveness in their day-to-day work with individuals.

Finally, and perhaps the most important of these factors to consider, is the client or the student – the consumer for whom you are providing a service. This may be in any setting and in any format (e.g., individual therapy, group therapy, family therapy, psychoeducation, classroom guidance, integrated medical care, assessments, consultation, and more). Ultimately, *they* want to know that what you are doing is working. They want to know that you are helping them reach their goals as you work with them. You owe it to them to be able to demonstrate, concretely, that you are an effective practitioner. First, let's take a simple example of what we mean. You have a mother who is bringing her adolescent child to you in an outpatient office setting. This child has been experiencing high levels of anxiety, to the point that she doesn't even want to leave the house. In what has taken at least an hour if not more, this mother has been able to get her teenage daughter to come and see you in your office, which is no small feat to say the least. Each time this youth comes to see you, it will be a huge effort for this mom. Mom has expressed willingness to do this – as long as what you are doing is working. She will be able to know what you do is working because she will see it. She will see the symptoms decrease, she will notice her daughter's anxiety lessen, and the ability for her to go to school or come to your office become easier week by week. While we can "see" symptomology decrease anecdotally, we also need to explore it empirically … through data … to show in numbers or subjective statements that what we are doing is working. Given how extreme this adolescent's anxiety is, her symptoms are not likely to decrease in one week. Her anxiety may not even decrease in a month or two. So, how do you help the mom (and the adolescent) know that what you are doing is working and that working to alleviate this elevated level of anxiety will take some time? You provide hard evidence of symptoms decreasing among previous clients. You provide data from research.

As another example, the population of many countries including the United States is becoming more racially and ethnically diverse (Zhou, 2003). Until recently, many of the interventions and theories guiding our work as practitioners have been focused on a Eurocentric view of clients and students. As the clients with whom we are working become more diverse, research is needed to ensure that ALL our clients' needs are being met, particularly if their cultural identities have not traditionally been represented by clinical research. One of the best ways to generate this research is for practitioners to engage in research in their own settings and to share their results.

All these individuals and organizations – your client or student, your boss, your employer, the place where you are receiving your income from, and you – all want to know that what you are doing is effective and working. This is where research comes into play. This is what research *does* for you and for the helping professions. It is how we know which treatments and interventions are most effective.

Are you convinced that research is vital to your clinical practice? Not yet? Okay, let's consider a more practical example. Picture yourself in your ideal position. Where are you? What are you doing? Now imagine you meet a client (or student or patient) for the first time. When this individual presents to you for treatment, what will you typically do? Usually, regardless of setting, we start by collecting information. In some settings, this may be through a formal, structured, intake interview, while in others it may be a series of brief questions to help you understand why that person sought your services. Some practitioners have information in a file prior to the first meeting, while others may not. Regardless, your goal in this first meeting is typically to gather information about your client.

As you can see in Figure 1.1, the scientific method connects well to clinical practice – regardless of setting. In this example of meeting a client and collecting some information,

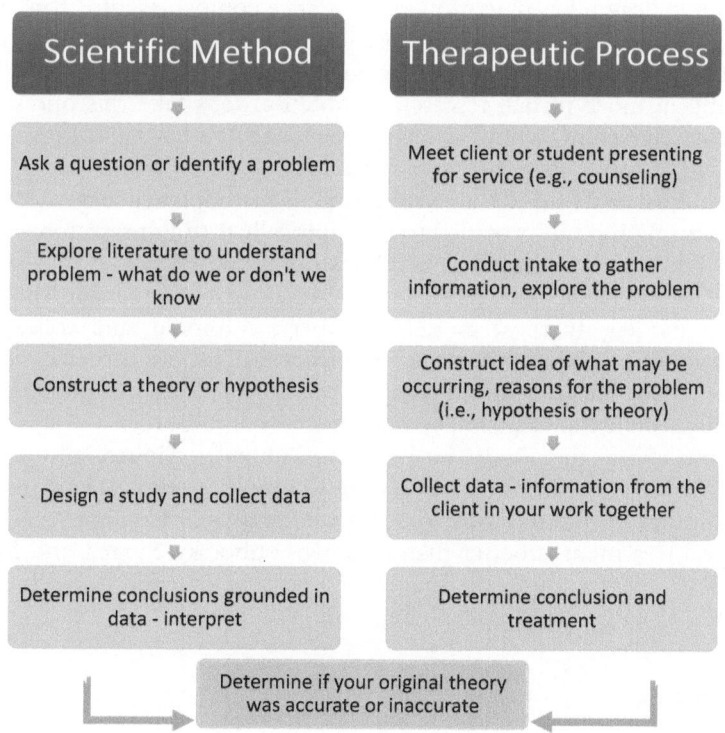

Figure 1.1 Scientific method aligned with clinical practice.

you are asking questions to determine the problem and then searching for an explanation to the problem through the questions you may ask this client.

After you have gathered some initial information, you will likely construct an idea of what you believe may be the client's presenting issue. For example, is the client having difficulties or presenting with symptoms due to depression, or anxiety, or relationship conflict, or substance use? Might this student have family difficulties in their home, or not have a good way of coping to manage their emotions or other problems? Typically, once you gather information from a client or student, you develop an idea of what you believe may be the underlying reason for the problem. This idea is what you would base your intervention or treatment on with this particular client – with the goal of helping that client reach a desired outcome.

Once you create an idea (or, in research language, a hypothesis), you continue to collect more information from the individual both before and while you implement the treatment intervention. This information helps you to test this idea or theory that you have. If your theory or hypothesis about the client is supported, you move forward with treatment implementation. But, if it was inaccurate based on the additional information you gather, you then move back to creating a new hypothesis about the underlying reasons that are driving the presenting concerns of this client.

Daily Knowledge

As we just discussed, you are already employing the scientific method in your day-to-day work with clients and students. You are already conducting informal research. You know there are several ways that research benefits those involved in your daily practice: your clients, yourself and your colleagues as practitioners, insurance companies, directors and larger organizations. If we genuinely want to broaden our lens, the world has benefited from science and research. Aspects of science and research play out in your daily practice, regardless of whether you are engaging in more formal research or not. But let's take this one step further and explore how research has impacted the daily knowledge you have and some everyday activities you engage in through your clinical practice.

Consider that most practitioners are very aware of the importance of the therapeutic relationship. This information was provided to us empirically through research via multiple studies (Frank and Frank, 1993; Lambert & Ogles, 2014; Wampold et al., 1997; Wampold, 2007). These researchers explored factors that led to client change, and then came up with common factors models. In these models, Lambert, Wampold, and colleagues found the therapeutic relationship is one of the most important factors in whether a client experienced change. Not only that, but they found that this relationship was also intertwined with theoretical orientation, client expectancies, and client external resources.

We also know about the Dodo bird effect (Luborsky, Singer, and Luborsky, 1975; Rosenzweig, 1936), which means that over time and multiple clinical trials no one treatment is better than another in the long run. Yet, this same research has shown us that counseling and psychological treatment is better than nothing (Luborsky, Singer, and Luborsky, 1975; Rosenzweig, 1936). These are just a couple of ways that research has influenced what you already know and how we conceptualize our work with clients.

Practitioner-Scientist

While we have spent some time focusing on *why* research is important to practitioners and how research has influenced practice, we haven't mentioned much about how practice influences science. Honestly, without practice, there really is not much use for mental health research. It is the practitioners who often influence researchers in terms of what questions need to be answered. As a practitioner, you more than likely have questions when a new student or patient walks into your office or presents with symptoms or behaviors with which you are less familiar. You may consider, "What do I need to know to better understand what is going on for Gina?" or "How might I best help Samuel?" These questions and considerations may be related to diagnoses or treatments. For example, they may be about whether an intervention should be in a particular format or for a particular length. Having these questions as a practitioner often helps lead researchers to answer these questions. Altering your programs or treatment methods with clients can create new questions. As a prime example, consider Marsha Linehan's dialectical behavior therapy (DBT) (Linehan, 1993). She created this theory and method of treatment due to her own experiences both as a client and, later, as a mental health professional. Once she created these treatments, researchers and clinicians alike immediately started to ask questions about the effectiveness of them, leading into decades of research among various client populations in various settings to determine if DBT worked, who it worked for, and what parts of it work in which ways. And this is just one larger example of how practice influences research.

In talking about science and practice, we tend to discuss these as separate entities. Do you engage in practice, or do you engage in research? Are you a researcher? Are you a practitioner? Yet, as we noted earlier in Figure 1.1, you technically engage in the scientific method daily with each person to whom you provide a service. Yet, we don't typically think of that as "research." Even when mentioning identity development, historically we have discussed the identity development of counselors or mental health practitioners separately from researcher identity development (e.g., Auxier et al., 2003). Very few have mentioned that these two identities (e.g., practitioner identity and researcher identity) can, in fact, be integrated. Talking about how these two identities can grow and develop together, having bidirectional influence, is important (Spengler and Lee, 2017). For example, Jorgensen and Duncan (2015) asked master's level counselors about their researcher identity. What they found was that researcher identity emerges and develops along with counselor identity development to some extent – that students reported developing their researcher identities through faculty modeling, external facilitators (such as on-site supervisors of their clinical work), internal facilitators (e.g., self-motivation, time management, research self-efficacy, thinking styles, curiosity), and through a conceptual learning about research. What is important, though, is that they did so when their counselor identity felt slightly more solid. The two interrelate. Spengler and Lee (2017) take this further to mention how, when a mental health professional has a practitioner identity combined with a researcher's identity, they ultimately practice differently. Being trained in research can influence mental health professionals in a way that they can approach their practice differently in terms of how they were able to see change, work with clients, and engage in treatment. Therefore, integrating both a practitioner and a researcher lens may be helpful in your practice, leading to bridging the scientist and practitioner gap, rather than seeing research and practice as separate behaviors.

So what does being a practitioner-scientist actually mean? Does this mean you have to collect data in your mental health practice? Well, we certainly hope you do, but it doesn't have to equate data collection or formal research (but we want to mention one more time … we hope that you do collect data to determine your own effectiveness). Ultimately, we see being a practitioner-scientist as multi-layered and containing three major tasks: consumption of research, application of research, and engagement in research (or conducting research).

Consume, Apply, Conduct

In asking counselors if they engaged in these research behaviors, Wester et al. (2006) discovered that unfortunately a large degree of counselors self-reported they did not. As can be seen from Figure 1.2, a maximum of 68% of counselors indicated they consumed professional empirical literature to inform their practice, with only 45% relying on what research may

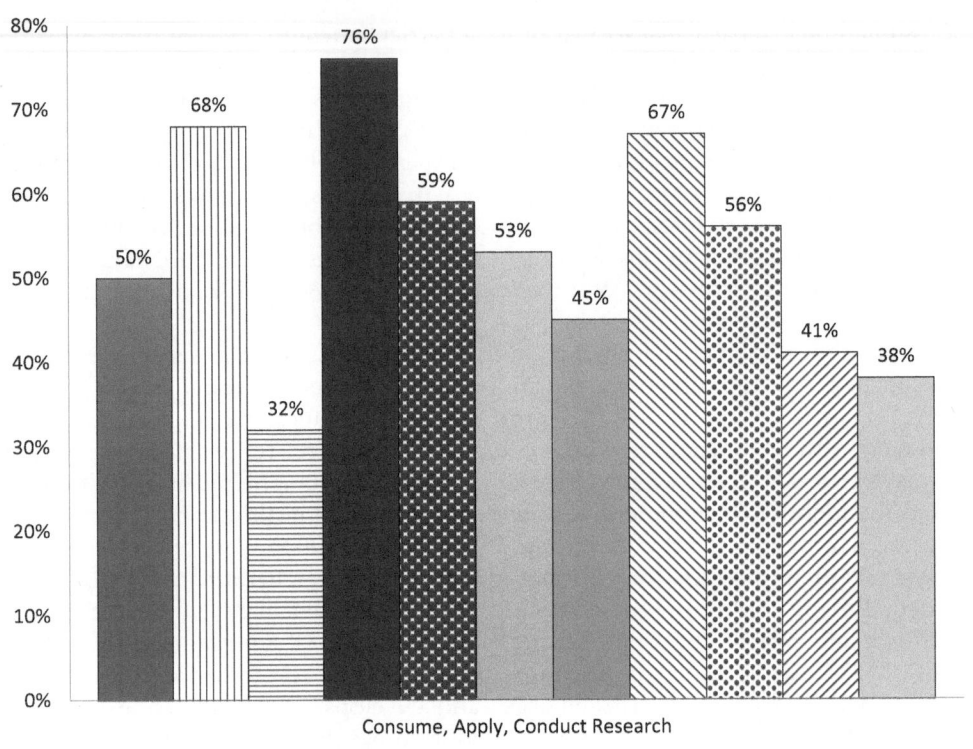

Consume, Apply, Conduct Research

■ Consume Literature to Support What I Do
▢ Consume Literature to Find New Empirically Supported Treatment
▤ Conduct Searches to Find Empirically Supported Treatment
■ Apply Info Learned From Consumption
▨ Recall Research When With Client
▢ Base Interventions on Empirically Supported Info
▨ Search for Empirical Treatment When Feel Stuck
▨ Use Professional Literature as a Guide
▨ Evaluate My Own Effectiveness
▨ Collect Data in My Practice on Client Change
▢ Collect Data Clt Sessions to Determine if Interventions/Techs Are Working

Figure 1.2 Percentage of counselors who consume, apply, and conduct research in their clinical practice (Wester et al., 2006).

suggest when they are stuck with a client. This leaves 32% of counselors indicating that they do not consume empirical research. This means that 32% of counselors are stating that they do not use what we *know* to be evidence based, because they are not reading up-to-date literature on what we know to be effective in work with clients. This is scary. Would you want to go to those mental health providers?

Of those counselors that consumed research (again, remembering that this is of the 68% of counselors who consume research) 53% to 76% reported that they apply what they have consumed. Fifty-three percent indicate they based their interventions on what they consumed, 59% reported they recalled what they read while they were with their clients, and 76% indicated they would apply the information learned with clients in their clinical practice. This is good news—most counselors who consumed research applied it. But, again, 32% of counselors did not consume research at all (thus they had nothing to apply) and of those that consumed research, 24% are not applying in practice what they are consuming. What is the reason counselors did not consume research or apply what they did consume? That is less clear. It could be that they believed it was not relevant to their practice. Or, maybe, it was difficult to consume or apply (as academic researchers do not typically write in language that is easy to immediately apply).

As expected, fewer counselors indicated that they actively engaged in research, or conducted research to determine if they were effective with their own clients. When asked, mental health providers typically overestimate their effectiveness with clients (Spengler & Lee, 2017); thus, asking clients about outcomes is important. But only 38% to 56% indicated they conducted research on their own practice. Thirty-eight percent reported collecting data on client sessions to determine effectiveness of interventions (this is a really low number by the way!), while 41% said they collected some form of data to determine their own effectiveness, and 56% indicated they evaluated their own effectiveness (with less clarity on how they evaluated this). So, approximately one-third to one-half of counselors in the study conducted by Wester and colleagues reported that they evaluate, in some format, whether they are effective. How do you think that would make their stakeholders feel? Are these practitioners that you would want to see if you knew they never collected information to determine if what they did worked? Are they practitioners that you would refer your loved ones to for services?

As you can see, the rate of research consumption is the highest, followed by a slightly lower rate of application of research knowledge, with an even lower prevalence of conducting research on one's practice. But, engaging in at least one of these research practices would lead to being a practitioner-scientist, with higher levels of practitioner-scientist proficiency being demonstrated by being engaging in all three forms of research in your practice.

Role of Evidence-Based Practice

In thinking about the role of research in clinical practice, it is difficult not to talk about evidence-based practice. Take a moment to consider what you believe evidence-based practice is before you continue to read.

Did you take a moment, or did you just read on? If you did not take a moment, seriously, pause to reflect on what you think of when you think about evidence-based practice. What do you consider to be the definition of evidence-based practice? Is it therapeutic interventions that are empirically supported by research? Is it specifically randomized clinical trials? Or is it generally empirically supported research? Is it somewhere in between those?

When someone has not read much about evidence-based practice or seen definition of evidence-based practice, they often believe that it equates solely to research-supported treatments, or even something as extreme as only the most manualized treatments. This is what the name sounds like, right? Wrong. That is only one component of evidence-based practice. Evidence-based practice is the integration of three things:

(1)   treatments and interventions that are supported empirically by the best available research
(2)   clinical expertise
(3)   client characteristics, culture, and preference.
                    (American Psychological Association [APA], Force, 2006)

Similarly, as noted by APA (Force, 2006), this definition of evidence-based practice is similar to that created by the Institute of Medicine (2001), which suggests that evidence-based practice is the integration of the best research evidence combined with clinical expertise along with patient values.

Let's take a moment to consider this. If, as a practitioner, you based your interventions, classroom guidance, psychoeducation or any other form of treatment solely on research, you lose the uniqueness and needs of each individual client who is sitting in your office. Also, you would fail to consider client factors, resources, and even their expectancy (or desire) to change – all of which are part of the common factors model (Lambert and Ogles, 2014; Wampold et al., 1997). So, more than likely, if you implement solely what researchers have found to be effective, even if you diagnose the symptoms correctly with your clinical expertise, the client may not change or reach their desired goal. At this point you have taken the client voice out of the process. That is not an effective way of establishing a therapeutic relationship (which, again, has been found to be one of the most important factors in the room!).

Now, let's say you do take client values, culture, and context into consideration. You inquire if they would like to engage in a 16-week, empirically supported, dialectical behavior therapy treatment (Linehan, 1993). The client agrees that she is willing to engage in all components of this 16-week DBT treatment and believes this would be helpful. You selected this treatment as you have deemed that the client is at risk of suicidal behavior and is depressed for a variety of reasons including ineffective relationships and lack of distress tolerance. At this point, you have incorporated both what researchers have supported (i.e., DBT 16-week program) along with client values and preferences. However, if you misdiagnosed the client, or your hypothesis about the underlying reasons for that diagnosis was incorrect, there is also the potential that the treatment will not work. For example, what if this client was depressed and suicidal because she watched her mother die by suicide a month ago and is traumatized and grieving? Or, what if the client is constantly under the influence of a substance but you are unaware of it or have neglected to assess for substance use or abuse? A lack of clinical expertise or the wrong diagnosis could lead to ineffective treatment. It is the integration of all three components, therefore, that is truly evidence-based practice (Figure 1.3). So, let's think through each of these pieces, what they look like in practice, and why they are important.

Let's start with empirically supported treatments. These are the interventions and approaches studied in ways that meet baseline requirements for rigor and shown a statistically significant degree of positive outcomes for clients. So, how do you find these treatments? There are several resources that are available for free – either through technology, through local libraries, or through clinically-affiliated organizations that may serve as information hubs. For example, online, a quick internet search may lead to sites like Google

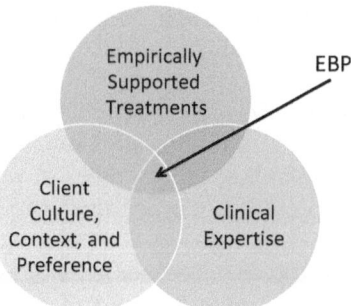

Figure 1.3 Evidence-based practice.

Scholar (https://scholar.google.com), NC Docks (https://libres.uncg.edu/ir/uncg/), or Open Education Resource Commons (https://www.oercommons.org/) that provide free access to a variety of academic and nonacademic resources that individuals may access. As open education resources are growing, some journals have been created that are truly open-access and accessible to anyone who can hop online for a few minutes. An up-to-date list of open access journals is currently available through the Directory of Open Access Journals, found at https://doaj.org/. Social media may also provide access to research, as individuals and groups use them as vehicles to distribute useful clinical research. Two examples are Mental Health Research, a United States–based Facebook page and The Mental Elf, a United Kingdom-based Facebook page. Both disseminate research on a variety of mental health–related topics of interest to practitioners.

Next Steps: Learning to Conduct Research

It is important to be able to locate studies relevant to the work that we do as practitioners through accessing research literature. Most of the research on empirically supported treatments that we rely on comes from randomized clinical trials. These studies typically emerge from the medical profession, but we can also get important information about empirically supported treatments from well-designed studies with a variety of methodologies that we will present in this book. Quantitative designs, in particular, are particularly well-suited to generating the type of research that will empirically support treatments, but qualitative methods can also give powerful insight into the ways that different interventions may be impacting our clients and students.

Doing a literature search is one way of learning about empirically supported treatments. Another way is to do research at your own clinical practice to contribute to the literature base. So, not only is research helpful for you (and all the other people who want to hear about how wonderfully effective you are), but it is also going to help other practitioners out there who are looking for ways to be as effective as you are!

Because of this you will also need to understand how to read and critique literature. This includes all parts of an article, including methods and results. Chapter 2 gives an overview of how to best consume and understand literature, so that you can truly integrate what you learn into your own clinical practice. After reading these first two chapters, we hope that you start thinking about how *you* can start to develop your own identity as a researcher. Chapter 3 talks about how to conduct research ethically and responsibly – something that is foundational to conducting research that increases what we know and also honors the trust that our clients have in us and our ethical standard to do no harm. Chapter 4 starts to introduce you to how to start thinking about conducting research, by digging into the details of survey design.

These first chapters form a foundation to then build your knowledge of a variety of different research methods and how they might naturally be suited to your work as a practitioner-scientist. While these are only a sampling of a number of research methods out there, they have been carefully selected to represent not only the methods that might be the most easily-suited to your work as a practitioner, but also several different philosophies of research. Many practitioners want or need to develop or select measures or assessments, and this information can be found in "Evaluating and Designing Surveys" (Chapter 4). Additionally, information from the in-depth qualitative exploration of a single client, group, or practice given by a case study (Chapter 6) to the more controlled implementation of a single treatment of the single case research design (Chapter 7), we hope to help you think through how even small numbers of clients can give you valuable information and insight when researched properly. From there, we start to look at larger groups of clients and how different client factors relate to each other in correlational-causal comparative (Chapter 8) and quasi-experimental (Chapter 9) designs. We then go to the tried-and-true gold standard of randomized control trials (Chapter 10). After discussing the highly controlled RCT method, we then shift gears to explore more client-driven emergent methods like content analysis (Chapter 11), which has both a qualitative and quantitative bent to it, and qualitative methods like phenomenology (Chapter 12) and photovoice (Chapter 13). Bridging the qualitative and quantitative realms is mixed-methods (Chapter 14), which allows practitioners to explore not only the numbers behind different behaviors, but also the nuances specific to individual clients. Every practitioner needs a baseline knowledge of program evaluation (Chapter 15) to take a critical look at their own practice or curriculum.

Each chapter will walk you through not only the basics of the research method, but also how it might be directly applied to specific questions or settings, to help you picture how you might be able to tailor the approach for your own practitioner-scientist needs. Each chapter also includes a practice-based application (see the following section) to help you apply the information you are learning. Further, each chapter is paired with a brief narrated PowerPoint that will give highlights of the method and, often, an additional example from a different setting. We recommend taking advantage of the text, videos, practice-based application, and reflection questions at the end of each chapter to guide your thinking about each method. This will support your development as a practitioner-scientist.

Practice Based Application

Given that each chapter walks through the basics of various methodologies or components of the research process, our intention with this book also is that you will begin to think about your own clinical practice through a researcher's lens. Throughout this book, we are going to ask you to apply what you have learned to your current and/or proposed clinical work – with a client, an organization, a specific presenting concern, or something else that you might wish to examine or explore related to clinical practice. At the end of each chapter, you will be asked to think through different questions related to the chapter's content as it relates to this current or proposed clinical work. So, before you start reading, take a few minutes to think about things that you are curious about related to your clinical practice. This may be related to a client or student that you've worked with, something that you've seen related to how your organization functions, a diagnosis or client presenting concern that has piqued your interest, or something else that is relevant to your work as a clinician. If you haven't had much client contact yet – or are struggling to think of something that feels particularly relevant right now, think about a movie, a book, a story you've seen in the media, or other content that has implications for clinical practice. So, take a moment and reflect on the following questions (we encourage you to write down your answers for reflection throughout the book):

1. What client-presenting concern, symptom, or situation left you needing or wanting more information? This could be something as specific as a presenting symptom, or a family dynamic present in the case. Or it could be wondering what intervention or treatment plan might be most effective with a particular population, demographic, or presenting concern. Take a moment and jot down your ideas, and if you are still struggling, consider free associating for 5 minutes about this question.
2. If what you jotted down for question 1 is extensive, or broad, that can be okay – but sometimes it is helpful to narrow it down a little further. Each chapter and methodology discussed will look at this topic or client from a different lens – requiring you to narrow the topic down to a specific question (or with some methodologies … to broaden it). But for now, out of what you have written – is there a specific group or population that you are interested in (e.g., adolescents, couples, families with teenagers, students with behavioral difficulties in the classroom, an individual presenting with cyclothymia)? And with the group or population you have narrowed it down to, what are you specifically interested in (e.g., factors that lead to a presenting concern, interventions that are most effective in treating the situation/symptomology, how to best create a therapeutic relationship, how to prevent the presenting symptomology)?

Now take the answers to these two questions and keep them for reflection as you read other chapters. The Practice-Based Applications section in each chapter will ask you to connect what you read in that chapter to your answers to these questions. Keep in mind that curious minds always wander, and you may want to know more, or something different, as you reflect and read each chapter – and that is perfectly okay. That is the mind of a researcher!

Questions for Further Review and Application

1 Do you believe that researcher identity and practitioner identity develop simultaneously or separately? Should they be integrated? Why or why not?
2 What do you think is needed at the practitioner level to feel confident in consuming, applying, and conducting research? Is something similar needed for all three or something different in terms of training and experience?
3 What is evidence-based practice? How will you know you are engaging in evidence-based practice in your own practice?

References

Auxier, C. R., Hughes, F. R., & Kline, W. B. (2003). Identity development in counselors-in-training. *Counselor Education and Supervision, 43*(1), 25–38.
Force, A. T. (2006). APA presidential task force on evidence based practice. *American Psychologist, 61,* 271–285.
Frank, J. D., & Frank, J. B. (1993). *Persuasion and healing: A comparative study of psychotherapy* (3rd ed.). Johns Hopkins University Press.

Institute of Medicine. (2001). *Crossing the quality chasm: A new health system for the 21st century.* National Academies Press.

Jorgensen, M. F., & Duncan, K. (2015). A grounded theory of masters-level counselor research identity. *Counselor Education and Supervision, 54,* 17–31. https://doi.org/10.1002/j.1556-6978.2015.00067

Lambert, M. J., & Ogles, B. M. (2014). Common factors: Post hoc explanation or empirically based therapy approach. *Psychotherapy, 51,* 500–504. http://doi.org/10.1037/a0036580

Linehan, M. (1993). *Cognitive-behavioral treatment of borderline personality disorder.* Guilford press.

Luborsky, L., Singer, B., & Luborsky, L. (1975). Comparative studies of psychotherapies: is it true that everyone has won and all must have prizes?. *Archives of General Psychiatry, 32*(8), 995–1008.

Rosenzweig, S. (1936). Some implicit common factors in diverse methods of psychotherapy. *American Journal of Orthopsychiatry, 6*(3), 412.

Spengler, P. M., & Lee, N. A. (2017). A funny thing happened when my scientist self and my practitioner self became an integrated scientist-practitioner: A tale of two couple therapists transformed. *Counselling Psychology Quarterly,* 1–19. http://doi.org/10.1080/09515070.2017.1305948

Wampold, B. E. (2007). Psychotherapy: The humanistic (and effective) treatment. *American Psychologist, 62,* 857–873.

Wampold, B. E., Mondin, G. W., Moody, M., Stich, F., Benson, K., & Ahn, H. (1997). A meta-analysis of outcome studies comparing bona fide psychotherapies: Empirically, "All must have prizes". *Psychological Bulletin, 122,* 203–215.

Wester, K. L., Mobley, K., & Faulkner, A. (2006, September). *Evidence-based practices: Building a bridge between researchers and practitioners.* Presentation provided at the Southern Association for Counselor Education and Supervision. Orlando, Florida.

Zhou, M. (2003). Urban education: Challenges in educating culturally diverse children. *Teachers College Record,* 105, 208–225.

2 Understanding Existing Literature

Amanda L. Giordano and Deborah L. Smith

Your newest client's case is unique. Although you have worked with this presenting concern before, there are novel variables to consider, including the client's distinctive cultural identities and a co-occurring disorder. You wonder how others have worked with similar clients and whether those clinical efforts were effective. What approaches have others employed with members of this cultural group, and what were the outcomes? Has anyone ever addressed these presenting concerns simultaneously? If so, how? Thankfully, you can find many of these answers by exploring existing literature in counseling and related fields.

Importance of Understanding Existing Trends in the Literature

The introduction to Section C of the 2014 American Counseling Association (ACA) *Code of Ethics* states, "Counselors have a responsibility to the public to engage in counseling practices that are based on rigorous research methodologies." Additionally, the American Psychological Association's (APA, 2010) *Ethical Principles of Psychologist and Code of Conduct* posits, "Psychologists' work is based upon established scientific and professional knowledge of the discipline" (2.04). Furthermore, the National Association of Social Workers' *Code of Ethics* (2021) asserts, "Social workers should routinely review the professional literature and participate in continuing education relevant to social work practice and social work ethics" (4.01). These ethical codes are designed to protect our clients and ensure we provide them with the highest standard of care. Therefore, it makes sense that clinicians of all fields are obligated to utilize counseling techniques and foster clinical environments that are supported by sound research studies. Consider the harm that could come to clients if we operated on instinct alone and failed to consult existing literature to identify empirically supported clinical approaches. Consider ways in which our own culture-bound worldviews may preclude us from considering alternative treatment options that may best serve diverse clients. Thankfully, we have access to hundreds of years of research and relevant literature upon which to ground clinical practice.

In 1995, a division of the APA (Division 12) created a task force (Promotion and Dissemination of Psychological Procedures) to empirically validate clinical techniques (La Roche & Christopher, 2009). The goal of the task force was to identify counseling approaches that were supported by rigorous research, particularly studies utilizing randomized controlled trials. The efforts of the Division 12 task force are relevant to you because they contributed to a growing emphasis on identifying and incorporating empirically supported treatment (EST) into clinical practice. Now you can utilize strategies that have demonstrated effectiveness, and thus you will be better equipped to provide appropriate care to your clients and

DOI: 10.4324/9781032706139-2

strong rationales to managed care organizations as to why your work is necessary (Sue & Sue, 2008). In addition to examining counseling techniques and approaches, APA Divisions 12 and 29 created a second task force to identify aspects of the counseling relationship supported by empirical research (Norcross & Wampold, 2011). This Evidence-Based Therapy Relationships Task Force determined that the therapeutic relationship contributed at least as much to the success of counseling as specific interventions and treatment methods (Norcross & Wampold, 2011). Thus, we now have evidentiary support for the fact that the strength of the relationships we build with our clients matters!

Despite the plethora of research available to clinicians, a gap exists between those generating research findings and the practitioners who would benefit most from the information. Indeed, Murray (2009) wrote, "For decades, however, the counseling profession has demonstrated a chasm between the knowledge developed by researchers and the practices used by clinicians" (p. 108). This research–practice gap can impede the progress, efficacy, and accountability of helping professions. What does this mean for you? One of your clinical responsibilities is to keep up with relevant research and apply it to your practice. To make reading research worth your time, researchers are charged with conducting studies that are relevant and meaningful to clinicians. Specifically, Wester (2011) stated that counseling research must have social validity or the potential to make a significant contribution to clinical practice, the counseling profession, or society at large. So those conducting research should be aware of the needs of clinicians and develop studies to address them. The next step is for practitioners like you to consume the research and let it influence your practice. Indeed, Balkin and Sheperis (2011) noted, "counselors must now be competent consumers of research conducted in the counseling profession and be able to make decisions about the applicability of research results" (p. 268). If researchers prioritize social validity and clinicians prioritize consuming the literature, the research–practice gap is likely to shrink.

Empirical Versus Nonempirical Literature

Sifting through existing literature can be a daunting task. There are many resources available such as peer-reviewed articles, book chapters, dissertations and theses, commentaries, magazine articles, blogs, and websites. How do you find credible, relevant sources? How do you differentiate between the many types of literature? What sources are the best match for your needs? To answer these questions, it is important to distinguish between empirical and nonempirical literature.

Empirical Literature

The word *empirical* simply means "originating in or based on observation or experience" (*Merriam-Webster's Collegiate Dictionary*, 2004, p. 408). Thus, empirical research seeks to verify or negate a specific question by collecting and analyzing data. You will notice that empirical research papers have a standard format including an introduction, a methods section, a results section, and a discussion of the implications (APA, 2019). These articles present findings from original quantitative, qualitative, or mixed methods investigations with the aim of contributing to the literature on a particular topic. Within the quantitative realm, researchers may conduct experiments, disseminate descriptive surveys, or utilize single-subject designs ($N = 1$), each of which you will be introduced to throughout the chapters in this book. Qualitative researchers, on the other hand, may conduct interviews or focus groups or engage in observations of members of a specific population in order to ascertain thick descriptions of a phenomenon. Both quantitative and qualitative studies seek to objectively examine constructs by employing standardized research techniques and analyzing the resulting data. Mixed methods design employs both quantitative and qualitative research methods in the same study (more about this in Chapter 14).

Nonempirical Literature

Conversely, rather than detailing a quantitative, qualitative, or mixed methods study, nonempirical research consists of literature reviews, practice pieces, and conceptual works (APA, 2019; Watts, 2011). When exploring a new topic, you may find a literature review particularly helpful, as it synthesizes all of the relevant literature and seminal works related to the subject. Baker (2016) noted that literature reviews should be free of bias, with clear inclusion criteria for the articles studied. Further, Pautasso (2013) purported that a quality literature review should be a focused summary of recent papers and original works pertaining to a designated topic. Literature reviews can provide a succinct overview of a construct so you can become familiar with the status of the topic in the field.

While literature reviews summarize many papers related to a given construct, practice pieces and conceptual works present new, original applications of a theory, technique, or clinical approach. For example, practice pieces describe the implementation of clinical interventions with new populations or provide specific details regarding the use of a novel counseling practice (Guiffrida et al. 2006). These papers often include a hypothetical case example or specific instructions describing how to alter a clinical technique for a specific purpose, such as a paper explaining how to apply acceptance and commitment therapy (ACT) to those with binge eating disorder (BED). You may find these "how-to" practice articles extremely relevant and applicable to your clinical work. Practice articles fall under the umbrella term *conceptual articles*, which Watts (2011) defined as papers that apply theoretical perspectives to particular clinical concerns, describe the use of a clinical procedure or intervention, discuss controversial or provocative issues in the counseling field, or respond to previously published works. Thus, broadly speaking, conceptual articles describe original, well-supported perspectives on current issues, clinical practices, or previous publications. Indeed, Balkin (2009) wrote that conceptual articles should be more than a synthesis of existing literature but instead offer innovative ways of applying theory or implementing clinical techniques.

Therefore, depending on your specific clinical needs, both empirical and nonempirical papers can be valuable resources. For example, suppose you just completed a training in motivational interviewing (MI) and want to know whether the approach is effective with Latino(a) (x) adolescents. Empirical research studies reporting outcomes of MI interventions with Latino(a)(x) adolescent clients may be most helpful in this situation. Once you know that MI is effective with samples of adolescents of Latin descent, howeyer, you may want to read a case example of how another clinician has used the approach. At this point, a conceptual piece detailing how to apply MI to a Latino(a)(x) adolescent client may be most useful.

How to Access Existing Literature

Now that you are familiar with the different types of literature, how do you go about accessing these resources? In our age of smart devices and Wi-Fi access, retrieving literature has never been easier. For those affiliated with a university, the school's library system is an excellent and cost-effective resource. There are numerous electronic research databases that affiliates of universities can access for free. For those who are not connected to a university, these databases are still very useful, yet you may need to purchase the articles for a fee (unless they are Open Access, described later). Following are descriptions of several research databases that may be of interest to you:

- **Academic Search Complete** (www.ebscohost.com/academic/academic-search-complete): This multidisciplinary database contains articles from topics including anthropology, psychology, women's studies, and multicultural studies.
- **ERIC** (Education Resource Information Center; https://eric.ed.gov/): This extensive database provides resources relevant to education from a variety of disciplines. The database is sponsored by the Institute of Education Sciences.
- **PsycINFO** (www.apa.org/psycinfo): This vast database is sponsored by APA and contains articles from a variety of fields including behavioral science, mental health, and sociology.
- **SocINDEX** (www.ebscohost.com/academic/socindex-with-full-text): This focused database showcases articles relevant to sociology including topics such as criminology, gender studies, and substance use.
- **MEDLINE** (https://health.ebsco.com/products/medline-with-full-text): This comprehensive database is sponsored by the National Library of Medicine and contains resources relevant to nursing, health care, and medicine.
- **Google Scholar** (https://scholar.google.com): This search engine is dedicated to directing interested readers to a wide array of scholarly journal articles, books, theses, and dissertations.

While many journals require a subscription or a fee to access articles, some journals offer Open Access, meaning that readers do not have to pay to access content (and they are open to the public). The Directory of Open Access Journals (DOAJ; https://doaj.org) is a good place to begin your search for free-to-access papers. Although Open Access is an effort to remove financial barriers to research by increasing accessibility of publications, there also exist predatory journals that publish articles (often at the author's financial expense) that are not peer-reviewed (meaning they are not reviewed by experts in the field and revised prior to publication) or not high-quality research (Elmore & Weston, 2020). Thus, when searching Open Access articles, it is incumbent upon the reader to ensure the research is rigorous and trustworthy (elements of which we will describe later in the chapter). Finally, another way to obtain research is through membership in a clinical association, which often comes with access to the organization's journal. For example, members of the Association for Spiritual, Ethical, and Religious Values in Counseling (ASERVIC) receive electronic access to the division's journal, *Counseling & Values*.

When utilizing research databases, it is important to consider your search terms and the many ways in which authors can describe any one topic. For example, if you are interested in finding scholarly articles related to substance misuse, you could search using the terms *substance use, problematic substance use, alcohol use, drug use, substance use disorder, dependence,* or *addiction*. Thus, if you vary your keywords, your searches will yield a greater breadth of papers. One way to help ensure you are not missing any important articles is to find a relevant paper and review the author's reference list. Rather than reinventing the wheel, you can begin your investigation on the subject by reading articles that another researcher deemed pertinent and helpful. Finally, another way you can access existing literature is to contact prominent researchers on the topic of interest (the majority of which will be flattered!) and request recommendations of essential books and articles. The extensiveness of counseling literature is a double-edged sword: On the one hand, we have research on almost every topic imaginable, but on the other hand, it can be difficult to know where to begin. Contacting a current expert in the field could be an efficient way to find a starting place for your investigation.

Consuming and Critiquing Empirical Research

Now you know how to access the literature, but that is only the first step. Indeed, Reynolds (2000b) offers five steps for applying existing research to clinical practice: (a) identify the specific clinical questions you would like to answer, (b) find existing research to address the question, (c) evaluate the quality of the research you found, (d) apply results of the research to your client, and (e) evaluate the outcomes. In this next section, we will focus on the third step of this process: how to evaluate the quality of research you find. Especially in an age with growing Open Access and the unfortunate existence of predatory journals, it is imperative to assess the quality of the research papers we consume. To help us do this, we will be examining a publication written by myself and a colleague, which explored cybersex addiction among college students (Giordano & Cashwell, 2017).

Evaluating Introductions

The purpose of the introduction is to present a case as to why the current study is needed. The authors of the article should summarize important existing literature and identify unanswered questions, areas of disagreement, or the need for replication. There should be a logical flow in the presentation of supporting research leading to the purpose statement, or identified need for the study. Just because a topic has not been studied before does not mean it should be. For example, there may not be any research on the correlation between nail polish color and symptoms of depression, but that does not mean the research is needed! Thus, the introduction should present a compelling argument as to why the topic deserves to be investigated, describe the social validity of the research project, and explain how the study fits within the broader scope of literature. By the time you finish reading the introduction, you should think, "of course we need this study!" (Giordano et al., 2021).

Additionally, the introduction should be free of bias. Researchers should describe supporting evidence, contradictory findings, and areas of disagreement and provide multiple perspectives on the topic. The presentation of material should be objective, and authors should refrain from trying to influence readers by presenting only one side of an issue. For example, in a research paper describing the need for a new treatment protocol for childhood trauma, the authors should speak to the strengths and limitations of treatment approaches that already exist. Furthermore, all major constructs in the research study should be discussed in the introduction with support from previous literature. Incomplete introductions may fail to describe a study variable, inadequately explain associations between primary constructs, or neglect to reference a theoretical orientation. You should be able to recognize these limitations and evaluate the extent to which the researchers investigated the phenomenon in question prior to beginning their study. Finally, as a critical consumer of research, you also must be able to evaluate the appropriateness of the resources cited in the introduction. Strong, quality articles utilize original rather than secondary sources, cite peer-reviewed articles rather than books or websites, and include the most recent references (Lambie et al., 2008b). By the end of the introduction, you should have a solid understanding of why the research article was written and the need for the study.

Let's consider the article that my colleague and I wrote about collegiate cybersex addiction. In the introduction of the article, we clearly explained the need for this particular study at this particular time. Specifically, we noted the social validity of the study. What this means is we stated the prevalence of cybersex addiction among the general population, the negative consequences of cybersex addiction, reasons why cybersex may be more prevalent among college students, gender considerations in the use of the internet for sexual activity, and the lack of prior research examining cybersex among college students. Given these realities, we claimed that this study was needed to better inform clinical practice, particularly among college counselors. We then identified the two research questions guiding our work: "What is the prevalence of cybersex addiction among college students?" and "Do significant differences exist between men and women on cybersex addiction?" to better inform clinical practice among college counselors (Giordano & Cashwell, 2017). Our goal was to have readers fully convinced by the end of our introduction that this study was needed and meaningful.

Evaluating Methods Sections

The methods section is something that most individuals who do not identify as researchers typically skim through or skip over altogether. This usually occurs because methods (along with results) sections are not as easily understood, yet it is one of the most important sections of an article to determine if the findings of the study are actually applicable to your clinical practice, specific clients in your practice, or students in your school. Therefore, becoming a critical consumer of empirical research means that you must evaluate the quality of the methods section. The methods detail the type of study design (e.g., experimental, phenomenological, descriptive, or correlational, which you will read about later in this book) and how the researchers conducted the study, including things like sampling procedures and instrumentation.

Sampling Procedures

Empirical researchers should describe how they selected the participants in their study. Accessibility, funding resources, and required sample size all influence the choice of sampling procedures. For example, in quantitative research, the type of statistical analysis and number of variables dictate the minimum number of participants needed in the study. Multiple-regression analysis, bivariate correlations, and analysis of variance (ANOVA) could have up to 100 or more participants depending on the specific elements of the research project. Qualitative research, however, typically requires much fewer participants because the goal is to *understand* a phenomenon. Therefore, qualitative studies may have eight to 50 participants depending on which qualitative tradition the researchers are using (Hays & Singh, 2011).

Probability sampling is the most rigorous form of obtaining participants and involves randomly selecting a sample from a population in such a way that each member of the population has an equal chance of being included in the study (Creswell & Creswell, 2022b; Sink & Mvududu, 2010b). For example, if you wanted to study the prevalence of students of color experiencing microaggressions in the middle school where you work, probability sampling would require that you list the names of all students of color enrolled in the school and randomly select a certain number to include in your study. There are many reasons why random sampling is not possible, however; thus researchers may use nonprobability sampling methods. Nonprobability sampling includes the solicitation of volunteers and utilization of the participants that researchers have access to (such as convenience sampling). For example, if you are interested in studying non-suicidal self-injury among women, you may elicit volunteers from among the female clients seeking services at your practice to assess for self-injury. Although this does not represent the entire population of female clients, it is a realistic, cost-effective, and achievable way to obtain participants (Sink & Mvududu, 2010b).

Consider again the study of cybersex among college students that we were talking about earlier. To employ probability sampling, we would have acquired the names of all undergraduate students from the registrar's office at my university, randomly selected several hundred, and called or emailed each one with an invitation to participate in the study. Although preferred, this would be logistically difficult and time consuming. Therefore, we utilized convenience sampling methods by emailing course instructors and asking if we could come to their classes to administer our survey to all consenting students in attendance. Although this form of sampling made the most sense for us, we still identified it as a limitation in our study, as we could not guarantee our sample was a true representation of all college students at the university.

So what does all of this sampling method information mean for you? When consuming literature, you should take the sampling method into account and evaluate whether the research will meet your clinical needs. For example, if the researchers used probability sampling to obtain results from a national sample of the United States, the findings may not be applicable to the Native American clients at your clinic in a small rural town in New Mexico. Conversely, if researchers used convenience sampling to assess clinical outcomes at a trauma center on a college campus, the results may not apply to your setting that serves largely older adult clients. Considering sampling procedures ensures that you are allowing the right type of research to influence your clinical work.

Another important sampling consideration is participants' demographics. What are the cultural identities of the participants included in the study? Can the results of this study generalize to other cultural groups? Before applying empirical research to your practice, you should consider the degree of similarity between the participants of the research study and your own clients. Was there evidential support that the technique or approach was effective for Asian male clients? For clients who identify as bisexual? For clients with disabilities? For clients in poverty? For clients who identify as multiracial? According to the ACA *Code of Ethics* (2014), researchers should "describe the extent to which results are applicable for diverse populations" (G.4.a, p. 16). Therefore, you should know whether the results of the empirical study are likely to apply to your particular client population. If the sample used in the empirical research study is majority White college students, you may need to adapt the intervention or approach to match the context of your clients from other cultural groups (Roysircar, 2009). In this way, you will offer culturally sensitive treatments. Indeed, Nagayama Hall (2001) noted that it is inappropriate to extract ESTs with privileged populations and apply them to marginalized group members. Instead, you should provide culturally sensitive treatment by tailoring evidence-based practices to reflect the cultural context of each unique client (Nagayama Hall, 2001). So it is recommended that you always read the sampling section in an empirical article so you can assess the relevance to your specific client or student population.

Returning to the study on cybersex, our convenience sampling procedures yielded a sample of 339 college students, of which the majority identified as female, White, and heterosexual. Although these demographics mirrored those among the students at the university, you would want to take caution when applying the results of our study to institutions with large numbers of students who identify in marginalized sexual orientation or racial groups, or for that matter even potentially to White male students, given the lower numbers of these individuals in the final sample.

Instrumentation

Another component of methods sections is a description of the instruments the researchers used to collect data. Typically, researchers consider a myriad of factors when determining instrumentation such as reliability, validity, cost, availability, number of items, and norming data. The authors should provide enough information so you can evaluate the quality and appropriateness of their measures. For example, researchers should report the reliability of the scores obtained for each scale. Reliability simply refers to the consistency of scores on a measure across time, conditions, and constructs (Creswell & Creswell, 2022b). If a measure has high reliability, it means that the scores from the instrument are relatively stable. For example, if an instrument claims to measure acculturative stress (AS), those with high levels of AS should score similarly on the instrument and those with low levels of AS also should score similarly (Heppner et al., 2016b). Additionally, reliable measures yield stable variable scores across situations, such that the individual with high AS will have high AS at the grocery store, at the gym, and on the school bus. Most often, reliability is reported in the form of Cronbach's alpha (ranging from 0 to 1), with higher alpha scores indicating greater levels of stability or reliability. Social science researchers tend to agree that Cronbach's alpha scores of .70 or higher indicate acceptable reliability. If reliability scores are lower than .70, you are unable to guarantee that your participants would report similar scores if they completed the measure at a different time or in different circumstances. This significantly limits the applicability of the research findings.

Let us return to the cybersex study. We utilized the Internet Scale of the Sexual Addiction Screening Test-Revised (SAST-R; Carnes et al., 2010) to assess college student cybersex addiction. The scale had six items with "yes" or "no" answer choices. Our Cronbach's alpha level for the scores we obtained was .694, which is acceptable yet lower than we hoped. This reliability score indicates only modest stability among scores (i.e., college students with cybersex addiction scored similarly, and those without cybersex addiction scored similarly); therefore, we noted the low alpha level in the limitations section of the article.

With regard to validity, researchers should report evidence detailing the extent to which the measures they used actually assessed the constructs of interest. For example, does the measure claiming to assess AS actually assess AS, or something else like fear, depression, or neuroticism? This is important to you as a practitioner for several reasons. If there is no evidence of validity, you cannot guarantee that the findings of the research study actually reflect the variables you are most interested in. Consider a researcher who claims to have developed an effective treatment for obsessive-compulsive disorder (OCD), yet he offered no evidence of validity for his OCD measure. Although the participants' scores improved, was the researcher really measuring OCD? Perhaps his measure was really assessing generalized anxiety disorder or a social phobia. The lack of instrument validity makes it very difficult for you to know who would benefit from this newly developed treatment.

So when you are reading a methods section, what are you looking for to ensure that the researcher's measures are valid? Researchers can support the validity of their instrumentation by describing how the scores correlate with other instruments that assess the same construct (construct validity), how the items on the measure assess all aspects of the construct (content validity), or how the scores on the instrument accurately predict scores of related measures in the appropriate direction (predictive validity; Creswell & Creswell, 2022b). For example, the SAST-R demonstrated validity by accurately differentiating between men in inpatient treatment for sexual addiction and college males or male clergy without sexual addiction (predictive validity). Also, the items on the measure assessed four components of sex addiction confirmed by principal component analysis, namely, (a) preoccupation, (b) loss of control, (c) affect disturbance, and (d) relationship disturbance (content validity). Finally, to demonstrate construct validity, scores on the original SAST significantly correlated with the Boundary Violation Index; an assessment that measured attitudes and behaviors of sexual misconduct (Swiggart et al., 2008). With all these forms of validity, it is safe to assume that the SAST in fact measures sexual addiction.

Establishing the validity of a measure gives credence to the researchers' claims about the implications of the results. Despite the importance of this information, sadly, evidence of validity was found to be absent in more than half of the measures used in articles published in the counseling flagship journal, the *Journal of Counseling & Development* (JCD; Wester et al., 2013). Therefore, when consuming existing literature, you must be wary of articles that do not provide support for the fact that their measures indeed assess the constructs under investigation.

Finally, along with reliability and validity, it is important for you to consider norming data when critiquing the instrumentation used in an empirical study. Researchers develop assessment measures by testing them on a particular population called a *norming sample*. It is important for researchers to describe the development and norming data of the instruments utilized in their study, as well as the extent to which the measures are appropriate for the current sample. For example, was the instrument developed using White, middle-class men? If so, to what extent is it appropriate to use with ethnically diverse low-income families? Cultural sensitivity in instrument selection is an important part of a research design because the meaning and experience of phenomena vary across cultural groups (Heppner et al., 2016b; O'Hara et al., 2021b). As you read empirical literature, consider whether the norming sample for the measures used in the study was appropriate for the researcher's participants. You can then take that one step further to consider whether the measure applies to your specific client population.

In the collegiate cybersex study, we utilized a subscale of the SAST-R, which Carnes et al. (2010) developed using samples of both male and female college students, clergy, and clients in treatment for sex addiction. The researchers found the measure to be reliable and valid across differing ages, occupations, and genders. In light of these findings, we were confident that we could utilize the SAST-R with both male and female college students. If Carnes et al. (2010) had developed the SAST-R using males only, we would have exercised caution employing the instrument with female college students. Investigating the development and norming process of the measure, how ever, gave us confidence to implement the SAST-R with multiple genders.

Examining Results

Although arguably the most meaningful, the results section of an empirical article can be the most intimidating. You may be experiencing anxiety symptoms just by thinking about the topic. But the results section can be your friend rather than your enemy. It is here that researchers detail the statistical analyses used to test the research questions and the results of those analyses. To critically consume existing counseling research, you must have a basic understanding of statistical methods and how to interpret outcomes. For example, one important consideration when critiquing a results section is whether the statistical analyses utilized in the study appropriately match the research question. You should be able to identify if the researchers used a group differences analysis when they were looking at variable relationships or vice versa. Once you determine that the researchers employed the appropriate analysis given the research question, you can then evaluate the statistical significance and effect size of the findings.

Statistical significance simply means that the researchers found an effect that did not happen by chance. That is an important first step to understanding the results of the study. However, statistical significance does not necessarily mean that the results are meaningful. Indeed, large sample sizes are likely to produce significant findings simply due to the volume of participants. Therefore, you must determine the *strength* of the observed significance, or the practical significance, by assessing the effect size. This value is what you may find most relevant to your clinical work, because it will help you determine which approach may be important to implement or not implement more than statistical significance will. The effect size reveals the magnitude of the effect that the researchers found. The units of measure for effect sizes are contingent upon the specific statistical analyses used, but small, medium, and large standardized benchmarks have been provided so we can interpret different units (Cohen, 1988b) (Table 2.1).

Now the meaning of the effect size depends on the specifics of the research study. For example, if you are examining the outcomes of a new treatment for depression compared to treatment as usual (TAU), a large effect size indicates that not only was the treatment statistically significant, the magnitude of the effect of the new treatment was substantially better than TAU. You then can conclude that the researchers found a high degree of practical significance in their study. So do small effect sizes mean that the findings were not worthwhile? Not necessarily. Remember, the interpretation of effect sizes depends on the specific research questions being investigated. If a team of researchers was studying the effects of a new medication on curbing the cravings of adults with opioid use disorder, even a small effect size would be important. Although the magnitude of the effect of the new medication was small, it still provided more relief to those with opioid use disorder than a placebo did. Therefore, given the opioid epidemic in the United States, these would be meaningful results.

In our cybersex study, we used descriptive statistical analyses and found that 10.3% of our sample met criteria for cybersex addiction and 89.7% did not. More men than women scored in the clinical range for cybersex addiction and this difference was statistically significant. Finally, we also noted the most endorsed cybersex addiction items on our measure, racial/ethnic differences in cybersex addiction prevalence, and differences based on sexual orientation.

Table 2.1 Research Questions and Corresponding Analyses

Research Question	Statistical Analyses
Do relationships exist between variables?	Multiple logistical regression, simple linear regression, bivariate correlation, path analysis, factor analysis
Do differences exist between groups?	Paired samples t-test, analysis of variance (ANOVA), descriptive discriminant analysis (DDA), chi-square, multivariate analysis of variance (MANOVA)

Evaluating Discussion Sections

The discussion section of an empirical article is where researchers interpret, evaluate, and make meaning of their research findings (Lambie et al., 2008b). Here, you will find authors reiterating whether the results of their study supported or contradicted the proposed research questions. If the researchers found support for their hypotheses, they should elaborate as to what those findings mean for the profession. If the researchers did not find support for their hypotheses, they should offer possible explanations for the unexpected findings. As a consumer of research, you should evaluate the extent to which the authors describe the implications of their findings. Do the researchers provide enough information in this section to answer your questions and help you contextualize the results? Do they provide practical implications for what their study means? Simply rewriting the results section without detailing how the findings fit within the broader scope of research does not meet the standard of social validity. On the other hand, overstating the findings and making generalizations beyond the scope of the study is misleading and potentially harmful to future clients. Consider a situation in which a researcher found that mindfulness-based cognitive behavioral therapy (MBCBT) had a statistically significant yet small effect on posttraumatic stress disorder (PTSD) symptoms among Black male combat veterans. Although the effect size was small and the study utilized only Black male veterans, this researcher claimed in his discussion section that all PTSD treatment centers should now begin using MBCBT. Do you see how misleading this would be? Researchers must find the delicate balance between describing the relevance of their results for clinicians while also staying within the bounds of their study.

Additionally, the discussion section should integrate the findings of the research study into previous literature. Did the researchers' findings confirm the results of previous studies? Did the results provide new information regarding a previously unexamined construct? How did this study advance the research in this area? What new questions are raised as a result of this study? A well-written discussion section should help you understand the constructs more fully, advise you as to how to use the findings in a practical way, and address the bigger picture.

Referring to the cybersex addiction study, we found that 10.3% of college students in our sample met criteria for cybersex addiction (indicating a problematic loss of control over online sexual activity). We found these results to be meaningful for several reasons: First, this percentage is larger than the prevalence rate of sexual addiction among the general adult population. Thus, there is reason to believe that the nature of college student development or characteristics of the collegiate setting increase the risk of cybersex addiction. Second, this substantial percentage of students with cybersex addiction has implications for clinical screening and training. Specifically, to what degree are college counselors assessing for problematic online sexual activity? Do they include items related to cybersex on their intake forms or mention it on their college counseling center website? Further, if compulsive cybersex is reported, to what extent do college counselors feel prepared to address the issue in counseling? What level of training have college counselors had pertaining to sex addiction, pornography addiction, and internet addiction? Third, our results were meaningful in that we found male college students were more likely to be addicted to cybersex than females were. How can we account for these gender differences? Is it merely biological, or are there societal norms that perpetuate addictive sexual behaviors among men? These considerations are presented in our discussion section, as we sought to apply our specific findings to the bigger picture of college student cybersex-related issues and describe practical implications for clinicians.

Finally, well-written discussion sections include a description of the study's limitations. Although no perfect study exists, you must review the limitations and determine whether they affect the practical significance of the findings. For example, a limitation may be the representativeness of the sample. Perhaps the researchers utilized convenience sampling methods and, as a result, 90% of the sample identified as female. How applicable are the findings to males? Are you able to generalize the findings across genders? Furthermore, a potential limitation could be insufficient sample size. To what extent does this affect the accuracy of the statistical analyses? Is there a large enough sample to truly identify an effect where one exists? Moreover, perhaps scores on the study instruments yielded low Cronbach's alpha levels. Can readers rely on the interpretation of data derived from unreliable and inconsistent measures? It is important that you consider the impact of the limitations on the strength, rigor, and validity of the study.

As I mentioned earlier, my colleague and I noted several limitations in our study of collegiate cybersex addiction. Along with a lower-than-desired Cronbach's alpha level and a predominantly female, White, heterosexual sample, we also noted that the sample came from one large public university in the southwestern United States. Therefore, we are unable to conclude if the same levels of cybersex addiction would be found in a small, Catholic, private school in New England. The generalizability of the findings is an additional limitation. By listing these shortcomings, we hoped to be as transparent as possible so readers could come to their own conclusions about the trustworthiness and applicability of our results (Table 2.2).

Table 2.2 Evaluating Existing Empirical Research

Manuscript Section	*Evidence of a Strong Study*
• **Introduction**	• Summarize important existing literature (recent literature and seminal works) • Logical flow to purpose statement • Compelling need for the study ("of course this study is needed!") • Bias free (provide multiple perspectives and differing opinions)
• **Methods**	• Appropriate sampling procedures (rationale for probability or nonprobability) • Participant demographics match population under study • Obtained required sample size • Reported evidence of instrument reliability ($\geq$ .70) and validity (construct, content, or predictive) • Norming sample of instrument matched sampled in research study
• **Results**	• Statistical analyses matched research questions • Reported statistical significance • Reported and interpreted effect size
• **Discussion**	• Provided meaningful interpretation of results • Described practical implications of the findings • Stayed within the bounds of the study • Accurately described study limitations

Applying Existing Research to Practice

Now that you are familiar with how to access and critique existing research, the final step is to apply what you discover to your own clinical practice. Recall that Reynolds (2000b) described the last two steps of the process of utilizing research as applying the findings to your clients and evaluating the outcomes. If the research article meets your standards of applicability (e.g., uses reliable and valid measures, matches your client's demographics, employs appropriate statistical analyses, yielded a desired effect size, detailed practical impacts, identified limitations), you may choose to let the research influence your clinical work. Once implemented, you are obligated to then assess the outcome. Did the services you provided based on the research lead to the expected effects? If so, should you continue? If not, should you adjust? Client reports or standardized assessments can help you ascertain whether or not the research you implemented was effective for your unique client's case.

It is important to note that the integration of evidence-based practice should influence and not determine your clinical work. Indeed, research is supplemental to the clinical judgement of the counselor. Reynolds (2000b) wrote, "clinicians should use their own clinical and professional experience in combination with the results of research based external evidence to make decisions about the care of their patients" (p. 258). Therefore, using both clinical judgement and evidence-based practice can help you provide the best care to your clients.

Ethical and effective client care should be your motivation to examine existing literature, because, let's face it, consuming research can be a daunting task. You will need to carve out sufficient time to identify, access, and read articles. You will need to think critically and evaluate whether the study meets your standards of applicability. Finally, after applying research to a particular client case, you must assess the outcomes to determine whether you should continue or adjust the services you provided. To facilitate the process and perhaps make it more enjoyable, consider forming a research group with other clinicians in your practice or local community. You can schedule regular times to meet and discuss current research, describe how you are applying results within your practice, and gain multiple perspectives regarding clinical outcomes.

Next Steps

This chapter provided an overview of accessing, critiquing, and applying existing literature in meaningful ways. There is much value and practicality in reviewing research in the counseling field. Perhaps you find yourself wrestling with an important question about the care of a client with a learning disability. Perhaps you are interested in starting a research project on client self-efficacy but do not know where to start. Perhaps you would like to begin a group counseling program in a school yet need to provide evidential support to the principal. Reviewing and evaluating existing literature can be a helpful strategy in each of these situations. As researchers continue to disseminate rigorous, relevant research and clinicians continue to consume and apply the research to their practice, the research–practice gap will diminish and the field of counseling will progress.

Practice-Based Application

Thinking again about the area of interest you identified in Chapter 1, consider the following questions:

- If you wanted to find current research about your topic of interest, what search terms could you use to identify relevant research articles to help you answer your question?
- When reviewing the literature related to your topic of interest, what would be the benefit of reading empirical literature? What about nonempirical literature?
- What are some practical ways you can keep up with current research trends related to your topic of interest?

Resources for More Information

Peer-Reviewed Journal Articles

Cohen, J. (1992). A power primer. *Psychological Bulletin, 112,* 155–159. https://doi.org/10.1037/0033-2909.112.1.155

Giordano, A. L., Schmit, M. K., & Schmit, E. (2021). Best practice guidelines for publishing rigorous research in counseling. *Journal of Counseling & Development, 99,* 123–133. https://doi.org/10.1002/jcad.12360

Lambie, G. W., Sias, S. M., Davis, L. M., Lawson, G., & Akos, P. (2008a). A scholarly writing resource for counselor educators and their students. *Journal of Counseling & Development, 86,* 18–25.

O'Hara, C., Chang, C. Y., & Giordano, A. L. (2021a). Multicultural competence in counseling research: The cornerstone of scholarship. *Journal of Counseling & Development, 99,* 200–209. https://doi.org/10.1002/jcad.12367

Reynolds, S. (2000a). Evidence based practice and psychotherapy research. *Journal of Mental Health. 9,* 257–266. https://doi.org/10.1080/713680248

Sink, C. A., & Mvududu, N. H. (2010a). Statistical power, sampling, and effect sizes: Three keys to research relevancy. *Counseling outcome Research and Evaluation, 1,* 1–18. https://doi.org/10.1177/2150137810373613

Wester, K. L., Wachter Morris, C. A., Trustey, C. E., Cory, J. S., & Grossman, L. M. (2021). Promoting rigorous research using innovative qualitative approaches. *Journal of Counseling & Development, 99,* 189–199. https://doi.org/10.1002/jcad.12366

Books

Cohen, J. (1988a). *Statistical power analysis for the behavioral sciences* (2nd ed.). Academic Press.

Creswell, J. W. & Creswell, J. D. (2022a). *Research design: Qualitative, quantitative, and mixed methods approaches* (6th ed.). Sage Publications.

Field, A. (2013). *Discovering statistics using IBM SPSS statistics* (5th ed.). Sage Publications.

Heppner, P. P., Wampold, B. E., Owen, J., Wang, K. T., & Thompson, M. N. (2016a). *Research design in counseling* (4th ed.). Sage Publications.

Sue, D. W., & Sue, D. (2022). *Counseling the culturally diverse: Theory and practice* (9th ed.). John Wiley & Sons.

Questions for Further Review and Application

1 Statistical significance is different than practical significance. How can you critique the practical significance of empirical research?
2 What are some characteristics of a sound, rigorous methods section? What errors may exist in the methodology of an empirical research study?
3 What is the difference between empirical and nonempirical literature? Provide examples of each type.
4 How would you describe a well-written, strong introduction section to an empirical research study? What would be the characteristics you would look for?
5 Are empirically supported treatments appropriate for all cultural groups? How do counselors ensure they are providing culturally sensitive treatments?

References

American Counseling Association. (2014). *ACA code of ethics*. www.counseling.org/knowledge-center/ethics

American Psychological Association. (2010). *Ethical principles of psychologists and code of conduct*. www.apa.org/ethics/code/principles.pdf

American Psychological Association. (2019). *Publication manual of the American Psychological Association* (7th ed.). Author.

Baker, J. D. (2016). The purpose, process and methods of writing a literature review: Editorial. *Association of Operating Room Nurses: AORN Journal, 103*, 265–269. https://doi.org/10.1016/j.aorn.2016.01.016

Balkin, R. S. (2009). Publishing a conceptual manuscript: An editorial perspective. *Journal of Professional Counseling: Practice, Theory, & Research, 37*, 1–2.

Balkin, R. S., & Sheperis, C. J. (2011). Evaluating and reporting statistical power in counseling research. *Journal of Counseling & Development, 89*, 268–272.

Carnes, P., Green, B., & Carnes, S. (2010). The same yet different: Refocusing the Sexual Addiction Screening Test (SAST) to reflect orientation and gender. *Sexual Addiction & Compulsivity, 17*, 7–30. https://doi.org/10.1080/10720161003604084

Cohen, J. (1988b). *Statistical power analysis for the behavioral sciences* (2nd ed.). Academic Press.

Creswell, J. W. & Creswell, J. D. (2022b). *Research design: Qualitative, quantitative, and mixed methods approaches* (6th ed.). Sage Publications.

Elmore, S. A., & Weston, E. H. (2020). Predatory journals: What they are and how to avoid them. *Toxicologic Pathology, 48*(4), 607–610. https://doi.org/10.1177/0192623320920209

Giordano, A. L., & Cashwell, C. S. (2017). Cybersex addiction among college students: A prevalence study. *Sexual Addiction & Compulsivity, 24*, 47–57.

Guiffrida, D., Schwitzer, A. M., & Choate, L. H. (2006). Publishing in the journal of college counseling, part II: Comments on disseminating college counseling knowledge through professional issues and innovative practice articles. *Journal of College Counseling, 9*, 29–32.

Hays, D. G., & Singh, A. A. (2011). *Qualitative inquiry in clinical and educational settings*. Guilford Press.

Heppner, P. P., Wampold, B. E., Owen, J., Wang, K. T., & Thompson, M. N. (2016b). *Research design in counseling* (4th ed.). Sage Publications.

La Roche, M. J., & Christopher, M. S. (2009). Changing paradigms from empirically supported treatment to evidence-based practice: A cultural perspective. *Professional Psychology: Research & Practice, 40*, 396–402. https://doi.org/10.1037/a0015240

Lambie, G. W., Sias, S. M., Davis, L. M., Lawson, G., & Akos, P. (2008b). A scholarly writing resource for counselor educators and their students. *Journal of Counseling & Development, 86*, 18–25.

Merriam-Webster's Collegiate Dictionary (11th ed.). (2004). Merriam-Webster.

Murray, C. E. (2009). Diffusion of innovation theory: A bridge for the research-practice gap in counseling. *Journal of Counseling & Development, 87*, 108–116.

Nagayama Hall, G. C. (2001). Psychotherapy research with ethnic minorities: Empirical, ethnic, and conceptual issues. *Journal of Consulting and Clinical Psychology, 69*, 502–510. https://doi.org/10.1037//0022-006x.69.3.502

National Association of Social Workers. (2021). *Code of ethics*. https://www.socialworkers.org/About/Ethics/Code-ofEthics

Norcross, J. C., & Wampold, B. E. (2011). Evidence-based therapy relationships: Research conclusions and clinical practices. *Psychotherapy, 48*, 98–102. https://doi.org/10.1037/a0022161

O'Hara, C., Chang, C. Y., & Giordano, A. L. (2021b). Multicultural competence in counseling research: The cornerstone of scholarship. *Journal of Counseling & Development, 99*, 200–209. https://doi.org/10.1002/jcad.12367

Pautasso, M. (2013). Ten simple rules for writing a literature review. *PLoS Computational Biology, 9*, 1–4. https://doi.org/10/1371/journal.pcbi.1003149

Reynolds, S. (2000b). Evidence based practice and psychotherapy research. *Journal of Mental Health, 9*, 257–266. https://doi.org/10.1080/713680248

Roysircar, G. (2009). Evidence-based practice and its implications for culturally sensitive treatment. *Journal of Multicultural Counseling & Development, 32*, 66–83.

Sink, C. A., & Mvududu, N. H. (2010b). Statistical power, sampling, and effect sizes: Three keys to research relevancy. *Counseling Outcome Research and Evaluation, 1*, 1–18. https://doi.org/10.1177/2150137810373613

Sue, D., & Sue, D. M. (2008). *Foundations of counseling and psychotherapy: Evidence-based practices for a diverse society.* John Wiley & Sons.

Swiggart, W., Feurer, I. D., Samenow, C., Delmonico, D. L., & Spickard, W. A. (2008). Sexual Boundary Violation Index: A validation study. *Sexual Addiction & Compulsivity, 15,* 176–190. https://doi.org/10.1080/10720160882055939

Watts, R. E. (2011). Developing a conceptual article for publication in counseling journals. *Journal of Counseling & Development, 89,* 308–312.

Wester, K. L. (2011). Publishing ethical research: A step by step overview. *Journal of Counseling & Development, 89,* 301–307.

Wester, K. L., Borders, L. D., Boul, S., & Horton, E. (2013). Research quality: Critique of quantitative articles in the Journal of Counseling & Development. *Journal of Counseling & Development, 91,* 280–290.

3 Research Ethics in Practice

Shreya Vaishnav, Jordan L. Austin, Kelly L. Wester, and Carrie A. Wachter Morris

We would guess that throughout your clinical training experiences, various aspects of ethics have been drilled into your head—doing no harm to the client, beneficence, engaging in effective practice, and even aspects about dual relationships or bartering with your client. However, did you know that almost all mental health professions have a code of ethics specific to research? You might have, but these are often discussed less frequently or skimmed over. Yet research influences our practice by informing us about what is considered to be evidence-based or empirically supported approaches. Research helps to provide new, updated information in order to move each specific discipline forward, and, truthfully, research *should* influence your practice on a daily basis.

While we all know that ethical behavior is important, what exactly is research ethics? Research ethics is the "study or science of right and wrong – of what one ought to do when confronted with conflicting values or obligations" (Steneck, n.d., p. 240). It is deciding right versus wrong when it comes to engaging in any aspect of research at any level. As you read in Chapter 1, one can engage in research at multiple levels, including reading existing research, applying what you have learned, and engaging in or conducting research.

Practitioners should be competent, and thus ethical, in their research behaviors – with the minimal level of this being the ability to consume, or read and critique, existing research (Wester & Borders, 2014). Consumption of research is important to be able to provide up-to-date, empirically supported and informative interventions to clients and students with whom you interact in your practice. Frankly, to not read and consume current research does your clients a disservice. In order to do this ethically, however, you need to know how to read and critique the current research you are consuming, as well as how to reflect upon the findings or implications from the research studies. An example of this would be considering or critiquing elements of the study, such as the participants, research analysis methods, and referenced implications in order to ethically consider the possible validity for use within your practice. Keep in mind, just because something is published doesn't necessarily mean that it is "good" or within research best-practices, nor does it mean that it applies directly to your clients or students. The information on how to read and critique existing research is covered in Chapter 2, so we wouldn't recommend skipping that chapter!

Another level of doing research as a practitioner is to *apply* what you are reading. Your efforts to stay up to date on the current practices will inform the questions, interventions, and treatments you should be offering, as well as the knowledge that has been generated about various diagnoses, symptoms, and behaviors that impact human beings in terms of daily functioning. When translating published research into practice, though, there is importance in making sure you are able to approach these decisions from a grounded and ethically informed perspective.

DOI: 10.4324/9781032706139-3

An example of this might be consideration of your current scope of practice when intentionally applying information you have consumed. If you are integrating a new intervention into your clinical skill set, what reflective practice measures might you put into place to ensure clients are benefiting from your efforts? Perhaps consultation with a supervisor or colleagues, as well as making sure you have a solid understanding of the approach.

At another level, research ethics also applies to *conducting* research – whether that be on a larger scale or within your own practice, even with one person. Many counselors may feel a bit of apprehension or trepidation about the idea of conducting research within practice. If this applies to you – pause, take a deep breath, and know that you'll feel more informed about research as you read along. We are going to focus a little more on how research ethics applies to conducting research in this chapter, although it is important to note that ethics would apply to all levels of research, including consumption, application, and engagement.

Okay, so let's jump off the soapbox temporarily about how ethical practitioners need to engage in research at the various levels (but don't worry, we will get back to that again!) and move into exactly what research ethics are when it comes to conducting research. We'll start with a case study that we will refer to throughout as we walk through various aspects of research ethics.

Zeke, a biracial male, comes to see you for therapy. He reports being angry and frustrated, has yelled at others, punched walls, and ultimately been difficult to be around given his mood and behavior. When asking additional questions, you also find that he has had past suicidal ideation, but nothing current and no intentions to hurt or kill himself. You also find that others have been bullying him. Other students have been making repeated jabs at him personally in ways that have made him question his confidence and efficacy in his daily tasks and activities, as well as feeling less clear about his interpersonal relationships.

Most mental health practitioners have ethical codes that state, while working with Zeke, you need to ensure that you are effective and knowledgeable in what you are offering in terms of interventions and treatment. Mental health practitioner ethical codes include, but are not limited to, the American Counseling Association (ACA, 2014), American Psychological Association (APA, 2016), and the National Association of Social Workers (NASW, 2017). These are just some of the organizations that require you to abide by their ethical codes if you are a member. But other governing bodies, such as licensure boards and divisions of larger organizations, include their own ethical codes as well. Let's step back to the first basic level of research – consumption. It is your ethical obligation to know how to provide Zeke services. That is, what is the most up-to-date knowledge that we have on bullying, anger, and potentially depression along with suicidal ideation? Let's think about some of the outcomes and consequences of bullying based on available literature and research findings. We know that while depression has specific symptoms noted in the *Diagnostic and Statistical Manual of Mental Disorders (DSM 5 TR; APA, 2022)*, researchers have noted a connection between anger and depression (Busch, 2009). We also know various behavioral and cognitive behavioral treatments have been found to be effective in working with individuals who exhibit depression (e.g.,Sturmey, 2009; Lopez-Lopez et al., 2019), as well as coping with the negative effects from being targeted with bullying behaviors (Association for Behavioral and Cognitive Therapies, 2017). However, the use of any of these treatments or interventions should depend on a critique of what you are reading. How would the treatment differ if your client was five years old versus 17 years old versus 39 years old? We would assume that treatment would be quite different, and the research would support that as well. Additionally, what is the setting that you are working in? Some settings allow for manualized, long-term treatment, while other settings do not (e.g., brief inpatient crisis treatment or school settings). So research *consumption* is where to begin when you consider what you are offering to clients or students as effective forms of treatment. Ethically, you would apply only what is most relevant to your clients, which, for this example, is Zeke.

Now let's get more into conducting research within your practice. In Zeke's case, maybe you have scoured the literature, yet have not found something that really fits his presenting symptoms and concerns, or maybe you have applied the various treatments and interventions without success. Maybe, through your years of experience, you have begun to formulate a new form of treatment that you have engaged in, combining or integrating different techniques or theories you have learned along the way. You think (based on anecdotal information from previous clients) that this "new treatment" works. In all of these cases, it may be time to conduct your own research to truly determine what works based on data rather than anecdotal information or simply your perception.

As you will read throughout this text, research can look different in terms of the various methodologies and designs you can select. Selecting a research design that will actually answer your question is one ethical consideration (Wester, 2011). Every step of the research process, from idea inception through methodological design and implementation of procedures all the way into publication and disseminating your results, entails ethical decisions (Wester, 2011). Bersoff and Bersoff (2008) even suggested that ethical decision making is a methodological issue, as you need to make decisions related to procedures throughout the entire research process that will often have ethical considerations. Given all this, let's step back for a minute and talk about research integrity, which is an overarching umbrella for research ethics. From there, we will get into more detail about which ethical principles are important to follow when conducting research.

Research Integrity

How many professional organizations are you a member of? One? Three? More than three? Take a moment and consider. Now that you have a list in your mind, do you know whether each of these organizations has an ethical code? If they do, are you aware of the ethical code of *each* organization and the indicated details around what you need to do when confronted with difficult situations in which right or wrong decisions could be made? In order to practice with integrity, you need to abide by all of the ethical codes of organizations that you are a member of, affiliated with, or employed by. Now take a moment and consider each of these organizations again – do their ethical codes include research ethics? In the same sense of using ethical codes within practice, knowledge of your organizations' research ethics is important in order to engage in research with integrity.

As stated, you need to abide by the ethical code of conduct for any professional organization of which you are a member. These codes likely include ethics governing both practice and research. Research integrity is defined as "a commitment to intellectual honesty and personal responsibility" (Institute of Medicine, 2002), in which you adhere to rules, regulations, guidelines, and commonly accepted professional codes or norms (Office of Research Integrity, 2000) of the organizations to which you belong and affiliate. Steneck (n.d.) specifically states this when talking about engaging in responsible conduct of research, or

conducting research in ways that fulfill professional responsibilities of researchers, as defined by their professional organizations, the institutions for which they work, and, when relevant, the government and public.

We would make the argument that all research you would conduct is relevant to the public given that individuals within the public are the clients to whom you are providing services – whether they be in outpatient or inpatient, hospital, medical, or K–16 settings. Each individual you work with and their families could either benefit or be harmed by the research you (or other mental health professionals) conduct.

When examining the various organizational ethical codes provided by ACA, APA, and NASW, they are more similar than they are different. Each one stresses the need to ensure participant safety, to allow for informed consent of participants to partake in research on their own volition, and to do no harm. Each also mentions aspects of publication, confidentiality, and ensuring engagement in responsible conduct of research. While each of these ethical codes goes beyond the basic principles required of conducting human-subject research, let's take a moment and focus on the minimal three principles that should always be considered when conducting research with humans: (1) respect for persons, (2) beneficence, and (3) justice. Each of these principles is inherent in the Belmont Report, which is considered one of the cornerstone documents of ethical procedures to assist in the protection of the rights of individuals participating in research.

Belmont Report

The Belmont Report was developed in 1979, by the National Commission for the Protection of Human Subjects of Biomedical and Behavioral Research, due to multiple atrocities in how human beings were treated as research subjects. The Belmont Report provided federal regulations to protect the rights of individuals that were, unfortunately, not being protected by researchers. Take a moment and consider any research studies that you have been a human subject in – do you recall getting informed-consent documents telling you about the study and what would be required of you, along with any potential risks that could be a result of participating in the research study? Did you receive any incentives? Did you feel coerced to participate? Hopefully, your answers to these questions reflect the pillars of ethical research of nonmaleficence, beneficence, and autonomy. Yes, you received an informed consent detailing what you were being asked to do, as well as the risks of participating, with an emphasis on your right to withdraw from the study at any time. Maybe you received incentives, but in the long run hopefully these incentives were not so bountiful that you felt coerced to participate in the research, even if you did not want to. These are all considerations that you need to think through when you are designing and engaging in research. Let's take a minute to walk through some pivotal moments in the history of research to determine *how* we even got to a place, mere decades ago, of needing regulations around engaging in research – and then we will talk through how these regulations impact you on a day-to-day or study-to-study level.

Across several historical examples, researchers executed studies involving human beings that led to suffering, pain, and death. In these studies, you will find that various components of beneficence, respect for persons, and justice are missing. In each of these studies, the behavior of the researchers and the subsequent consequences and harm that came to the participants led to the principles noted in the Belmont Report and, ultimately, the protocols that institutional review boards (IRBs) use to evaluate research today.

Nazi Medical War Crimes

The Nazi Medical War Crimes is regarded as one of the most infamous and horrendous research studies publicly known. In World War II, Nazi physicians performed medical experiments on thousands of prisoners in concentration camps to study how the human body reacts to various stressors, such as viruses, extreme temperatures and conditions, and the injection or ingestion of poisons, gasoline, and other contaminants. The results of these studies were suffering and death for the prisoners forced into participation. Ultimately, the Nazi physicians were tried for crimes against humanity; however, that did not undo the cruelty and deaths that had already been caused by their studies.

Tuskegee Syphilis Study

The Tuskegee Syphilis Study, conducted for 40 years spanning from 1932 to 1972, was one of the longest-running studies in the United States. The stated goal of this study was to specifically explore the impact of syphilis on the human body. However, many horrific acts occurred within this study, including but not limited to lack of informed consent. Participants were deceived about the nature of the study, and they were not informed of risks of participation. Furthermore, the researchers failed to disband the study once known risks emerged. Ultimately, the researchers of this study enrolled 600 Black males, 400 of whom were infected with the syphilis virus and 200 who were considered controls. The participants were deceived by being provided with misinformation that they would receive "free treatment" through their participation in the study; however, the researchers knowingly provided interventions that would do nothing to alleviate or cure the syphilis virus. By 1936, and within four years of starting this study, it was clear from the data that the 400 males with syphilis had a greater number and severity of symptoms and complications compared to the males without syphilis – therefore, the researchers were aware of the risks existing without proper treatment. Even armed with this information, the researchers neither informed participants nor did they alter their "treatment interventions." Within 10 years of the start of the study, it was obvious that the death rate for participants with syphilis was at least double that of the controls, yet nothing was done at this point to terminate the study *and* the study continued until 1972 – an additional 30 years. To make matters worse, penicillin was introduced in the 1940s, but researchers of the Tuskegee Syphilis Study did not inform participants or provide penicillin as a treatment option.

Willowbrook Study

From 1956 to 1971, a study designed to explore the effects of hepatitis on children within a controlled environment was conducted in the Willowbrook State School, a school originally developed for children who were "mentally defective." Parents who tried to enroll their children in the school were informed that the school had limited spaces available, so consenting to allow their child to be injected with the hepatitis virus was the only way to enroll a child in the school. Parents were provided no other information other than statements provided to assuage any fears, stating that all children would likely contract the virus anyway given the crowded and unclean nature of the school facilities. The information provided to parents could be incorrectly deemed "consent" in some ways, but it ultimately included misinformation and inaccurate details. Furthermore, it was coercive in nature, as the school did have vacancies but was only admitting children of parents who agreed to allow their children to be injected with hepatitis. Additionally, parents were not provided with information about the long-term chronic liver disease that would develop later in life due to the virus.

Jewish Chronic Disease Hospital Study

While the Willowbrook and Tuskegee Syphilis studies were continuing, researchers in the Jewish Chronic Disease Hospital in New York began a study in 1963 to determine if the human body could reject cancer cells or, if due to other medical illnesses or ailments, fighting off cancer cells was improbable. The researchers recruited participants by asking if they would like to engage in a treatment intervention, however, they did not indicate what this treatment intervention was nor the risks associated with it. Ultimately this "treatment intervention" was injecting live cancer cells into participants' bodies. There was no informed consent and no written documentation of the procedures. When confronted with cruelties performed on the patients, the researchers stood by their actions, indicating that they did not inform patients about the live cancer cells because they believed it would frighten patients. Though it can be noted that written documentation for medical procedures was not common in this era, it is also possible there were additional ethical concerns related to this decision. This behavior and belief maps onto what Bersoff and Bersoff (2008) suggested as a reason why ethical breaches in research occur – when researchers see human participants as a means to an end and no longer view them as individual people.

The accumulation of horrors that each of these studies created led to the Belmont Report, a document written to protect human subject participants by outlining basic ethical principles and responsibilities of researchers. The Belmont Report outlines the three ethical principles that all researchers should follow in the design and follow-through of their studies. These principles include respect for persons, beneficence, and justice for all participants. So, you might be asking, what do these actually mean?

Respect for Persons

Respect for persons entails two components: (1) autonomy and (2) protections for vulnerable populations. Any individual who is being considered as a participant for a research study needs to be treated as an autonomous agent in their own right (National Institute of Health [NIH], 2002), meaning that they have the ability to make decisions for themselves and that their thoughts, opinions, and choices should never be ignored, obstructed, or disrespected by the researcher. Additionally, certain populations, such as prisoners, inpatient populations, children, elderly, individuals with mental incapacities, and pregnant women (due to their unborn children) are considered vulnerable populations. Thus, special caution must occur to make sure steps are taken within the consent process to respect the rights of these individuals who may have less autonomy and freedom as other individuals to decline to participate in a research study.

How does this play out in research? First and foremost, the idea of autonomy and protections occurs within the informed consent. With the informed consent process, you are providing your clients, students, or research participants with enough information for them to make an informed decision about whether they would like to participate in this study. To make an informed decision, individuals need to know what they will be asked to do in the study (e.g., complete survey questionnaires about a particular topic, press buttons, engage in exercise, receive a clinical treatment, take medication), how long this process may take (e.g., 15 minutes, one hour a week for 12 weeks), and the risks of participation (e.g., emotional distress, pain, embarrassment, illness). Individuals should also be made aware of whether the information they provide will be confidential or even anonymous or whether the information can be known by people outside the study (e.g., in publications, presentations, other clinicians).

Knowing this information allows for individuals to make an informed choice as to whether they believe that the risks of participating outweigh the benefits of participating.

Respect for persons also includes ensuring that participation in research is voluntary and that individuals can withdraw at any time. Additionally, it is important that no coercion is occurring – or unjust persuasion to participate in the study. Coercion is dependent on the situation, the population, and the context. For example, you can see how incarcerated individuals are a vulnerable population – do they have the ability to voluntarily make a decision to participate in the study, or are they forced to do so because the study is being implemented prison-wide? Context can lead to coercion by a lack of ability to decline participation in a study. Incentives can do the same thing. For example, let's suggest that we ask you to take part in a study, and we offer you $20. Would this entice you to participate? You may say "yes" … or maybe your response is "it depends." It may depend on whether we are asking you to answer a packet of questionnaires that may take you 30 minutes or if we instead indicated that we needed you to drive to a specific location 40 minutes away one time per week for four weeks. We may even ask you to ingest a pill. You can see how in one case an incentive may be enticing – although not enticing enough to be coercive – while in another scenario it may not be worth it at all. Take this same $20 incentive, and now imagine a family who is struggling to make ends meet or put food on the table for their children. This same $20 might become more coercive, as it meets a life need that isn't otherwise met. You can see how this family, as an example, might engage in more risk-taking behaviors in a study for the same $20 incentive. Studies have resulted in participant death due to the nature of the incentive or the perceived lack of choice (Wolf, 2009).

Now that we've introduced the concept, let's apply this idea of respect for persons to Zeke, considering that you are wanting to collect data and study whether your "new treatment" is effective in decreasing symptoms of depression and anger. Zeke is a client with whom you would like to not only apply the treatment but also begin collecting information and data. Hypothetically, you can actually apply the treatment or intervention and never collect data – as long as you are abiding by your professional organizations' ethical codes of providing effective treatments and doing no harm to your client, you can continue to offer this treatment. Collecting data from Zeke, however, adds a new layer. You now need not only to ask him if he would like to participate in the treatment, but you also need to ask him if he is willing to participate in the research side of this by providing you with data (e.g., answering questionnaires, providing information through interviews in your sessions, allowing you to use your behavioral observations). You need to provide Zeke with informed consent to participate in research that is separate from his consent to engage in treatment with you generally. He needs to know:

1 That this is a research study, which is separate from the actual treatment.
2 That his choice to provide you with data is voluntary, and that he would be able to receive the treatment even if he said "no."
3 What he would need to do (e.g., participate in treatment, answer questionnaires five times throughout treatment) if he decided to participate.
4 That he can withdraw from providing you with study data at any point in time without penalty (e.g., fees wouldn't go up, treatment would still be offered).
5 What the risks are to participate (e.g., would information be released, confidentiality questioned, would he not receive another form of treatment, would he experience emotional distress in answering questions).

6 What the benefits are to participate in the research (e.g., would he receive free treatment, would he gain anything – incentive not included).
7 Are there incentives to participate (e.g., typically defined as monetary or material in nature but could be other things as well)?

Once he has all of this information, Zeke can make an informed choice of whether to participate. This is all, of course, assuming that Zeke is considered an adult who can make decisions on his own, and that he is not a member of what is considered to be a vulnerable population. If, for example, he is under the age of 18, he is considered to be a minor; you not only have to gain parental consent with all of the information provided earlier, you still need to gain Zeke's assent as well – and talk to him about your research using developmentally appropriate vocabulary. Additionally, if Zeke was residing within a prison, then you have different considerations to make sure he is not coerced into the study. Those might include that this study was not being inflicted on him as a prisoner because of "easy access" to him and that it was a study that truly needed a prison population to answer the question.

Beneficence

The ethical principle of beneficence refers to the responsibility that you have as a researcher to "do good." Essentially, is the result of your study going to enhance knowledge or add quality information to the topic or discipline area? We stated that, ethically, research should be enhancing and expanding our knowledge within our (or other) disciplines, and, thus, each study should have an element of social validity. Rosenthal (2008) went further to state that conducting research with no social validity and that does not lead to influential outcomes is ultimately unethical. What he means by this is that the risks and costs to participants in terms of their time, money, and energy expended to participate in this study outweigh the benefits (or lack thereof) to the knowledge gained. We would hope that if you are conducting research, you have an intention behind it – such as wanting to know if you are effective, desiring to gain understanding about the impact of a new treatment method or technique, or seeking to provide better comprehension about a particular symptom, behavior, or diagnosis.

Under the principle of beneficence, you need to consider all aspects of your study prior to even implementing it. This means considering each decision well in advance before asking your clients or students to participate. You have to consider and plan for all possible scenarios that might occur and the risks that individuals might experience. According to the American Counseling Association (2014), as a researcher, you are responsible for designing, planning, conducting, and reporting research.

Let's apply this particular ethical principle to Zeke. The intervention and engagement in research needs to have minimal interference in Zeke's life and daily functioning, including in the treatment you are offering. While you believe you are offering an effective treatment to him, you have to acknowledge (a) if there is a better treatment out there for his diagnosis, symptoms, or behavior, or even for Zeke, specifically; or (b) if you realize in the middle of treatment this is not working for Zeke, that you need to abandon your research study with Zeke and offer him a treatment that might be more effective for him.

While beneficence may seem to be common sense, the difficulty with it is there is no "right way" to determine if the benefits outweigh the risks for each participant, as each person is different. Beneficence tends to be subjective to some extent. However, it should be noted that this judgment should not simply be made one time in the research process, such as at the beginning of the study. Rather, this evaluation should be continual throughout the process and should be based on each individual. Some have even questioned whether those providing a service should be the evaluators of that service (Coyle & Olsen, 2005), suggesting that bias may be an inherent flaw in making beneficence judgment calls. Wanting the data to demonstrate a positive outcome could potentially lead to coercion or ignoring of negative outcomes. It is believed that you can conduct research on your own practice, but you need to be cautious or pull in a collaborator who does not have a conflict of interest in the study to help you see when you may be violating ethical boundaries.

Justice

The principle of justice deals with objectively evaluating fairness to participants of the research study. Justice lends itself to inquiring if the benefits outweigh the risks in the study. This does not just mean outweighing them generally but ultimately asking the question of "who bears the burden of risks and who receives the benefits?" Risks include threatening participant safety, interfering with day-to-day life, methods used for sampling or selecting participants, and ensuring participants receive what they are promised (i.e., incentives, benefits of the study, interventions and treatments, outcomes). In this principle, if the participant experiences all of the risks and none of the benefits, then justice does not exist – even if the benefits would be expanding knowledge in the field. Not all participants may experience a benefit in the immediate future, but the risks should not drastically outweigh the benefits. An example may be that participating in a 30-minute survey about depression with no immediate benefits (e.g., no free intervention or training, no immediate outcome) may not have a large differential for someone to participate when comparing participant risks to benefits. The risks here are likely not high. However, in an extreme example, being injected with the hepatitis virus with no benefit does lack justice.

Other aspects of injustice that can result in a study would be to claim that participants would receive $5 upon completion, and somehow one participant does not receive this $5. In this case, injustice has occurred. Another aspect to consider is whether traveling to your office for one hour per week for 12 weeks is even feasible for a client, and, if not, then the client's life may be impacted by participating in the study. Finally, considering who to include in your study is important, as is how you ask the questions or collect information. For example, in the case example study exploring this new treatment, is there a reason why you may include Zeke (a biracial male) in your study, but you may not include Lauren (an 18-year-old White female) or Micah (a 47-year-old Black male)? You may also consider identities of your participants and clients, especially marginalized identities, including but not limited to religion, sexual orientation, nationality, disability, and several others. The National Institute of Health (2002) speaks to the selection of human subjects, stating that selection of research participants needs to be equitable. In conducting your study, you need to consider from whom you need information (e.g., age group, sex, gender) based on who the particular study is designed for with the knowledge that no population should be overburdened to participate in research without benefits, and no population should be excluded without good reason (NIH, 2002). Additionally, no person should be a research participant unwillingly, nor should individuals be selected solely due to convenience and access. Justice (though respect and beneficence can be argued here as well) also includes the types of questions and information you collect from individuals. Various organizations have developed competencies and standards of care when researching marginalized or vulnerable populations. One recent example of this is the Standards of Care for Research With Participants Who Identify as LGBTQ+ (Griffith et al., 2017), which was developed by individuals affiliated with the Association for Lesbian, Gay, Bisexual, and Transgender Issues in Counseling and the Association for Assessment and Research in Counseling.

Institutional Review Board

This is a lot of information to remember and balance when conducting research. That said, we cannot overstate the importance of thinking through all of these things from the beginning and considering them not only when you are developing your idea but also when you are designing it and carrying it out. The good news is that most researchers do not have to do this on their own. Checks and balances exist in most systems – at least when you are first designing and proposing your study. All institutions that have any federal funding typically have (or have access to) an institutional review board (IRB). An IRB is a group of individuals (typically around five or more) from various disciplines that assists with ensuring respect, beneficence, and justice of all human participants by examining and evaluating your study before you can conduct it (Leedy & Ormrod, 2005). Their task is to weigh the risks versus the benefits to determine how your client, student, or participant will be directly impacted. The IRB will examine the safeguards you have put into place regarding the risks that you have identified, and the board will determine if there are risks inherent in your study that you haven't identified. They will explore the way in which you are gaining informed consent to determine if this meets all respects for persons in terms of autonomy, along with taking into account any vulnerable populations, oversampling of populations, or inappropriate exclusion of other populations. But what happens if you are working with an agency that does not have federal funding or access to an immediate IRB? There are other ways to make sure you have oversight. For a fee, commercial IRBs do exist, or you can partner with another researcher who is at an institution with access to an existing IRB (Rice, 2008). Most schools, universities, and hospitals have IRBs within their organization and would have easy access.

You may think that with the creation of the Belmont Report and the oversight of the IRB, research is free from misconduct. Or even if there is occasional misconduct, all research follows the guiding principles of respect, beneficence, and justice. Unfortunately, you would be incorrect in those assumptions. In a study exploring counseling professionals (including educators, students, and practitioners), 24% to 45% of participants self-reported the likelihood that they would deviate from the responsible conduct of research with specific behaviors (Wester et al., 2008). More specifically, 24% reported they would be likely to use deception to persuade individuals to participate in their study, while 4% reported they would be likely to report false data to gain grant funding. In another study (Wester et al., 2010), 7% of counseling practitioners reported they wouldn't get parental consent before approaching a vulnerable population of children to participate in a study, and 3% reported publishing before removing identifying information about participants. These irreparable actions violate client confidentiality and research participant rights.

In another recent study funded by the National Institutes of Health, researchers explored babies born prematurely at 24 to 27 weeks. At this preterm birth, babies are typically at risk for death or eye disease. This study was designed to divide babies into two groups: One group receiving higher amounts of oxygen and the second receiving lower amounts of oxygen. This study resulted in the death of 221 out of 1,163 babies across both groups (Macklin, 2015). While the study was not found to be unethical, the Office of Human Research Protections determined that the informed consent documents lacked information about the consequences of using varied levels of oxygen with this at-risk population, which resulted in the inability of the parents to make an informed choice.

Another recent case that resulted in legal allegations is the example of *Taus v. Loftus*. In this example, a researcher had produced – with client permission – video recordings of her as a child, again in her late teens, and finally as an adult. These videos revealed the process of repressed memory that can occur in the case of child sexual abuse. The video recordings had been used, with client permission, in educational training and had been written about professionally in peer-refereed articles, with the original authors removing all identifying information. However, another researcher (Loftus), who had a desire to combat the statements behind repressed memories from the initial author, hired a private detective to dig into and collect information about the client's personal life and history (Kluemper, 2014). While Loftus was not the clinician of the client, she was in the role of a researcher. Others have reflected on the role that Loftus had – given that she was not the client's clinician and thus was not bound by the same ethics of confidentiality of mental health practitioners (Koocher, 2014). What can be determined, though, is that Loftus did not abide by the basic principles of respect, beneficence, and justice. Ultimately, she never asked for permission to dig into the life of this client by utilizing a private detective and to then disclose personal and identifying information in the public domain through presentations and publications. Additionally, the data was flawed, and only one side was provided without doing a thorough unbiased analysis (Koocher, 2014), thus inhibiting beneficence. Only harm came from the outcome of this research without a quality product.

Ultimately, the takeaway message we have for you is that research ethics must be considered from the start of your idea and should be considered throughout the entire research process. It should underscore the design of your study and procedural decisions, as well as the analyses and dissemination of your research findings. When you are both the mental health provider and researcher, an added layer is required to ensure that your client or student always receives adequate and ethical care; your research study does not supersede this care. This may look similar in some instances and different in others when it comes to qualitative and quantitative research designs, but ultimately, you should always consider the three overarching ethical principles of *respect for persons, beneficence,* and *justice.*

Practice Based Application

Think about the client-presenting concern, symptom, or situation as well as the population/group that you identified in Chapter 1, and use that to answer the following questions:

- How do the three overarching research principles laid out in the Belmont Report (respect for persons, beneficence, and justice for all participants) relate directly to the topic and population/group that you identified in Chapter 1? Provide an example of how you would engage in each of these research principles in your potential study.
- What are some situations related to research ethics that you may need to keep in mind as you pursue answers to your question(s) about this topic?

If you were to conduct research on this topic, whom would you need to contact within your institution to review your ethical procedures and receive approval to begin your study? Identify the website and contact information.

Resources for More Information

Peer-Reviewed Journal Articles

Wester, K. L. (2011). Publishing ethical research: A step-by-step overview. *Journal of Counseling and Development, 89,* 301–307.
Wester, K. L., & Borders, L. D. (2014). Research competencies in counseling: A Delphi study. *Journal of Counseling & Development, 92,* 447–458.

Books and Other Resources

*Your discipline's, organization's, or place of employment's ethical codes regarding research.Ethics in Mental Health Research. (n.d.). *Ethics in mental health research.* Retrieved November 8, 2017, from http://emhr.net/

Office of Research Integrity. (2000). *Office of research integrity policies.* Retrieved November 9, 2017, from https://ori.hhs.gov/ori-policies

Wester, K. L. (2005). *Conducting research responsibly: Cases for counseling professionals. Handbook and DVD.* NBCC.

Questions for Further Review and Application

1   What are the three main principles for ethically conducting research?
2   What committee typically has oversight to assess the risk versus benefits to research participants?
3   What is the reason the Belmont Report was created?
4   When considering conducting research in your own practice, what are some of the questions you need to consider in order to make sure you are abiding by the three ethical principles?

References

American Counseling Association. (2014). *ACA code of ethics.* Author.

American Psychological Association. (2016). Revision of ethical standard 3.04 of the ethical.

American Psychiatric Association. (2022). *Diagnostic and statistical manual of mental disorders* (5th ed., text rev.). https://doi.org/10.1176/appi.books.9780890425787

Association for Behavioral and Cognitive Therapies. (2017). *Bullying.* Retrieved November 14, 2017, from www.abct.org/Information/?m=mInformation&fa=fs_BULLYING

Bersoff, D. M., & Bersoff, D. N. (2008). Ethical perspectives in clinical research. In D. N. Bersoff (Ed.), *Ethical conflicts in psychology* (pp. 387–389). American Psychological Association.

Busch, F. N. (2009). Anger and depression. *Advanced in Psychiatric Treatment, 15,* 271–278.

Coyle, A., & Olsen, C. (2005). Research in therapeutic settings: Ethical considerations. In R. Tribe & J. Morrissey (Eds.), *Handbook of professional and ethical practice for psychologists, counsellors, and psychotherapists* (pp. 249–262). Brunner-Routledge.

Griffith, C., Akers, W., Dispenza, F., Luke, M., Farmer, L. B., Watson, J. C., Davis, R. J., & Goodrich, K. M. (2017). *Standards of care for research with participants who identify as LGBTQ+.* Retrieved November 14, 2017, from www.algbtic.org/standards-of-care.html

Institute of Medicine. (2002). *Integrity in scientific research: Creating an environment that promotes responsible conduct.* National Academy of Sciences Press.

Kluemper, N. S. (2014). Published case reports: One woman's account of having her confidentiality violated. *Journal of Interpersonal Violence, 29,* 3232–3244.

Koocher, G. P. (2014). Research ethics and private harms. *Journal of Interpersonal Violence, 29,* 3267–3276.

Leedy, P. D., & Ormrod, J. E. (2005). *Practical research: Planning and designing.* Pearson.

Macklin, R. (2015). Can one do good medical ethics without principles? *Journal of Medical Ethics: Journal of Institute of Medical Ethics, 41,* 75–78.

López-López, J. A., Davies, S. R., Caldwell, D. M., Churchill, R., Peters, T. J., Tallon, D., … & Welton, N. J. (2019). The process and delivery of CBT for depression in adults: a systematic review and network meta-analysis. *Psychological medicine,* 49(12), 1937–1947.

National Association of Social Workers. (2017). *Code of ethics of the National Association of Social Workers.* Author.

National Commission for the Protection of Human Subjects of Biomedical and Behavioral Research. (1979). *The Belmont Report: Ethical principles and guidelines for the protection of human subjects of research.* Retrieved from https://www.hhs.gov/ohrp/regulations-and-policy/belmont-report/index.html

National Institute of Health. (2002). *Responsible research: A systems approach to protecting research participants.* National Academies Press.

Rice, T. W. (2008). How to do human subjects research if you do not have an institutional review board. *Respiratory Care, 53,* 1362–1367.

Rosenthal, R. (2008). Science and ethics in conducting, analyzing, and reporting psychological research. In D. N. Bersoff (Ed.), *Ethical conflicts in psychology* (pp. 390–397). American Psychological Association.

Steneck, N. H. (n.d.). *ORI introduction to the responsible conduct of research.* Office of Research Integrity. Retrieved November 14, 2017, from https://ori.hhs.gov/ori-introduction-responsible-conduct-research

Sturmey, P. (2009). Behavioral activation is an evidence-based treatment for depression. *Behavior Modification, 33,* 818–829.

Wester, K. L., Willse, J., & Davis, M. S. (2008). The responsible conduct of research measure: The initial development and pilot study. *Accountability in Research, 15,* 87–104.

Wester, K. L., Willse, J., & Davis, M. (2010). Psychological climate, stress, and research integrity among counselor educators. *Counselor Education and Supervision, 50,* 39–55.

Wolf, L. E. (2009). IRB policies regarding finder's fees and role conflicts in recruiting research participants. *Ethics and Human Research, 31,* 14–19.

4   Evaluating and Designing Surveys

W. Bradley McKibben

Throughout this book, you are exposed to a variety of methodologies that can be used to answer important research questions. Many of the methodologies discussed in this book, including quantitative and experimental designs, may utilize surveys as part of the study. Have you ever thought about where these surveys come from, how a survey is created, or whether a survey is actually a good one? There is an old saying that a worker is only as good as one's tools, and this holds true for survey-based research as well. The conclusions we draw from responses to a survey are only as good as the extent to which those responses are valid and reliable. The purpose of this chapter is to familiarize you with the process of designing a survey so that you have the tools to develop your own survey should the need arise. You will learn how surveys are typically used in counseling research, what surveys are designed to do, and the steps you need to take in designing a survey. Because this chapter merely scratches the surface of survey design, the chapter will conclude with additional resources that can further guide you through the process.

Introduction to Survey Design

Surveys are a common tool that practitioners and other helping professionals use to gain information about human behavior, thoughts, emotions, personality traits, and more. Whereas researchers in natural sciences such as biology, chemistry, or physics can observe and study physical phenomena more directly, behavioral scientists such as counselors, social workers, marriage and family therapists, or psychologists tend to study occurrences that are difficult to observe directly because they exist in the psychological realm rather than the physical world. For example, a chemist can study the molecular composition of cells through carefully organized experiments and observations. Because a cell is a physical object, the cell and its components can be studied directly. Now, consider the cognitive-behaviorally oriented practitioner who is interested in negative thought patterns. Many people likely would agree that such thought patterns exist, but they cannot be observed directly in the physical world. We cannot observe negative thought patterns in a vial or under a microscope.

A fundamental way that behavioral scientists come to understand psychological phenomena is by understanding how people express and experience them. By understanding people's experiences and expressions of psychological phenomena, we develop and test theories that describe and explain the human condition (e.g., behaviors, thoughts, emotions). There also might be differing definitions or theories of such phenomena, depending upon who you ask. These phenomena, often referred to as constructs, can be defined in ways that we can systematically study them.

DOI: 10.4324/9781032706139-4

Constructs, theories, and ideas about the human condition are often where surveys come into play. In the behavioral sciences, where counseling lies, the survey is one of our microscopes or vials, metaphorically speaking, to measure aspects of the human condition not directly observable by physical means. A survey allows us to gather information from people about their experiences with, expressions of, reactions to, or opinions about a construct of interest. A construct is how we operationally define something we are interested in knowing more about and need to measure, such as negative self-talk, happiness, or depression. A well-designed survey allows a practitioner to get as close as possible to measuring the construct of interest in a valid and reliable way. And it is this point, the idea of measuring a construct as purely as possible, that drives the design of any new survey.

When to Design a Survey

A good litmus test of when it is time to design a survey is when you have a question you want to answer or a construct you are interested in, but you cannot find a way to measure it. Although innumerable surveys exist already, the human psyche, the human condition, society, and culture are infinitely complex and ever evolving. Further, as practitioners and other behavioral scientists continue to learn about people, the theories and conceptual frameworks that inform our understanding will be refined or debunked, and new ones will be developed. Thus, it is very possible that you will stumble upon a question or hypothesis about people through your work with clients that someone else has not developed a way to measure.

When you want or need to measure something and there is no (good) way to do it, then survey design may be appropriate. However, in order to design a survey, you need to know enough about your construct of interest to be able to operationalize it for measurement. That is, you need to be able to define your construct conceptually based on theory, and you need to be able to define the construct in a way that it can be studied. If you do not have enough information to do this, you may need to do further reading and research to better define your construct. Alternatively, you may wish to start with qualitative research studies, some of which are described in other chapters in this book, that can help you better understand people's experiences with the phenomena you are seeking to study and measure.

Sample Research Questions in Survey Design

Because survey design, as discussed in this chapter, has a specific purpose (i.e., developing and testing a new survey), this means that a practitioner is trying to answer specific questions about how well a new survey measures what it is supposed to measure (e.g., validity) and how reliable the information gained from clients is on the survey. For example, if a practitioner wants to develop a new survey (or even evaluate an existing survey) to measure depression, some of the first questions that need to be answered are how well does the new survey actually measure depression (validity), and how consistent is the new survey at producing accurate information about depression (reliability)? Because such questions are very specific, the research questions may look different from other methodological approaches you read about in this book. Survey design tends to follow a series of steps in which you first develop the survey itself, and then you have clients (or students, if you work in schools) complete it so that you can research how well your survey holds up statistically. Research questions for survey design are usually honing in on those statistical tests with the sample of clients who completed the survey. This process is explained later in the chapter. Examples of research questions when designing a survey might include:

- To what extent is there evidence for construct validity?
- To what extent is there evidence for reliability among the subtests used to specify factors?
- To what extent is there evidence for convergent validity?
- To what extent is there discriminant validity?
- Is there evidence for social desirability or inattentive responding among individuals completing the survey?

If these research questions sound extremely specific and statistical, they are. However, they are not as intimidating as they may seem at first. Remember, when you design a survey, you are essentially creating a test of some aspect of the human condition that you hypothesize to exist (e.g., behaviors, thoughts, emotions, personality traits, relational processes) but typically cannot immediately be observed by you. The research questions and accompanying statistical tests are designed to provide you with evidence for how well your survey *actually* captures what you *think* it captures.

Tackling Survey Design: The Case of Meredith

To illustrate how surveys are designed and tested, consider the case of Meredith (she/her), a professional counselor working in a community mental health center. Meredith specialized in working with clients who engaged in non-suicidal self-injury (NSSI; e.g., cutting, burning, scratching), and she noticed that many of her clients discussed using NSSI as a way to cope with overwhelming, negative thoughts and feelings. A pattern seemed to emerge in which clients would experience a wave of thoughts (e.g., "I am worthless," "My life will never get better") and/or emotions (e.g., sadness, anger, panic/anxiety), and these thoughts and emotions were experienced so intensely that clients could not bear them. As a result, Meredith's clients would use NSSI to relieve the intensity, and many reported feeling better after engaging in self-injury.

Meredith wanted to better understand these thoughts and feelings that seemed to spur NSSI behavior so she could help her clients learn to recognize and de-escalate them with healthier coping strategies, thereby releasing the perceived need to use NSSI. She recognized that she had no way to assess for these thoughts other than verbal self-report from her clients, which could sometimes be difficult for them to articulate aloud. She also wondered if other practitioners might encounter similar phenomena when working with clients who engage in NSSI. A survey might help her gather information from clients quickly, and it could help her study whether overwhelmingly negative thoughts and emotions prompt NSSI behavior.

Important Steps in Survey Design

This section breaks down the steps to designing a survey, and we will use Meredith's case as an example throughout the steps. There is no one way to design a survey, but there are some very important steps to take to do it correctly. In this chapter, we will draw from steps outlined by DeVellis and Thorpe (2021): (1) determine what to measure, (2) generate an item pool, (3) determine the format for measurement, (4) submit survey for expert review, (5) consider validation items, (6) administer items to a development sample and evaluate, and (7) optimize scale length.

Determine What to Measure

A seemingly obvious yet highly important first step in survey design is clearly establishing what will be measured by the survey. It is not enough to develop a survey to measure a construct without first clearly defining what the construct is. The challenge is that many of the phenomena of interest to practitioners may have different definitions. For example, some people define depression in cognitive terms characterized by negative thought patterns (e.g., Beck, 1979), while others may categorize it as an emotional experience (e.g., Greenberg & Watson, 2006) or as a diagnostic cluster of symptoms (American Psychiatric Association, 2022). No single definition or theory can capture a construct completely, and sometimes varying definitions overlap (see Figure 4.1). Some definitions cover the breadth of a construct, while others narrow in to capture the depth of a construct.

How you define a construct has implications for what goes on your survey, because survey items that are irrelevant to your defined construct will not help you better understand, define, and study the construct, yet too narrow a view of a construct really limits one's understanding of what may be occurring. With our depression example, if you are focused on measuring depression from a cognitive perspective, then including items on your survey that measure emotions will not necessarily help you understand thought patterns. If you cannot clearly articulate what you want to measure, not only is it unlikely that people who might complete your survey would understand it, but ultimately you may find that the results you get are not actually about what you had been trying to study.

The key to clearly defining what you want to measure, particularly in capturing breadth versus depth, is to use a theoretical framework. This might be a counseling theory, but it can be broader than that. Professionals in many disciplines use theories to define, predict, and explain things, and you may find a theory from a separate discipline best captures what you want to measure. A helpful guide to developing or discovering a theoretical framework is *Reason & Rigor: How Conceptual Frameworks Guide Research* (Ravitch & Riggan, 2017). Overall, the goal of this stage is to be able to articulate how your construct of interest can be measured by a survey. As mentioned previously in this chapter, if you struggle with this process, you might need to delve back into the professional literature to help you better understand the best way to operationalize your construct and what may need to be included on your survey.

In Meredith's case, she was interested in overwhelming thoughts and emotions that triggered clients to engage in NSSI behavior. If she thoroughly reviewed the available literature, she could find that other scholars and researchers have addressed this phenomenon (e.g., Chapman et al., 2006; Wester & McKibben, 2016), and she could use the conceptual

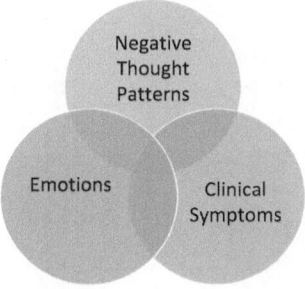

Figure 4.1 Theory-Based Perspectives of Depression.

frameworks and research to operationally define these thoughts and emotions in which she was interested. If we break down Meredith's interest in NSSI as we did with depression, there are two constructs at hand: Overwhelming thoughts and overwhelming emotions. As with depression, these two constructs are likely not the sole definition of NSSI, and they also could overlap in different ways (see Figure 4.2).

In order for Meredith to concretely determine what her survey should include, she needs to decide how broad or how narrow she wants her survey to be. She can start by defining what exactly overwhelming thoughts and overwhelming emotions are. She can likely identify this easily from reading what researchers have found and from her own experience working with her clients. Meredith also needs to consider more nuanced aspects related to capturing the depth of these experiences on her survey, such as what makes a thought or emotion overwhelming. How is intensity defined? At what point does a thought or emotion go from salient or distressing to overwhelming? Meredith also might wish to measure how frequently the overwhelming thoughts and emotions occur, as well as any precipitating events that evoke these thoughts and emotions. With these thoughts in mind, Meredith could better articulate the breadth (i.e., thoughts and emotions) and depth (i.e., intensity, frequency) of her constructs of interest, which would be a huge help as she develops items for her new survey.

Generate an Item Pool

After clearly defining what you want to measure, it is time to start developing items for the survey. This can be a tedious task to do correctly, and it is helpful to think of each item as a miniature test of the construct being measured. To that end, a helpful guide during item generation is Heppner et al.'s (2016) MAXMINCON principle for research. Your overall goal is to *maximize* true score variance, *minimize* error variance, and *control* for as many confounds as possible. In classical test theory, an individual's response to any given item on a survey is assumed to consist of their true score plus an error score (Allen & Yen, 2002). Error in an individual's response may stem from a variety of sources (e.g., environmental distractions, ambiguous or confusing items, motivation to participate), and error obscures practitioners from measuring and observing the construct of interest in its purest form.

Try as we might, we cannot control all aspects of the research process. Thus, we cannot completely eliminate sources of error from survey responses. Nevertheless, there are steps you can take in survey design that can help maximize the true score variance and minimize the error variance across individuals' responses. DeVellis and Thorpe (2021) recommended several useful strategies, such as choosing items that reflect the survey's purpose, writing

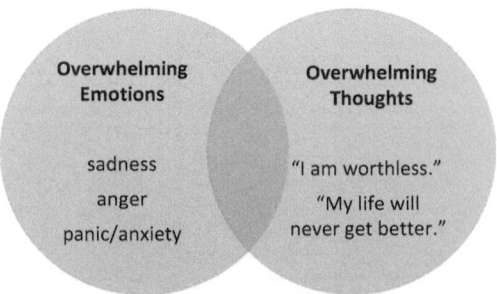

Figure 4.2 Venn Diagram Illustrating Meredith's Constructs of Interest.

items that are clear and concise, ensuring items are written at the appropriate reading level, and avoiding confusion in item wording (for examples of these strategies with a creativity survey, see Table 4.1).

Although it may seem obvious, you want to make sure that the items you draft are related to the construct(s) you are trying to measure. This can become more nuanced as your constructs of interest become more specific. For example, it seems obvious to say that Meredith should generate items related to NSSI, but what she needs to focus on is capturing the emotional and cognitive processes or experiences of NSSI. An item that is not related to these particular experiences would not help her test the notion of overwhelming emotions and thoughts. Meredith also needs to make sure she has a clear picture of what these emotions and thoughts look like so that her items are relevant and specific. Meredith will also want to generate as many relevant items as she possibly can at this phase. In this early phase of survey design, it is a good idea to generate as many relevant items as possible, even if some seem redundant, and the scale can be shortened later (DeVellis & Thorpe, 2021).

Another consideration in maximizing true score variance is making sure your items are clear and free of ambiguity. The more a client has to guess or infer what you are asking, the more likely their response will contain error. Remember: What you think you are asking is not always what is interpreted by clients (this is true in counseling practice and in survey research!). This point relates to another – try to make items as concise as possible. Wordy items can make

Table 4.1 Examples of Poorly and Strongly Worded Survey Items for Overwhelming Emotions in NSSI

Issue	Poorly Worded	Strongly Worded
Reflect the survey's purpose *The poorly worded item is asking about a person's views on NSSI as a mental health need, which is unrelated to Meredith's goal of measuring overwhelming thoughts and emotions.*	"I believe that self-injury is a valid mental health issue that needs to be addressed in mental healthcare."	"When I feel extremely anxious, I engage in self-injury."
Item clarity *The poorly worded item is long, wordy, and it is unclear whether it is measuring emotions or behaviors.*	"When you're really upset, do you ever injure yourself on purpose without suicidal intent as a way to cope with emotions that are too much to handle?"	"I self-injure when I feel extremely overwhelmed by my emotions."
Appropriate reading level *The poorly worded item uses needlessly complex, clinical language that could confuse some clients.*	"I engage in self-injury as a maladaptive coping mechanism when experiencing affective dysregulation."	"When my feelings get too big, I self-injure."
Double barrel item wording *The poorly worded item asks about two emotions at once: Stressed and upset. Which one should the client think about when answering this item?*	"I engage in self-injury when I am stressed or upset."	"I engage in self-injury when I am stressed."
Biased/leading item wording *The poorly worded item is assuming a client agrees with the statement or is encouraging them to agree. This may yield data favorable to the counselor's views but may not reflect reality.*	"How much do you agree with this statement: For some people, self-injury may be the only viable coping skill they have in difficult moments."	"At times, self-injury feels like a viable coping mechanism for me."

it more difficult for a client to decipher what they are responding to, which again poses a risk for error. Notably, ambiguously worded items may not only confuse clients, but they may also increase risk for socially desirable responding (Fleming, 2012), a type of nonrandom error discussed later.

In seeking to reduce ambiguity, it is important to ensure that items are written at a level that is appropriate for the intended audience. For example, a survey written for children ages five to eight years will have items at a reading level different from a survey written for adults over 18 years. Culturally, it is important to consider the language and dialect of the population being studied. If English is not the primary language spoken, then it may be necessary to translate items into the language spoken by participants. Additionally, you want to avoid a common mistake of a double-barreled item. A double-barreled item contains two ideas within one item, and it is impossible to know which idea is being endorsed in a client's response.

Although intentionality is required to develop strong items, there is no right or wrong process for generating items. Some people may find it helpful to map out the theory or conceptual framework driving the survey design and then develop items from there. Others may wish to brainstorm as many items as possible before going back and evaluating them. It is also a good idea to talk to other practitioners, particularly those with experience or expertise in your construct of interest, to get ideas for generating items. Although it may not be feasible to seek ideas or feedback from your clients directly, it can be helpful to seek ideas from those who might ultimately take your survey. Meredith, for example, might try to locate a few people who engage in NSSI, and she could potentially host a focus group to get feedback on the items she has been developing, to ask for new item ideas, or both. The key is to work from your strengths and to engage your own creativity. Find what works for you and use that to be productive.

Determine Measurement Format

In addition to generating items, you must decide how individuals will respond to the items. Measurement formats are often referred to as scales, and there are a variety of options from which to choose. The most important factors in selecting a scale are that it fits with the wording of your items and that it provides you with the information you are seeking. Some of the more common measurement scales include Likert scales, binary scales, and visual analog scales (see Table 4.2 for examples of each). On a Likert scale, an individual is asked to indicate the extent of their agreement or disagreement with items. Accordingly, items written along

Table 4.2 Examples of Common Measurement Formats

Sample Item	Scale Example					
"I am a nice person."	Likert	Strongly Disagree 1	Disagree 2	Neutral 3	Agree 4	Strongly Agree 5
	Binary*	Yes	No		True	False
	Visual Analog	Very Like Me				Not at All Like Me

|—————————————————————————————————|

Note: Two examples are offered for binary scales in this table: Yes/No and True/False.

with a Likert scale are declarative statements rather than questions. The practitioner also must determine what the numbers on a Likert scale mean. A binary scale offers a person two options in response to an item (e.g., true/false, agree/disagree, yes/no). This type of scale is used when a practitioner is trying to concretely classify information into two categories. With a visual analog scale, a person is asked to indicate the extent of their agreement or disagreement with an item along a continuum with two end points. For a more comprehensive review of measurement format options, see the books in the Additional Resources list at the end of the chapter.

Expert Review

Once the items and the measurement format have been developed, it is a good idea to have other people look over the newly designed survey and provide feedback. When you are in the process of developing a survey, it can be easy to get "too close" to the topic, a bias that might limit a broader or more critical perspective. That is, you can easily spend a good deal of time reading, trying to narrow down and define your construct, writing out items, and arranging items with a response scale. All of that investment may make it difficult to see when something is not quite right on the survey, when you have overlooked something, or when something might make sense to you but not to others. Extra pairs of eyes from professionals with expertise in your topic of interest can help uncover potential biases or blind spots you might have.

There is no standard for how many experts should review a survey under development, but more than one seems minimally necessary so that you can triangulate feedback from more than one source. The more experts that can review the survey the better; this may just create more work to integrate the feedback and possibly confusion about what to do if experts offer conflicting feedback. Ultimately, you must decide how to integrate expert feedback to improve your survey.

There are a few aspects to consider in the expert review process. First, you need to determine what constitutes an *expert* in the area(s) addressed on your survey. Who is qualified to offer substantive feedback that can help you improve or tweak your survey? Start by using more objective criteria to identify content experts, and then narrow in to people you might know who meet the criteria. For example, Meredith might start with criteria such as a licensed mental health practitioner with at least ten years of experience working with NSSI, or who has published at least five research studies on NSSI. Next, before you contact experts, clarify what you want feedback on and how they can assist. Common questions for experts are:

- Readability: Do the items make sense? Are any items confusing? How could any items be reworded for clarity? Will the population(s) likely to take this survey be able to understand the items?
- Validity: Do the items appear to relate to the construct(s) being measured? Do the items encompass all aspects of the construct(s)? Do any of the items contain biased, leading, or double-barreled wording?
- Instructional clarity: Do the survey instructions make sense?
- Measurement format: Is the selected measurement format appropriate for this survey? Can people respond to the items using the measurement format? Does the measurement format help me better understand my construct?
- Addition/Removal: Is there anything that should be added to or removed from the survey?

Validation Items

Previously, we discussed generating items in a way that maximizes true score variance and minimizes error variance, thereby gleaning information as purely as possible via a survey. Sometimes, a survey (or any study for that matter) can be solidly designed, yet despite best efforts, additional error can be introduced by individuals completing the survey. A common source of error is socially desirable responding, which occurs when someone attempts to present themselves in an overly positive way on a survey (Bäckström & Björklund, 2013). Depending on what a survey is attempting to measure, socially desirable responding may look like over- or underinflated scores. The problem with this is the information being provided on the survey is not accurate and can potentially lead practitioners to draw invalid or unreliable conclusions.

For example, it is possible that some of Meredith's clients deal with intensely aversive emotions that prompt them to engage in NSSI. However, when they take Meredith's new survey, they might respond to items by indicating that the intensity of their emotions is lower than what they actually feel. This could be for any number of reasons, including that they do not want to admit to themselves that their emotions are intense and negative or because they do not want Meredith to know the true intensity of their aversive emotions. Regardless of the motivation, these clients have produced scores on Meredith's survey that are artificially lower than is actually the case. As a result, Meredith might draw inaccurate or unreliable conclusions from the data.

Unfortunately, you cannot read a person's mind to know for sure if they are accurately representing themselves on a survey. Because we cannot know for sure if someone is responding accurately, we cannot fully eradicate instances of social desirability. What we can do is try to detect it, and a common way to do that is by including a measure of social desirability. There are several popular, free social desirability scales available that have been used in hundreds of studies, including the Marlowe-Crowne Social Desirability Scale (Crowne & Marlowe, 1960) and its short forms (Reynolds, 1982). By including a social desirability scale along with your new survey when you administer it (in the next step), you can correlate scores on your survey with scores on the social desirability scale to see if there is a significant correlation. A significant result may indicate that social desirability is an issue in your data, and you should use caution in interpreting the results of your survey. For a more nuanced discussion of social desirability, as well as another common source of error variance called inattentive responding, see McKibben and Silvia (2016) in the additional resources at the end of this chapter.

Administer a Development Sample and Evaluate

At this point, you have clearly defined what you want to measure, you have developed items and an accompanying measurement format, you have had the items reviewed by experts and made any edits you deem necessary, and you may be including some validation items or scales to detect potential error. You are now ready to administer your survey to see just how well it holds up. Before sending out your survey for people to complete, an often overlooked yet notable consideration is the aesthetics of your survey. That is, how does the survey look? Is it easy to read? Is the layout visually appealing? A plain or convoluted survey layout may dissuade people from taking the survey or may make their process more difficult, which can increase the chances for error.

There are a few quick ways that you can check the aesthetics of your survey informally. You might hand out the survey to clients individually or in a group (or to a group of students in a classroom) and ask them to comment on the overall look and feel of the survey. If you work in an office that has a waiting area, then you might distribute your survey to clients who are waiting for their appointments. Assume, for example, that Meredith facilitates a dialectical behavior therapy skills group with some of her clients who engage in NSSI. Either prior to the group starting or at the end of a group, she might hand her survey to her clients in the group and ask them to give her some feedback on how her survey looks. Notably, this could also be an opportunity to ask clients some of the questions asked of experts during expert review, particularly around readability, instructional clarity, and measurement format.

Administering your survey to people is an exciting, and sometimes anxiety-inducing, step in the survey design process because you are putting your hard work out there for people to complete. This process is yet another vital and complex step in the overall survey design process, and it requires careful attention to do correctly. First, you need to select a population of people that you can sample with your survey. It is important to be intentional in defining to whom you will administer your survey. For whom did you design the survey? Is it for a broad audience or a more specific group? Who is most qualified to respond to the items on your survey? The answer(s) you come up with should be who you recruit. For example, Meredith's survey has grown out of her work at her community mental health center with clients who engage in NSSI. A good population for her to test her survey with would probably be people who engage in NSSI.

As a quick note on defining the most optimal population to sample, some researchers rely on convenience samples (i.e., a group of people that are easy to access, even if not the most relevant to the study), but this can be problematic if a group of people has no knowledge of or exposure to the content of a survey. In Meredith's case, she might have an easier time gathering a large number of people by partnering with a professor at a local university who could distribute her survey to college students. However, for those students who have not engaged in NSSI or who have not sought counseling services, they may be confused by Meredith's survey, and their responses to the survey may not be particularly useful. Responses from people with no knowledge of Meredith's constructs of interest are essentially noise that can complicate and distort the conclusions she can make about her survey's performance. Again, remember Heppner et al.'s (2016) MAXMINCON principle – selecting a group of people who are most qualified to speak to what your survey is about will help you maximize the true score variance on your survey.

Once you define your target population, you need to sample individuals from that population. The number of people you need depends on the statistics you plan to use to evaluate a survey (which have even deeper measurement theory guiding the statistical approaches), and there are varying perspectives on how many people are "enough" to adequately test factor structures. A common statistical approach in survey design is factor analysis, which is based in classical test theory. Although a comprehensive discussion of factor analysis and classical test theory exceeds the scope of this chapter, a common way to determine a sample size for factor analysis modeling is to calculate a sample size-to-variable ratio. Essentially, the more items on a survey, the more people you need in a sample to sufficiently evaluate the factor structure with factor analysis. Again, researchers and measurement theorists vary on an ideal ratio, but a ratio of 10 to 20 people to every one item may be appropriate (Crockett, 2012; Mvududu & Sink, 2013). Researchers also tend to agree that at least 200 people are needed to conduct factor analysis modeling (Crockett, 2012; Mvududu & Sink, 2013), even if there are only a handful of items. Another school of thought in evaluating surveys comes from item response theory (IRT), which involves a more nuanced evaluation of items. The implication for sample sizes is similar in IRT approaches – large sample sizes are required.

Once a survey has been administered and the data are in, you are ready to analyze the data. This step relates directly to research questions described near the beginning of this chapter. Evaluating a survey involves tests for evidence of validity (e.g., construct, convergent, discriminant) and reliability. In essence, how well does the statistical evidence support the theoretical structure and utility of your survey? Evaluating a survey often requires access to statistical software and proficiency at interpreting statistical output. If you are employed in a setting that does not have access to statistical software, or if you do not feel confident to evaluate a survey yourself, you may wish to seek assistance from a measurement expert. There are many statistical tests you could conduct to evaluate your survey; some of the more common approaches are listed in Table 4.3.

A quick note about testing for evidence of validity and reliability that may seem like semantics but is actually an important distinction: It is not uncommon in peer-reviewed journal articles involving survey design to see researchers state that they found evidence (or not) that the *survey* is valid or reliable. This is a misnomer. As Elmore (2010) pointed out, what is valid or reliable is not a statistical result itself but rather the conclusions that one infers from the result. Applied to survey design, a survey itself is not valid or reliable. Rather, validity and reliability refer to the conclusions one makes based on the survey responses. If this sounds unclear, remember that a survey is essentially a test of a hypothesized construct. By extension, each time you use a survey, you are basically retesting how well that survey performs in measuring the construct(s) with a new group of people. Each test with a new sample is an opportunity to infer conclusions about the human condition under study. In sum, what are valid and reliable (or not) are the decisions you make as the practitioner, not your survey. It is an inanimate object after all!

Optimize Scale Length

Assuming that your survey holds up under tests for validity evidence, a final step is to try to shorten the survey if possible. Before you do this, heed this word of caution: It is almost never worth dropping an item from a survey if doing so will impact the validity or overall reliability of your survey. You can make informed decisions about whether an item should stay or go by consulting results from an item analysis (see Table 4.3).

The statistical program SPSS (IBM Corp., 2022) offers useful and reader-friendly output that you can use to evaluate items, such as item–total correlations. EZAnalyze (n.d.), which was originally designed for school counselors, offers a free add-on to Microsoft Excel that all practitioners may find useful for this step. An item–total correlation essentially estimates the degree to which people's responses on any given item are related to all other items on the survey or subscale on a survey (Howard & Forehand, 1962). A weak correlation (e.g., less than .2 [Everit, 2002]) signals that an item may not really relate to other items and can probably be deleted. An additional piece of information that SPSS provides is a "Cronbach's alpha if item deleted" value. As noted in Table 4.3, Cronbach's alpha is an estimate of internal consistency of the survey (or subscale) items as a whole – that is, how well the items converge on a unidimensional construct. If you already know the Cronbach's alpha value for your survey and/or any subscales on the survey, you can consult the Cronbach's alpha if item deleted for each item to see if dropping the item will impact the overall internal consistency of your survey.

Table 4.3 Common Statistical Tests in Survey Design

Statistical Tests	What It Does	Provides Evidence For	What to Look For	Software Programs
Item analysis	Helps you identify statistically weak items and the normality of data	Data normality	Item means and standard deviations	SPSS (IBM Corp., 2022)
Item strength/ weakness	Item skew and kurtosis			
	Item–total correlations			
Exploratory factor analysis (EFA)	Tells you how well items load onto your constructs/scales (CFA) or how well items load on scales that are extrapolated from the data (EFA)	Construct validity	Model fit indices	Mplus (Muthén & Muthén, 1998–2017)
	Factor loadings	Amos (Arbuckle, 2014)		
Confirmatory factor analysis (CFA)	Residual values	SPSS (IBM Corp., 2021)		
		LISREL (Scientific Software International, Inc., 2021)		
Item response theory (IRT) models	Evaluates items as a function of item difficulty and people's ability to answer items	Construct validity	Model fit indices	ConQuest (Adams, Wu, & Wilson, 2015)
Item characteristic curve	R (R Core Team, 2023)			
Pearson product moment correlation (r)	Tells you the extent to which scores on your survey overlap with scores on a theoretically similar or distinct survey	Convergent validity	A correlation is considered statistically significant if $p < .05$. Also examine r for strength of correlation and whether r is +/–	SPSS (IBM Corp., 2022)
Discriminant validity				
Cronbach's alpha (α)	Tells you the extent to which item scores relate to one another in converging on an underlying construct	Internal consistency reliability	α values at or above .8 are considered evidence of good to strong internal consistency among items	SPSS (IBM Corp., 2022)
Kuder- Richardson Formula 20 (KR-20)				

Chapter Summary

Survey design is a robust area in counseling, and in many ways, it serves as the foundation for much of the research (particularly quantitative) and applied work that practitioners do. The steps outlined in this chapter, though not the sole authority on how to design a survey, can help start you on the path to designing a quality survey. By designing surveys that reliably measure what they are intended to measure, practitioners can make informed decisions about the work they do and about the clients they serve.

Practice-Based Application

Think about the client-presenting concern, symptom, or situation that you identified in Chapter 1, and use that to answer the following questions:

1. Think about a topic or client population that you are interested in. When would it be appropriate to consider survey design? What do you need to know about that topic or population to determine if survey design is needed in this area?
2. Imagine you wanted to develop a new survey to address an area you identified in Chapter 1. Try to develop a few items for this survey. What would those items look like? What are they trying to measure? How would clients respond to those items (i.e., what would the measurement format be)?

Resources for More Information

Peer-Reviewed Journal Articles

Crockett, S. A. (2012). A five-step guide to conducting SEM analysis in counseling research. *Counseling Outcome Research and Evaluation, 3,* 20–47. https://doi.org/10.1177/2150137811434142

Elmore, P. B. (2010). Reporting standards for research publications. *Counseling Outcome Research and Evaluation, 1,* 19–29. https://doi.org/10.1177/2150137810386108

Leech, N. L., Onwuegbuzie, A. J., & O'Conner, R. (2011). Assessing internal consistency in counseling research. *Counseling Outcome Research and Evaluation, 2,* 115–125. https://doi.org/10.1177/2150137811414873

McKibben, W. B., & Silvia, P. J. (2016). Inattentive and socially desirable responding: Addressing subtle threats to validity in quantitative counseling research. *Counseling Outcome Research and Evaluation, 7,* 53–64. https://doi.org/10.1177/2150137815613135

Mvududu, N. H., & Sink, C. A. (2013). Factor analysis in counseling research and practice. *Counseling Outcome Research and Evaluation, 4,* 75–98. https://doi.org/10.1177/2150137813494766

Books

DeVellis, R. F., & Thorpe, C. T. (2021). *Scale development: Theory and applications* (5th ed.). Sage.

Dillman, D. A., Smyth, J. D., & Christian, L. M. (2014). *Internet, phone, mail, and mixed-mode surveys: The tailored design method* (4th ed.). Wiley-Blackwell.

Fink, A. G. (2012). *How to conduct surveys: A step-by-step guide* (5th ed.). Sage.

Ravitch, S. M., & Riggan, J. M. (2017). *Reason and rigor: How conceptual frameworks guide research* (2nd ed.). Sage.

Questions for Further Review and Application

1   What is the MAXMINCON principle, and how does it play into the survey design process? Why is it important that counselors adhere to this principle in survey design?

2   What are potential sources of error that can show up in survey scores? How can counselors try to prevent/address these during the survey design process?

3   What factors should one consider when administering and evaluating a newly designed survey?

References

Adams, R. J., Wu, M. L., & Wilson, M. R. (2015). *ACER ConQuest: Generalised Item response modelling software, Version 4* [Computer software]. Australian Council for Educational Research.

Allen, M. J., & Yen, W. M. (2002). *Introduction to measurement theory*. Waveland Press.

American Psychiatric Association. (2022). *Diagnostic and statistical manual of mental disorders* (5th ed., text rev.). Author.

Arbuckle, J. L. (2014). *Amos, Version 23.0* [Computer software]. IBM SPSS.

Bäckström, M., & Björklund, F. (2013). Social desirability in personality inventories: Symptoms, diagnosis, and prescribed cure. *Scandinavian Journal of Psychology, 54*, 152–159.

Beck, A. T. (1979). *Cognitive therapy and the emotional disorders*. Meridian.

Chapman, A. L., Gratz, K. L., & Brown, M. Z. (2006). Solving the puzzle of deliberate self-harm: The experiential avoidance model. *Behaviour Research and Therapy, 44*, 371–394. https://doi.org/10.1016/j.brat.2005.03.005

Crockett, S. A. (2012). A five-step guide to conducting SEM analysis in counseling research. *Counseling Outcome Research and Evaluation, 3*, 20–47. https://doi.org/10.1177/2150137811434142

Crowne, D. P., & Marlowe, D. (1960). A new scale of social desirability independent of psychopathology. *Journal of Consulting Psychology, 24*, 349–354.

DeVellis, R. F., & Thorpe, C. T. (2021). *Scale development: Theory and applications* (5th ed.). Sage.

Elmore, P. B. (2010). Reporting standards for research publications. *Counseling Outcome Research and Evaluation, 1*, 19–29. https://doi.org/10.1177/2150137810386108

Everit, B. S. (2002). *Cambridge dictionary of statistics* (2nd ed.). Cambridge University Press.

EZAnalyze . (n.d.). *Excel-based tools for educators*. Retrieved from www.ezanalyze.com

Fleming, P. (2012). Social desirability, not what it seems: A review of the implications for self reports. *The International Journal of Educational and Psychological Assessment, 11*, 3–22.

Greenberg, L. S., & Watson, J. C. (2006). *Emotion-focused therapy for depression*. American Psychological Association.

Heppner, P. P., Wampold, B. E., Owen, J., Thompson, M. N., Wang, K. T. (2016). *Research design in counseling* (4th ed.). Cengage.

Howard, K. I., & Forehand, G. A. (1962). A method for correcting item-total correlations for the effect of relevant item inclusion. *Educational & Psychological Measurement, 22*, 731–735.

IBM Corporation. (2022). *SPSS statistics for windows, Version 29.0* [Computer software]. Author.

McKibben, W. B., & Silvia, P. J. (2016). Inattentive and socially desirable responding: Addressing subtle threats to validity in quantitative counseling research. *Counseling Outcome Research and Evaluation, 7*, 53–64. https://doi.org/10.1177/2150137815613135

Muthén, L. K., & Muthén, B. O. (1998–2017). *Mplus user's guide* (8th ed.). Author.

Mvududu, N. H., & Sink, C. A. (2013). Factor analysis in counseling research and practice. *Counseling Outcome Research and Evaluation, 4*, 75–98. https://doi.org/10.1177/2150137813494766

R Core Team. (2023). *R: A language and environmental and statistical computing* [Computer software]. R Foundation for Statistical Computing. https://www.R-project.org

Ravitch, S. M., & Riggan, J. M. (2017). *Reason and rigor: How conceptual frameworks guide Research* (2nd ed.). Sage.

Reynolds, W. M. (1982). Development of reliable and valid short forms of the Marlowe-Crowne social desirability scale. *Journal of Clinical Psychology, 38*, 119–125.

Scientific Software International, Inc. (2021). LISREL (Version 12) [Computer software]. Author.

Wester, K. L., & McKibben, W. B. (2016). Participants' experiences of non-suicidal self-injury: Supporting existing theory and emerging conceptual pathways. *Journal of Mental Health Counseling, 38*, 12–27. https://doi.org/10.17744/mehc.38.1.02

5 Quantitative Data Analysis and Interpretation

W. Bradley McKibben and Arianna Alverio

Variables. Sampling. Z-scores. Reliability. Validity. These are concepts that often conjure distant traumatic memories from an undergraduate statistics course and strike fear in the hearts and minds of many future helping professionals. Nevertheless, as this book has made clear in other chapters, research informs best ethical practice. Therefore, it is not just a good idea to know something about research, but in order to be a competent mental health professional, it is critical to understand how data are collected and analyzed and how to draw valid and reliable conclusions from data. In this chapter, we will address the basics of quantitative data analysis and interpretation, including how to define and measure variables, sampling strategies, instrumentation considerations, reliability and validity, and basic descriptive statistical concepts. To make the material a little less academic and a little more clinically relevant, we will examine these concepts within the context of a hypothetical scenario.

Kai (they, them) is a licensed professional counselor working as the clinical director for a community mental health center. They oversee a clinical team of ten counselors, clinical social workers, and marriage and family therapists. Through conversations with the clinical team, Kai realizes that many of the clients served by their agency are experiencing significant levels of depression and anxiety, which appear to be impacting the clients' overall well-being. Kai wants to investigate this further by collecting some data from clients at the agency. Specifically, they are interested in answering: To what extent are our clients' levels of depression and anxiety related to clients' overall well-being? To answer this question, Kai needs to follow the scientific method (refer back to Chapter 1 discussion on the scientific method) by carefully defining their variables of interest, identifying a strategy for collecting and analyzing data, and interpreting their findings.

Defining and Measuring Variables

The first step Kai should take is to clearly identify and define the variables they wish to study so that they can measure them as accurately as possible. A variable can be just about anything that – as the name suggests – varies. Characteristics or features can vary across groups of people, within a person over time, or both. For example, a person's race is essentially unchanging, but race can vary across groups of people. Similarly, age will change for each person over time, and it also varies across groups of people. In Kai's case, depression, anxiety, and well-being may vary across the population of clients serviced by their agency, and each variable may also vary within each client over time as levels wax and wane for individuals.

As mentioned in Chapter 4 on designing surveys, when it comes to studying things in the psychological and social realms, we are usually studying things that cannot be observed directly. A biologist researching bacteria can directly observe and study that bacteria because

DOI: 10.4324/9781032706139-5

it is a physical object. However, we do not have the ability to directly observe and study most psychological phenomena (e.g., thoughts, emotions, values, culture). We cannot extract a thought from a person's mind, place it under a microscope, and look at it. Similarly, there is no mathematical formula to explain a person's values. One exception is behavior, which can be observed directly, thus making it a popular source of data for some researchers.

Because we often study these nonphysical concepts indirectly, it is important that we clearly define the "thing" we want to study so that we can measure it accurately. Researchers call this operationalizing a variable, or defining a variable in a way it can be measured (Goertzen, 2017). Take Kai's interest in studying depression as an example – what constitutes the experience that we label depression? If Kai utilized the *DSM-5-TR* (APA, 2022) definition, then depression might be a complex cluster of mood-related symptoms. If they go by Beck's cognitive triad definition from cognitive therapy (Beck et al., 1987), then depression might be defined by cognitive errors that drive negative emotions and behaviors. With either definition, Kai can start to ask people about their symptoms or their cognitions, emotions, and behaviors and quantify these experiences for research purposes. How a variable is defined operationally depends on the theory used to make sense of that variable, which is why researchers like Kai must consult the existing literature for theoretical and empirical guidance on how variables have been defined and studied previously.

Levels of Measurement

Researchers measure variables by assigning numbers to them, and there are various levels of measurement (Stevens, 1946). Some numbers may be assigned simply for identification or classification purposes (e.g., 1 = man, 2 = woman, 3 = agender, 4 = genderfluid), referred to as a nominal or categorical variable. Nominal data do not have any mathematical value; for example, genderfluid (4) is not twice the amount of woman (2), that makes no sense. Kai and their team might use numbers to classify demographic information about the clients at their agency who participate in their study, such as sex, gender, race, ethnicity, and religion or spirituality. Each of these would be nominal variables that they can sum to see how many are represented.

Other variables may have numbers assigned to them that do have mathematical value and that allow for measuring how much of something exists. Kai is interested in the extent to which clients' levels of depression and anxiety relate to well-being. To answer this, they need some way to measure how much depression, anxiety, and well-being exist for each client participating in the study, and numbers classify amounts for each variable. There are three levels of measurement to consider here: ordinal, interval, and ratio. Ordinal-level data allow for rank ordering amounts, but the distance between the amounts is not known. Many surveys and questionnaires in behavioral science research utilize Likert scales to measure variables (see Table 5.1 for examples). What does it mean for depression to go from 1 (mild) to 2 (moderate) or from 2 (moderate) to 3 (severe)? Is the distance between 1 (strongly disagree) and 2 (disagree) the same as the distance from 2 (disagree) to 3 (neither agree nor disagree)? Not only are these distances unknown, but people might also have differing perceptions of what the numbers of a scale mean and of the distances between the numbers. One person's "mild" anxiety might be another person's "severe" anxiety. Because of this subjectivity, ordinal data can be rank ordered in terms of amount or magnitude, and we can calculate median or range values (discussed later), but that is about as far as we can infer information from this level of measurement. For Kai, measuring depression, anxiety, and well-being at the ordinal

Table 5.1 Examples of Likert Measurement Scales

1 Mild	2 Moderate	3 Severe				
1 Strongly Disagree	2 Disagree	3 Neither Agree nor Disagree	4 Agree	5 Strongly Agree		
1 Not at All Like Me	2 Not Like Me	3 Somewhat Not Like Me	4 Neutral	5 Somewhat Like Me	6 Like Me	7 Very Much Like Me

level would allow them to rank order client participants from lowest to highest on each variable.

Interval level measurement implies that data are ordinal and that there are equal distances between values. Most standardized tests yield interval level data. Scores on the SAT test range from 400–1600 and increases or decreases in scores are equidistant. Temperature measured in Fahrenheit and Celsius is another example as changes in temperature are equidistant in terms of degree. Although most quantitative data in the behavioral sciences are ordinal, many researchers treat it as interval by assuming that distances between scores on variables are equidistant.

Ratio level measurement implies that data are interval and that there is a meaningful zero point. Variables measured at the ratio level include weight, age, and money. Weight has equal intervals of measurement (e.g., the distance from 10 to 11 pounds is the same as 11 to 12 pounds) and zero pounds is a meaningful zero point. Unlike Fahrenheit and Celsius scales, temperature measured on the Kelvin scale has a meaningful zero point that refers to zero heat being present. In the behavioral sciences, ratio data is essentially nonexistent because meaningful zero points are very difficult to define. What does it mean to have zero depression, anxiety, or well-being? Many Likert scales do not start at zero, making a person's score on a survey impossible to equal zero, but even if they did, it does not mean that a score of zero is useful or understandable.

Independent and Dependent Variables

In addition to levels of measurement, Kai needs to identify which variables are independent and dependent. These terms can be confusing, but essentially independent variables are reasoned to assert some influence on dependent variables (Mitchell & Jolley, 2013). In other words, changes in dependent variables depend, at least in part, upon changes in independent variables. Consider Kai's question of whether depression and anxiety are related to well-being. The way Kai is thinking about this implies that depression and anxiety are independent variables because the amount of depression or anxiety a client has is reasoned to occur independently of well-being. Because Kai wants to know if well-being increases or decreases as depression and anxiety increase or decrease, this makes well-being a dependent variable because they assume its magnitude depends to some degree on the magnitude of the other two variables. Whether variables are independent or dependent depends upon the research question guiding the study and what existing literature supports as a logical way to study the variables.

Instrumentation and Measurement

Once variables are defined operationally, researchers must consider the mechanism for collecting data from participants. Kai needs to consider how they plan to collect data on depression, anxiety, and well-being. In the behavioral sciences, this often is accomplished with some form of a survey. Surveys typically contain statements that participants respond to and rate or questions that participants answer. Most surveys are self-report, meaning that participants complete the survey about themselves, though some might be other-report in which a participant completes a survey about another person.

Thousands of surveys exist that measure many different constructs or variables, and an in-depth review of different surveys is beyond the scope of this chapter. A researcher should utilize surveys that measure their variables as they have been defined operationally. If Kai believes that depression is best defined with *DSM-5-TR* (APA, 2022) criteria, then it may make sense to utilize a symptom inventory that aligns with diagnostic criteria for depressive disorders. This type of survey would allow Kai to measure depression in terms of how frequently symptoms occur within a specific timeframe. If Kai goes with the cognitive therapy conceptualization of depression, then it may make more sense to utilize the Beck Depression Inventory (BDI-II; Beck et al., 1996).

Another method for measuring variables is through direct observation, which is commonly used to measure behaviors. To do this, a researcher might utilize an observation form or checklist to track and record behaviors. Regardless of the mechanism, the key is that the mechanism used to measure variables needs to align with how the researchers define the variables operationally. Otherwise, the data will not make much sense.

Participant Populations and Samples

Whereas defining variables refers to what is being studied, identifying populations and samples refers to who is being studied. Kai needs to think through who should participate in their study, how many people they need to include, and how they will recruit clients to participate. Ultimately, decisions made about sampling should help researchers answer their research questions guiding the study. In this section, we review sampling strategies for recruiting participants and explore how to determine an adequate sample size.

Sampling Strategies

A population, or target population, is the group that researchers want to know something about. Sometimes, a target population is fully known and accessible. In Kai's case, they can reasonably know all the clients receiving services at their agency. They may even get lucky and all clients would agree to participate in their study, allowing Kai to study the entire population. There also may be times when a population is not completely known or is not accessible. It is far less feasible to identify all adults in the United States who have depression or anxiety (or both), and even if this information were known, it is not possible to include all of them in a study.

When a population is not fully known or accessible, the solution is to identify a smaller group from within the target population, commonly called a sample, and study that group. The goal is to learn information about the sample and attempt to generalize knowledge learned from the sample to the larger target population. To generalize from a sample to a population, research participants in the sample should be representative of people in the target population as much as possible. Representativeness refers both to demographic representation and to the variables being studied. For Kai, they should be aware of the demographics of clients served at their agency so that they can recruit a sample that represents this population. For example, if more women are seen at the agency than men, then it makes sense that their sample would include more women participants. Larger, less accessible populations may present a challenge for researchers because detailed demographic information may not be available. However, demographic representativeness is critically important because many counseling interventions and treatment approaches have been developed by, and researched with, White individuals but have been generalized to and imposed upon Black, Indigenous, and People of Color (BIPOC) communities without adequate research.

There are a variety of strategies one might choose to select a sample from a larger population, and which one is most appropriate depends in large part on answering the research questions being investigated. Random sampling, a method in which everyone has an equal chance of being selected to participate (Novosel, 2023), is often considered a gold standard in quantitative research because this method will often yield a representative sample. Kai could use random sampling by generating a list of all clients served by their agency, assigning each client a number, and using a random number generator to randomly select clients to recruit for participation. The website random.org has a free random integer set generator that researchers can use to identify participants at random. Although this method is likely to yield a representative sample, the target population needs to be known and accessible to the researchers for everyone to truly have an equal chance of being sampled.

Another sampling option is systemic sampling, which refers to simply choosing people in a certain order from a list and recruiting them to participate. Kai might use their list of clients and select every other person, or perhaps every third person, depending upon how many participants they need, and ask them to participate in their study. This approach is easier for researchers to do, but the potential risk is that the resulting sample will not be representative of the target population. Kai might end up with a sample that is exclusively women or with clients who are mostly low in depression or anxiety. In these cases, the researchers' ability to generalize knowledge gained from the sample back to the target population will be limited.

Stratified sampling is a more sophisticated approach that can overcome the limitations of systemic sampling. Stratified involves dividing people into groups and then using either systemic or random sampling to identify participants. This approach is often used when researchers identify important subgroups within the target population that they want to sample independently. Perhaps Kai wants to group clients by gender and sample a certain number of clients from each group. Alternatively, perhaps Kai wants to ensure that they equally sample clients from each clinician's caseload, so they decide to group clients by clinician and sample a certain number from each group. Once people are stratified into subgroups, researchers can use either random or systemic sampling to identify participants within each subgroup.

Finally, convenience sampling involves sampling people who are most accessible to the researcher. Kai might utilize a convenience method by putting up flyers about the study throughout the agency's building, and clients who read the flyers can reach out to participate in the study if they choose. Other convenience methods include posting information about a study on email listservs, social media, websites, or other spaces where participants might reasonably see the information; sending out emails to people known to the researchers; or verbally asking people known to the researchers. If you ever took an undergraduate introductory psychology course that required you to complete a certain number of research participation hours as part of the course, you were part of a convenience sample for researchers. Although convenience sampling is the least rigorous, it is the easiest method and sometimes the only feasible option. In terms of rigor, researchers are more likely to end up with a nonrepresentative, or biased, sample that will limit generalizability to the target population. Sometimes, though, it is simply not feasible to use the other sampling methods, particularly if the target population is not accessible.

Sample Size

Having reviewed sampling strategies, a common question one might ask is, "How many participants do I need?" As is often the case in mental health professions, it depends. Sample size depends on three primary things: How many variables the researcher is studying, the statistical analyses being used, and how strongly independent and dependent variables are related to one another. Generally, the more variables a researcher plans to study and the more complex the statistical analyses, the larger the sample size needs to be. This is called statistical power, or having enough participants in a study to be able to observe an effect or relationship between variables if such an effect or relationship truly exists (Schneck, 2023). Researchers need enough power to be able to conduct their study and draw reliable and valid conclusions from data. If this is confusing, think of it this way: participants provide data, and data are observations of variables being studied. We need enough observations to be able to see what we are trying to study. If we do not have enough observations, then we run the risk of concluding that variables are not related to one another when they actually may be. The problem is that we did not have enough data to see the relationship clearly. This is called type II error, or a false negative (Carlin et al., in press).

When the relationship between two variables is strong, we need fewer participants to be able to observe that relationship. Conversely, when the relationship between two variables is weaker, we need more participants to observe that relationship. This speaks to something called effect size, or the magnitude of the relationship between variables (Balkin & Lenz, 2021). Imagine trying to view something under a microscope. The larger the specimen you are looking at, the less you need to zoom in, but the smaller the specimen, the more you need to zoom in to see it clearly. In research, more participants provide us with more data, which are more observations to be able to "zoom in" and examine relationships between variables.

The challenge is that researchers do not always know how strongly variables are related before they conduct a study. One way to estimate effect size is to consult published research, if it exists, to see what has been previously observed. Researchers can also use programs like G*Power (Faul et al., 2007), a free computer program that will estimate a sample size based on the number of variables, statistical analysis to be used, and an estimate of effect size (i.e., small, medium, large). Importantly, just as there is a such thing as too much pizza, there can be too much of a good thing with participants as well. A very large sample size can result in finding significant relationships between variables even if they are not truly related. This is called type I error, or a false positive (Carlin et al., in press). In this instance, the metaphorical microscope has zoomed in too far and everything looks relevant. Ultimately, researchers need a sample size that is large enough to allow them to answer their research question, but not so large that everything looks significant if it truly is not.

Reliability and Validity

Earlier in the chapter, we discussed instruments (e.g., surveys) that a researcher might use to measure a variable. Let's assume that Kai decided to use a depression symptom inventory with a Likert scale to measure depression in their study. Each time a participant responds to an item on that survey by selecting a number that represents their depression symptoms, we call each of those responses an observed score because it is the score we can see. However, a logical question is just how accurate are those observed scores that the participants provided? Were they being honest? Are they self-aware enough to know about their depression symptoms? Were they fully alert and attentive when taking the survey or were they distracted?

Did they read and really think about each item, or did they just mark something down? Did they understand the survey instructions, item wording, and scale?

As you can imagine, a study with multiple surveys containing multiple items across a sizeable sample of participants is likely to contain some inaccuracies, referred to by researchers as measurement error (Traub, 1997). Therefore, researchers often operate under an assumption that observed scores are biased and contain participants' true scores plus some degree of error (Charter & Feldt, 2002). In Kai's study, all those scores on the depression survey likely contain people's actual level of depressive symptomology plus some error. Just how much error there is, and where it comes from, across a sample of participants, we often do not know for sure and there is no way to measure it definitively. However, it makes sense that we would want minimal error and maximal true score variance to draw conclusions from data that are valid and reliable.

Sometimes, error is random, such as a participant simply not knowing how to answer an item and providing the "best possible" response that they could or a participant who skipped their morning coffee and had a distracting migraine when they took the survey. Other times, error is not random, such as researchers using a poorly designed survey, recruiting participants who are not representative of the target population or who are not a good fit for the study, or utilizing the wrong statistical analyses. We cannot anticipate, control, or eliminate every source of error – and no study is completely free from error – but too much error limits our ability to draw reliable or valid conclusions from data. What we can do is estimate reliability of scores across participants or across time, and we can take steps to ensure we draw valid conclusions.

Reliability

Reliability refers to the consistency and stability of data collected. When participant responses are reliable, we see consistent results over time across different observations or instruments. For example, if participants in Kai's study provide generally consistent scores across items on the depression symptom inventory, then we might consider them reliable scores that closely measure participants' true score of depression symptoms. Alternatively, we might expect participants' total depression scores to be consistent over time, assuming that depression levels truly stay the same. There are many ways to measure reliability (see Table 5.2). Reliability

Table 5.2 Measures of Reliability

Test-retest	Assesses the consistency of a measure over time by administering the same measure to the same group of participants on separate occasions and examining the correlation between their scores.
Internal consistency	Measures the consistency of a measure by examining the correlation of each item to all other items on the measure.
Split-half	Assesses the consistency of a measure by dividing the measure into two halves and examining the correlation of scores for each half. Related methods that average all possible split-half combinations of a measure include Cronbach's alpha (continuous data) and Kuder Richardson (binary data).
Parallel forms	Measures the consistency of a measure by having participants complete similar measures of the same construct and examining the correlation between the two measures.
Interrater	Measures the consistency of observations made by different raters, which ensures that different observers are consistently interpreting the data in a similar way. Used for observations rather than surveys.

helps ensure that the findings are dependable and not influenced by random error, and the best way to maximize reliability is to minimize error because the more we are able to measure participants' true scores, the more reliable those scores will be.

Validity

Whereas reliability refers to consistency, validity refers to the accuracy of decisions made from data. It is possible for data to be reliable, but for a researcher to reach an invalid conclusion. For example, if a scale is off by two pounds, then it will offer a reliable reading of your weight each time you step on the scale, it will just be reliably wrong. On the other hand, if the scale provides accurate measures of your weight, then the measures will be reliable also. This is also the case in quantitative research; when researchers draw valid conclusions from data, then the conclusions will also be reliable.

Historically, researchers thought of validity as containing several different forms – such as content, construct, and criterion validity – all of which assess different aspects of accuracy (see Table 5.3). Today, validity is more of a unidimensional idea. Like reliability, validity is impacted by random and nonrandom error. The more error hiding in a study, the less valid our conclusions will be, and the overall usefulness of the study will be limited. However, because no research study is perfect and there will almost always be some degree of error, no study will yield findings so pure that conclusions are perfectly valid.

Making Sense of Data: Descriptive and Inferential Statistics

Assume that Kai uses three surveys to collect data from 110 clients at their agency: One survey each for depression, anxiety, and well-being, respectively. If each survey contained just ten items each, that would be 1,100 data points per survey and 3,300 data points total. This is a lot of data to comprehend! Descriptive statistics are a set of tools that researchers can use to make sense of large datasets like these. In this section, we will review three types of descriptive statistics: Score distributions, measures of central tendency, and measures of variability.

Score Distributions

Distribution refers to how frequently scores occur across participants in a sample. In Kai's study, if each of the three ten-item surveys are scored on a one to five Likert scale, then the minimum score on each survey would be a ten and the maximum score would be a 50.

Table 5.3 Domains of Validity

Content	Content validity is the extent to which an instrument covers the full range of the concept being measured. It assesses whether the items or questions on a survey or test adequately represent the content domain of interest. For example, does Kai's depression symptom inventory measure all DSM–related symptoms of depression?
Construct	Construct validity refers to how well an instrument accurately measures the theoretical construct or concept it was intended to measure. For example, to what extent does Kai's depression symptom inventory actually measure depression?
Criterion	Criterion validity refers to the extent to which an instrument can accurately predict or relate to an external criterion or established standard related to the construct being measured. For example, do people with higher scores on Kai's depression symptom inventory also meet diagnostic criteria for a depressive disorder?

Across a sample of 110 participants, survey scores may fall anywhere between these values. Examining score distributions can help Kai see which scores occur more or less frequently. One method is to generate a table that displays frequency counts for each observed value. This may be somewhat helpful, but the table may be lengthy if there are many different scores across 110 people.

Score distributions are commonly examined with a type of bar graph called a histogram in which observed scores are plotted on the x-axis and the frequency of those observed scores are plotted on the y-axis (see Figure 5.1). This allows researchers to quickly discern trends in how participants' scores are distributed in a sample. Do the 110 clients in Kai's study tend to report low depression scores? High anxiety scores? Do scores for well-being tend to be average, with fewer low or high scores? Histograms offer a graphical representation of scores so that researchers can identify such trends.

Let's assume that most of the 110 clients in Kai's study did report average levels of well-being. That is, many of the clients tended to report scores around 30. Perhaps some were slightly higher and some slightly lower, but there were very few clients who reported very low (i.e., close to 10) or very high (i.e., close to 50) levels of well-being. If these scores were graphed using a histogram, it might look similar to Figure 5.1, and we would consider this a fairly normal distribution of scores.

Next, let's assume that many of the 110 clients reported low levels of depression, meaning that many of the participants' depression survey scores are closer to ten than 50. A histogram of these scores might look like Figure 5.2, and we would refer to this as a positively skewed distribution. The term positive skew refers to the direction the tail is pointing on the x-axis, which in this case is pointing to the right or the positive direction of the x-axis. Finally, let's assume that many of the clients reported high levels of anxiety, meaning that many of the participants' anxiety survey scores are closer to 50 than ten. This histogram might look like Figure 5.3, which is called a negatively skewed distribution because the tail is pointing in the negative direction on the x-axis.

Examining score distributions matters because researchers can compare their observed distribution of scores to a theoretical distribution called a Gaussian or normal distribution. In a normal distribution, data points cluster symmetrically around the mean. The values on either side of the mean follow a bell curve shape (see Figure 5.1). Many phenomena that we

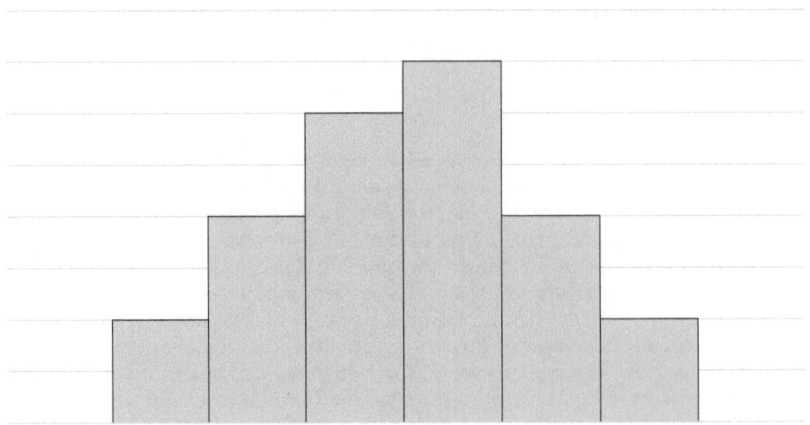

Figure 5.1 Histogram.

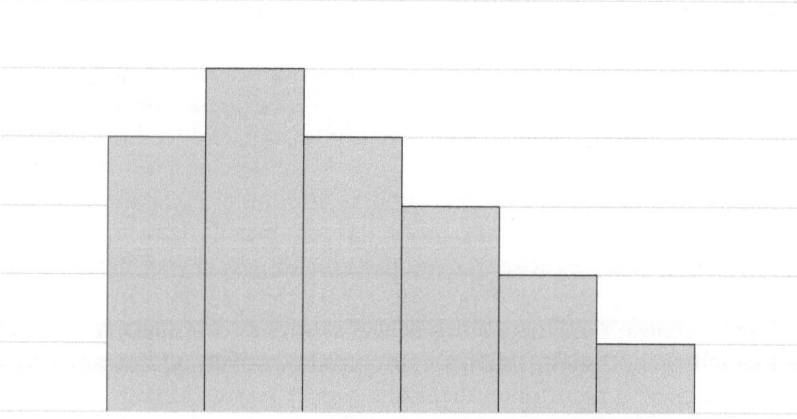

Figure 5.2 Histogram.

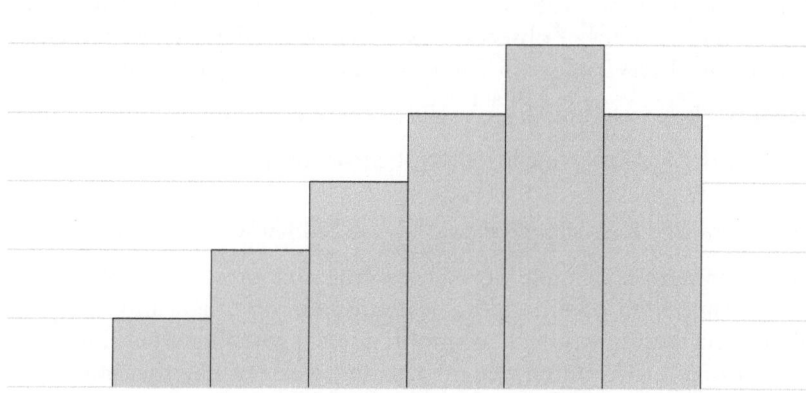

Figure 5.3 Histogram.

study in the behavioral sciences tend to show this kind of distribution. A normal distribution is based on the central limit theorem, which states that as sample size increases, the distribution of sample means approximates a normal distribution, even if the original data is not normal (Rouaud, 2013). In other words, if Kai hypothetically were to sample different groups of people and measured their depression, anxiety, and well-being over and over again to infinity, then the sample means would likely take the classic bell curve shape of a normal distribution. When Kai conducts a single study with one sample of 110 clients, they can compare the distribution of scores on the three surveys to a hypothetical normal distribution to determine whether the current observed data appear normally distributed or not.

Measures of Central Tendency

Central tendency refers to the central or typical value for a probability distribution or dataset (Weisberg, 1992). It aims to provide a single value that is a "best" representative summary of all the data values. There are three common measures of central tendency: Mean, median, and mode. The mode is the easiest to identify because it does not involve calculating anything. The mode is the value that occurs most frequently in a dataset, and a dataset can have more than one mode if several values tie for highest frequency. The mode may not be very useful for survey data, but it can be useful for nominal data. For Kai, the most frequently occurring anxiety score may not be as useful to them as modes for client demographic information.

The mean, or arithmetic average, is calculated by summing all data values and then dividing by the total number of values. For example, Kai can obtain the mean depression value by adding up all the depression survey scores and then dividing that sum by 110. This would tell Kai what the average value was for depression across the sample of clients. The mean is a popular measure of central tendency, but it is also sensitive to outliers (e.g., uncharacteristically high or low scores) and skew. When we discussed positively and negatively skewed score distributions previously, we mentioned that skew happens when lower or higher scores occur more frequently. When this happens, the mean will be lower or higher as well.

Just like a median on the highway refers to a divider in the middle of the road separating oncoming lanes of traffic, the median in statistics refers to a middle value that separates the higher half from the lower half of a dataset. For Kai to find the median value for depression, they would first need to rank order all 110 survey scores and then locate the middle value. When there is an odd number of observations, it is easy to identify the middle value because an equal number of observations will fall above and below that value. Mathematically, the middle value would be located at: $\dfrac{N+1}{2}$. When there is an even number of observations, as is the case for Kai, the median value is located halfway between $\dfrac{N}{2}$ and $\dfrac{N+2}{2}$. The median value for depression with Kai's sample would be located halfway between $\dfrac{110}{2}$ and $\dfrac{110+2}{2}$; that is, halfway between the 55th and 56th value in the rank ordered list of scores. Because the median relies on rank ordering scores, it is less sensitive to outliers and skew than the mean, making it a more accurate measure of central tendency when data distributions are skewed. When data are normally distributed, the median and mean will be the same.

Measures of Variability

Variability refers to how spread out the values are in a dataset. It indicates scatter around central tendency measures such as the mean and median. If all scores are tightly clustered, there is low variability. A wider scatter of scores indicates high variability. Three common measures of variability are range, variance, and standard deviation.

Range is the simplest measure of variability and refers to the difference between the minimum and maximum values in a dataset. It measures the total spread of scores, but it is a limited indicator of variability because it only incorporates two values and ignores distribution shape. The primary advantage is ease of computation and understanding. Recall that Kai's surveys for depression, anxiety, and well-being each yield scores between 10–50. If the highest participant score for well-being was 48 and the lowest participant score was 12, then the range for well-being with this sample would be 48 – 12 = 36.

Variance is a much more complex concept, both to calculate and to interpret. Basically, variance is a measure of how close scores are to the sample mean. Variance is calculated by squaring the difference of each value from the mean, totaling the squared values, and then dividing by $n - 1$. A larger variance indicates that scores tend to be more spread out from the sample mean, whereas a smaller variance indicates that scores tend to be closer to the sample mean. Because variance is reported in squared units, it can be hard to interpret, so standard deviation is often used.

Mathematically, standard deviation equals the square root of the variance, which converts the value to the same units as data. Standard deviation gives an absolute sense of average dispersion of scores around the mean (Hinkle et al., 2003). For example, let's assume that across the 110 clients in Kai's study, the mean score on the anxiety survey was 32 and the standard deviation was four. What this standard deviation tells us is that, among scores in this sample, scores varied above or below 32 by about four points on average. Circling back to the concept of a normal distribution, about 68% of normally distributed values fall within $+/-1$ standard deviation from the mean, 95% fall within $+/-2$ standard deviations, and 99.5% fall within $+/-3$ standard deviations. Assuming that anxiety scores are mostly normally distributed in Kai's study, we can assume that 68% of clients' scores are between 28 and 36, 95% of scores are between 24 and 40, and 99.5% of scores are between 20 and 44.

The information that a standard deviation offers is helpful for understanding variability around the mean, but we are still somewhat limited because we cannot say for certain how far a raw survey score is from the mean exactly. For example, we know that an anxiety score of 29 likely falls within one standard deviation below the mean of 32, but how far from the mean exactly? To find out, we need to standardize scores into something called a z-score, which allows a researcher to directly compare scores relative to the mean, even if the original units of measurement are different. To translate that anxiety survey score of 29 into a z-score, we subtract the mean from that value and then divide by the standard deviation: $\frac{29-32}{4}$. This z-score of $-.75$ tells us exactly how far a score of 29 is from the mean of 32. Standardization allows researchers to compare observations more clearly and directly across participants in a sample and to compare multiple samples from multiple studies. That is, if Kai wanted to compare participant scores from their sample to other samples that have completed similar measures, standardized scores allow for such comparisons.

Inferential Statistics

Inferential statistics are methods that researchers use to examine relationships among variables and/or among groups of people. Recall that Kai's original research question was about the extent to which clients' levels of depression and anxiety relate to clients' overall well-being. After collecting data, Kai can utilize inferential statistical tests to answer this question. Inferential statistics also allow researchers to infer conclusions about target populations based on data gathered from samples. That is, Kai can use statistics to learn from their sample of 110 clients and attempt to generalize that knowledge to all clients served by their agency.

There are many types of statistical tests to choose from, and selecting the most appropriate test depends on the research question(s) being asked, the level of measurement for the variables (see Table 5.4), and the number of variables being studied. Some statistical tests, such as correlations and regressions, are designed to test relationships among continuous variables (i.e., ordinal, interval, ratio). These tests are most applicable to Kai's research question because they are interested in the relationship between depression, anxiety, and well-being. A correlation analysis can only measure the relationship between two variables at a time: One independent and one dependent variable. Thus, Kai would need to run two different correlation analyses to answer their question: One correlation testing the relationship between depression and well-being and another testing the relationship between anxiety and well-being.

Table 5.4 Common Statistical Tests

Statistical Test	IV #	The IV Is ...	DV #	The DV Is ...
T-Test	1	Categorical	1	Continuous
Univariate ANOVA	2+	Categorical	1	Continuous
Multivariate ANOVA	1+	Categorical	2+	Continuous
Correlation	1	Continuous	1	Continuous
Univariate Regression	2+	Continuous	1	Continuous
Multivariate Regression	1+	Continuous	2+	Continuous

Kai could also use a multiple regression analysis, which would allow Kai to test whether depression and anxiety together (rather than separately) predict well-being.

Statistical tests such as t-tests and analysis of variance (ANOVA) allow researchers to compare group differences (i.e., nominal variables) in relation to some other continuous variable. For example, early in this chapter we discussed how Kai might use numbers to classify demographic information about clients at their agency. If Kai wanted to test whether there are significant gender differences (e.g., 1 = man, 2 = woman, 3 = agender, 4 = genderfluid) in well-being among clients at their agency, then an ANOVA would allow them to test whether such group differences exist based on the data they collected with their sample. An ANOVA is most appropriate for Kai in this example because ANOVAs are used when there are more than two groups being compared within the independent variable. If Kai were interested in sex-based differences (e.g., 1 = male, 2 = female), then a t-test would be appropriate (see Table 5.4).

In these examples, what Kai is doing with statistics is hypothesis testing. Hypothesis testing involves drawing conclusions about whether relationships differ from what we would expect by random chance alone, which allows researchers to make inferences about whether patterns seen in samples reflect true effects versus being coincidences. That is, just because we find that a set of variables are related to each other (e.g., as depression levels get higher, well-being levels get lower) within a sample of clients, that does not mean that the relationship between these variables is a true effect within the broader population. The observed relationship could be random, or it could be caused by error. A common indicator that an observed pattern reflects a true effect is statistical significance, which refers to the probability that the results observed in a study are not just due to chance. Statistical significance helps researchers determine whether relationships between variables or differences between groups reflect actual effects versus random variation.

For example, if Kai finds that higher levels of anxiety relate to lower levels of well-being, they want to know if that same effect exists only in their sample of 110 clients or if there is a true relationship in the broader population of clients served at their agency. Statistical significance gives the probability the found connection would occur by coincidence alone if no real relationship was present. Typically, a statistical significance level, or p-value, evaluates the chance of coincidence (often $p < .05$ or 5%). If the p-value of a statistical test exceeds .05, the observed result is considered to lack statistical significance, meaning it could reasonably happen randomly even if in reality no relationship exists in the broader population. If the significance level is at or below .05, then we can infer significant relationships likely exist at the population level also.

Chapter Summary

Throughout this chapter, we have explored a variety of important research topics, including how to define and measure variables, how to sample participants for a study, how to evaluate reliability and validity, how to understand data with descriptive statistics, and how to examine variables with inferential statistics. This chapter just scratches the surface of many of these concepts, and there are other related statistical concepts that we did not cover in this chapter. Nevertheless, the concepts covered here offer a foundation to understand what researchers are trying to do in quantitative studies and how we make sense of data that we gather from participants. Information in this chapter also sets you up to understand quantitative research designs covered in future chapters, such as correlational/causal-comparative, quasi-experimental, randomized controlled trials, and single-case research designs.

Practice-Based Application

Think about the client-presenting concern, symptom, or situation that you identified in Chapter 1, and use that to answer the following questions:

- What variables can you identify? How might you define these variables operationally in a way that you could measure them?
- If you were to study those variables, who would be the target population? Which sampling strategy makes the most sense if you were to try to study this population and why? What are some of the limitations of the sampling approaches?
- Choose one variable and see if you can locate an existing survey that measures this variable. Look at the items and the scoring format. Do the items seem to measure your variable comprehensively? Why or why not?

Resources for More Information

Peer-Reviewed Journal Articles

Elmore, P. B. (2010). Reporting standards for research publications. *Counseling Outcome Research and Evaluation, 1*, 19–29. https://doi.org/10.1177/2150137810386108

Kalkbrenner, M. T. (2023). Alpha, omega, and *H* internal consistency reliability estimates: Reviewing these options and when to use them. *Counseling Outcome Research and Evaluation, 14*(1), 77–88. https://doi.org/10.1080/21501378.2021.1940118

Leech, N. L., Onwuegbuzie, A. J., & O'Conner, R. (2011). Assessing internal consistency in counseling research. *Counseling Outcome Research and Evaluation, 2*, 115–125. https://doi.org/10.1177/2150137811414873

Liu, X. S. (2013). Comparing sample size requirements for significance tests and confidence intervals. *Counseling Outcome Research and Evaluation, 4*(1), 3–12. https://doi.org/10.1177/2150137812472194

Sink, C. A., & Mvududu, N. H. (2010). Statistical power, sampling, and effect sizes. *Counseling Outcome Research and Evaluation, 1*(2). 1–18. https://doi.org/10.1177/2150137810373613

Books

Cooper, H., Coutanche, M. N., McMullen, L. M., Panter, A. T., Rindskopf, D., & Sher, K. J. (Eds.). (2023). *APA handbook of research methods in psychology* (2nd ed.). American Psychological Association.

Pasque, P. A., & Alexander, E. (Eds.). (2022). *Advancing culturally responsive research and researchers: Qualitative, quantitative, and mixed methods.* Routledge.

Walliman, N. (2021). *Research methods: The basics* (3rd ed.). Routledge.

Electronic Resources

1. Analysis Toolpak, a free add-in to Microsoft Excel for computing descriptive statistics: https://www.excel-easy.com/examples/descriptive-statistics.html
2. Free online randomizer tool (e.g., for randomly selecting participants): https://www.random.org/integers/
3. G*Power software for estimating statistical power: https://www.psychologie.hhu.de/arbeitsgruppen/allgemeine-psychologie-und-arbeitspsychologie/gpower

Questions for Further Review and Application

1   What are the four levels of variable measurement, and what are the similarities and differences across the four levels?
2   Many research studies relevant to the mental health professions rely on convenience samples. What are some potential strengths and limitations of convenience samples in mental health research?
3   What types of reliability and validity evidence might mental health researchers report in their studies and what do they tell you about error and the conclusions drawn from the data?

References

American Psychiatric Association. (2022). *Diagnostic and statistical manual of mental disorders* (5th ed., text rev.). Author.

Balkin, R. S., & Lenz, A. S. (2021). Contemporary issues in reporting statistical, practical, and clinical significance in counseling research. *Journal of Counseling & Development, 99*(2), 227–237. https://doi.org/10.1002/jcad.12370

Beck, A. T., Rush, A. J., Shaw, B. F., & Emery, G. (1987). *Cognitive therapy of depression*. Guilford Press.

Beck, A. T., Steer, R. A., & Brown, G. K. (1996). *Manual for the Beck Depression Inventory-II*. Pearson.

Carlin, M. T., Costello, M. S., Flansburg, M. A., & Darden, A. (in press). Reconsideration of the type I error rate for psychological science in the era of replication. *Psychological Methods*. https://doi.org/10.1037/met0000490

Charter, R. A., & Feldt, L. S. (2002). The importance of reliability as it relates to true score confidence intervals. *Measurement & Evaluation in Counseling & Development, 35*(2), 104–112. https://doi.org/10.1080/07481756.2002.12069053

Faul, F., Erdfelder, E., Lang, A. G., & Buchner, A. (2007). G*Power 3: A flexible statistical power analysis program for the social, behavioral, and biomedical sciences. *Behavior Research Methods, 39*, 175–191.

Goertzen, M. J. (2017). Introduction to quantitative research and data analysis. *Library Technology Reports, 53*(4), 1–9. https://doi.org/10.5860/ltr.53n4

Hinkle, D. E., Wiersma, W., & Jurs, S. G. (2003). *Applied statistics for the behavioral sciences* (5th ed.). Houghton Mifflin.

Mitchell, M. L. and Jolley, J. M. (2013) *Research design explained*. Cengage Learning.

Novosel, L. M. (2023). Understanding the evidence: Non-probability (non-random) sampling designs. *Urologic Nursing, 43*(5), 245–247. https://doi.org/10.7257/2168-4626.2023.43.5.245

Rouaud, M. (2013). *Probability, statistics, and estimation: Propagation of uncertainties in experimental measurement*. Author.

Schneck, A. (2023). Are most published research findings false? Trends in statistical power, publication selection bias, and the false discovery rate in psychology (1975–2017). *PLoS ONE, 18*(1), 1–18. https://doi.org/10.1371/journal.pone.0292717

Stevens, S. S. (1946). On the theory of scales and measurement. *Science, 103*, 677–680. https://www.jstor.org/stable/1671815

Traub, R. E. (1997). Classical test theory in historical perspective. *Educational Measurement: Issues and Practice, 16*(4), 8–14. https://doi.org/10.1111/j.1745-3992.1997.tb00603.x

Weisberg, H. F. (1992). *Central tendency and variability*. Sage.

6 Case Study

Holly Downs

When doing research, inevitably someone will ask, "What do you want to research?" usually followed by the question, "How do you plan to do that?" In tackling a research project, one of the most challenging topics is how to get started in the design of the study. Qualitative designs are typically used in research to provide in-depth descriptions of a specific program, practice, or setting (Denzin & Lincoln, 2011). One of the most popular types of social science research related to qualitative inquiry is case study. Although not always solely qualitative, case study does seek to provide an in-depth view of a case or phenomenon. According to one of the leading case study researchers, Robert Yin (2014), doing case study research "remains one of the most challenging of all social science endeavors" (p. 3). While this sounds daunting, one of the rewards of doing a case study well is that you are given insights into your data that otherwise would have remained uncovered; much like an iceberg in the ocean, case study can help reveal what is under the surface of the water that is not as readily evident at first glance. This chapter will review case study research, including an introduction to case study research, when to use case study research, an example of a case study, case study methodology including case study designs, analysis activities, and presentation of case study findings to provide you with guidance as you design your own case study.

What Is Case Study?

The definition of case study research is not as simple as one would think because the term has been bandied about at times incorrectly. Before talking about what case study is, it is important to dispel some myths by covering what case study is not.

Case Study Is Not Solely Used in One Field of Study

Case study is not field specific, as case studies have been used in counseling (Hill, Carter, & O'Farrell, 1983; Wester, Downs, & Trepal, 2016), psychology (Cosmides & Tooby, 1989), traditional and online education (Cann, 2005; Downs, 2014; McAdams, Hess, & Viteritti, 1999), health (Luo & Wang, 2003; van Oort, Schröder, & French, 2011), engineering (Wieringa, 2014), and business (Berson & Avolio, 2004; Eisenhardt & Graebner, 2007; Garrett & Vogt, 2003; Perren & Ram, 2004) as well as others. Even though fields may privilege or favor one type of data collection or analysis over another, case study is valuable to all fields when the researcher seeks to do deeper exploration of a topic.

DOI: 10.4324/9781032706139-6

Case Study Is Not Just *Qualitative Data and Analysis*

Case study is also not solely qualitative, as some believe. Rather, it includes many different data collection techniques and analysis strategies that are both qualitative and quantitative in nature. While most are familiar with the common qualitative data sources like interviews and observations that are potentially rich data sources for a case study, omitting numeric data and analysis is shortsighted. Many case study authors assert that having both qualitative and quantitative data actually increases credibility (Bickman & Rog, 2009; Korzilius, 2010; Yin, 2014), as it creates "a strong evidentiary base." With that base, "methodically analyzing these data using qualitative or quantitative methods will then lead to more defensible findings and solutions" (Bickman & Rog, 2009, p. 279).

Case Study Does Not Have to Be a Single Case

Case study can be a single case or multiple cases. One of the most prominent case study researchers, Robert Stake, says case study "is the study of particularly and complexity of a single case, coming to understand its activity within important circumstances" (p. xi) that is driven by the interest of the researcher in the case (Stake, 1995). While Stake emphasizes a single case being the focus of a study, others talk about the possibilities of including in-depth exploration of multiple cases for more comparative purposes and richer findings. Linda Chmiliar (2010)asserts that multiple-case design is "more powerful than single-case designs as it provides more extensive descriptions and explanations of the phenomenon or issue" (p. 583).

Regardless of whether single- or multiple-case studies are used, at the heart of a good case study is that it is "an empirical inquiry that investigates a contemporary phenomenon (the 'case') in depth and within its real-world context, especially when the boundaries between phenomenon and context may not be clearly evident" (Yin, 2014, p. 18). It is the depth of the study that truly defines the value of what quality case study research should do and be.

When to Use Case Study

A number of factors may suggest that case study is appropriate for a research method for your study. Ultimately, the best way to determine the type of research to do, regardless of whether it is case study, is by positing the research questions you want to answer (which is discussed in the next section). However, there are several general characteristics agreed upon by most case study researchers. Yin (2014) asserts that a case study design should be specifically considered when the researcher (a) seeks to answer "how" and "why" research questions, (b) will not manipulate the behavior of those involved in the study, (c) wants to fully explore the context because it is relevant to the phenomenon being studied, or (d) cannot separate the case from the context. For instance, conducting a case study on how graduate students are making decisions on their dissertation research methodology might result in very different findings depending on factors like their personal experience, coursework, and dissertation advisor preferences. Without considering the full context, it would be impossible for this case study researcher to have a true picture of the case without it.

Research Questions Best Suited for Case Study

As suggested by the National Research Council, posing carefully designed, significant questions that can be tested is the first guiding principle in conducting rigorous, quality research regardless of the approach (Shavelson & Towne, 2002). Looking across the literature,

Table 6.1 Types of Research Questions for Case Studies

Research Question Purpose	Definition	Research Question Example
Descriptive	This question is for informational purposes that seeks to answer, "What is happening or has happened?"	How are graduate students trained on research methods?
Process	This question is for process purposes that seeks to answer, "How or why did something happen?"	How do graduate students decide what type of research methods to use for their dissertations?
Issues	This question is for raising attention to potential issues that seeks to answer, "What are some potential problems that might be important to explore?"	How does the power structure of the graduate advisor and graduate student influence the decisions on the types of research methods they use?

typically case study is used to answer "how" or "why" questions that fit into three different category types and purposes, including descriptive, process, or issue questions (see Table 6.1). The first two purposes are the typical purposes in almost all research projects (Shavelson & Towne, 2002). First, **descriptive questions** come from the need to pose questions for informational gathering purposes. Next, **process questions** look more deeply into how or why something happened to try to find associations or factors that may have influenced the outcome. The third type is **issue questions**, which may be posed to get at more cause-and-effect relationships, but this can sometimes be controversial given the case study nature of the design. Stake (1995) talks about the need to raise issue questions, which are used in order to "force attention to complexity and contextuality ... identification of issues draws attention to problems and concerns" (p. 16). He goes on to describe issue questions as "intricately wired to political, social, historical, and especially personal contexts" (p. 17).

Case Study of Digital Online Degree Programs

To illustrate the application of the methodological concepts, an example of a study that undertook a multiple-case study approach to probe how three prominent science, technology, engineering, and mathematics (STEM) programs with entirely online graduate degree programs were evaluating their programs (Downs, 2014). This case study included a combination of document review, surveys ($n = 107$), and interviews ($n = 27$) with program administrators, faculty, and students from the three established STEM online master's degree programs, including the departments of natural resources and environmental sciences (NRES), crop sciences (CRSC), and mechanical science and engineering (MechSE) at a midwestern university. The study probed the core research question of:

How are the online graduate programs from the various STEM fields discerning the quality of their programs?

Case Study Methodology

This section will discuss the characteristics and common designs used when implementing case study research and specifically how these applied to the case study of the aforementioned three STEM online degree programs. Design and data analysis considerations are also discussed.

Characteristics of Case Studies

In case study research, a few key elements across all case studies are fundamental to their success that almost all researchers agree upon regardless of their field of study. Some of the most important elements to consider include the concepts of bounding a case, defining case study type and design, and determining the unit of analysis.

Bounding a Case

A critical early step in conducting a case study is to define or bound the "case" that is going to be studied (Creswell, 2009; Stake, 1995; Yin, 2014). This is more than the sheer identification of a general topic area, it is truly looking to define the boundary between the case and with other phenomena surrounding it. For instance, several authors have suggested bounding a case by (a) time and activity and uniqueness (Stake, 1995), (b) time and place (Creswell, 2009), (c) definition and context (Miles & Huberman, 1994), or by (d) other factors like unit of analysis, group, organization, or geographic area (Yin, 2014). Bounding the case will not only help strengthen the understanding of the case but will also guard against the scope of the project becoming too broad or too big, which is important to all researchers but particularly to novices. Stake (1995) also recommends considering the historical background, the economic, political, and legal contexts, and the multiple stakeholder groups that make up the case.

For the STEM study sample mentioned earlier, it was important to establish the boundaries of the cases, particularly since it was in the digital realm. In order to be a part of this study, programs needed to meet five criteria, including being (a) an online degree program affiliated with the midwestern university in the fall of 2009, (b) a complete master's degree program, (c) an established program housed in a department for at least five years at the main campus at Midwestern University, (d) one of the nine STEM departments identified by the National Science Foundation, and (e) an online program in which **all** of the content is delivered online (Downs, 2014). Thus, the cases were bounded by the degree requirements, departments, and time.

Defining the Case Study Type and Design

A second critical piece in conducting a case study is to define the type of case study that is going to be used. Some cases can be more complex, and therefore it is harder to define what type of case study is being done. While choosing an individual might be an easy way to define the case, case study research involving multiple people like in a program, organization, population, clinic, or geographic region can be more difficult to define. First, it is important to identify the type of case study a researcher is undertaking, which is closely related to a researcher's overarching purpose. Stake (1995) categorizes the types of case study research as intrinsic and instrumental, while Yin (2014) categorizes these as explanatory, exploratory, or descriptive. Evident from Table 6.2, these case study types for research purposes are distinct, but they also overlap and can be used in tandem.

Further, these case study types can primarily be further separated into two design categories of either single- or multiple-case study designs. In deciding between single- or multiple-case studies, it is important to understand what they are. A single-case study is comparable to single-subject experimental research designs in which the individual him or herself is the focus of the study and the focus of analysis (Bickman & Rog, 2009; Creswell, 2009; Egel & Barthold, 2010). Typical justifications for doing single-case studies include if the case seems to represent a critical test to existing theory, an extreme case, a typical case, or a longitudinal case

Table 6.2 Case Study Types for Research Purposes

Case Study Types	Use If a Researcher ...
Intrinsic	Has an interest in the particular case chosen because it illustrates a particular trait or issue of interest; the case is of primary interest. For instance, the case is explored because the researcher seeks deeper knowledge of the case itself.
Instrumental	Wants to provide insight into an issue or support for a theory in which the case is of secondary interest. For instance, the case is explored because it helps the researcher pursue knowledge of an external interest.
Explanatory	Seeks to explain causal links in interventions (in experimental and quasi-experimental designs). For instance, the case is explored because it has outcomes set, and the study seeks to explain how the process links with the outcomes. This also can include pre–post designs in which two time points are separated by some critical event.
Exploratory	Desires to explore cases in which the outcomes in interventions are unknown. For instance, the case is studied to explore and identify what the outcomes are.
Descriptive	Aspires to describe an intervention or phenomenon and the real-life context in which it occurred. For instance, the case is explored primarily to describe how it exists and interacts with the environment and immediate context.

(Yin, 2014). However, some researchers suggest that doing single-subject research is limiting (Cook & Campbell, 1979), but researchers like Stake (1995) posit that this perceived limitation is precisely the strength of this design – it maximizes what we can learn about this single case without trying to force the assertions to be applied or generalized to other cases.

Multiple-case studies are the other overarching option in case study design and give the researcher the option to explore similarities and differences within and between cases. In other words, multiple cases are oftentimes done for replication to find similar results (sometimes referenced as direct or literal replication) or contrasting results for anticipated reasons (theoretical replication; Yin, 2014). It is believed that

> Multiple-case design allows examination of processes and outcomes across many cases, identification of how individual cases might be affected by different environments, and the specific conditions under which a finding might occur. It may also help to form more general categories of how the specific conditions might be related.
>
> (Chmiliar, 2010, p. 583)

While the evidence created from a multiple-case study design can be more robust and reliable than just looking at one case, it can be more time consuming and expensive to conduct because it deals with multiple sites. For instance, rather than doing extensive data collection with one site, doing this with multiple sites usually requires more researcher time to do the data collection and analysis.

The second limitation of multiple-case studies is that there are no quick rules or tests like power analysis to justify the sample size or number of cases in a multiple-case study. Qualitative research specialists like Merriam and Tisdell (2015, p. 101) admit,

> Unfortunately for those with a low tolerance for ambiguity, there is no answer. It always depends on the questions being asked, the data being gathered, the analysis in progress, and the resources you have to support the study. What is needed is an adequate number of participants, sites, or activities to answer the question posed at the beginning of the study.

Yin (2014, p. 61) recommends,

> [Y]ou may want to settle for two or three literal replications when your theory is straight-forward. … However, if your theory is subtle or if you want a higher degree of certainty, you may press for five, six, or more replications.

Ultimately, it is up to the researcher to decide and justify the design decisions and assertions that they make. In other words, the more contentious your case, theory, or assertion, the more evidence or support you will need to justify your findings so that other people find the evidence compelling and credible. For instance, the STEM example referenced before was done for descriptive purposes utilizing a multiple-case study design. In many ways, it would have been easier to just focus on one online class or program, but because the study sought to build not only an understanding but also a model for meta-analysis that could be applied to more than one program, focusing on just one program was insufficient for the assertions, so three entire degree programs were chosen. Moreover, the digital delivery was different, so using one program would not have given the breadth and depth of information that was required to deliver a more compelling in-depth study of the programs.

Determining the Unit of Analysis

After the type of research design is established, it is then important to determine the unit of analysis (Patton, 2015). Because both single- and multiple-case designs may have one to several units of analysis depending on the findings and the research questions, case study researchers usually describe the unit of analysis as either *holistic* or *embedded* (Berg, 2004; Gall, Borg, & Gall, 1996; Yin, 2014). For a case study using a holistic unit of analysis, this means that you can choose a single or main unit for analyzing the overall case or cases. A case study using an embedded unit of analysis translates into looking at the main unit as well as other subunits for the analysis of the case. For instance, if you wanted to look at a single case such as a single leadership training program in one school or a single unit within multiple cases such as the same leadership training program within different schools, then this would be a holistic unit of analysis. However, if a case is the training program and the researcher also wanted to investigate individual subunits such as participants in the program by demographics such as gender, then this would be an embedded unit of analysis. It's much like looking at an onion – you could either look at the onion in its entirety or multiple whole onions in their different contexts (like from homes, gardens, and stores), or you could look at the onion and the different sublayers in that single onion or those sublayers in multiple onions. For the STEM example, each program was looked at individually, so it was a multiple-case study design with a holistic unit of analysis. If the researcher would have looked at individuals or subunits within the three programs, this could have been an embedded unit of analysis, because the overall program and subunits within would have represented multiple layers of analysis.

Additional Design Considerations

In addition to the considerations mentioned, within any case study design, some additional decisions should be made including deciding whether to develop a formal theoretical framework and considering the quality of the case study research, including the concepts of validity and reliability.

Deciding Whether to Develop a Formal Theoretical Framework

Similar to the other topics that we've discussed on case study, the use of theory is driven by the design and purpose decisions you make. Theory can help you complete the other important steps like developing your research questions, bounding your case, making your design decision, or defining the unit of analysis that you're interested in exploring (Yin, 2014). Additionally, it is the hope that this will benefit the precision and the ability of others to replicate the analysis to yield similar findings on other similar research. However, having an initial theoretical map or perspective about your case may not fit directly with your purpose. For example, having an initial theoretical perspective about metrics of success in a training program might be very helpful to know at the onset of a study in order to attempt to build, extend, or challenge this framework and your study in order to support hypothesis testing. However, it is the belief of some case study researchers that this may limit your ability to make discoveries about the case in its individual context and may bias the researcher to focus too much on one aspect of the picture. This does not mean that preparation work is not necessary, but it means that it might take a more generalized or exploratory approach to preparing to do systematic data collection (Stake, 1995). The general advice that one should take is that if you are looking to convince others that your study has produced findings that contribute to your field, developing a theoretical framework is advisable and necessary.

Considering the Quality of Case Study

Despite the commonness of using case study research, there is trepidation about using case study as a method of choice because of the question of the credibility or "trustworthiness" of the method, the instruments, the data, and the findings. Quality case study research should be done by using systematic procedures in terms of case study data collection and analysis procedures. If anyone tells you that case study research is "easier" because you can "just do it," they are sorely mistaken. While a number of concepts have been offered for judging the quality of any research, two main concepts are common for judging social science research and should be addressed in case study research: Validity and reliability (see Figure 6.1).

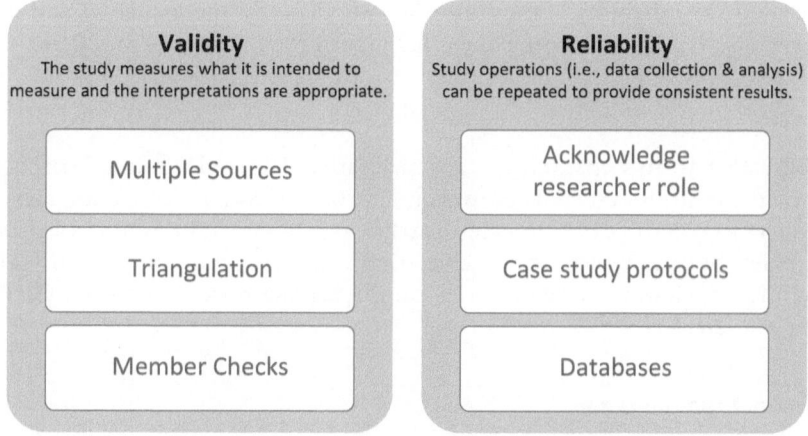

Figure 6.1 Strategies to Increasing Validity and Reliability in Case Study Research.

Validity refers to the extent to which the study measures what it is intended to measure (Cho & Trent, 2006; Maxwell, 1992; Miles & Huberman, 1994; Patton, 2015) and the interpretations are appropriate, meaningful, and useful (Messick, 1989; Patton, 2015; Stake, 1995). Important to all research, validity in case study can be particularly difficult to justify. Qualitative data and findings may be suspect of researcher bias, instrument weakness, and individual interpretation, which limit confirmatory replicability (Mertens, 2010; Patton, 2015). However, strategies have been proposed by case study researchers to strengthen the validity of findings in case study, including:

- Collecting multiple sources of evidence,
- Checking data to see if methods support a single conclusion, known as triangulation,
- Inviting persons who were sources of data to review the data collected and reports, known as member checking,
- Utilizing multiple data sources for triangulation,
- Using replication logic in multiple cases.

(Denzin & Lincoln, 2011; Maxwell, 2013; Patton, 2015)

Reliability is the extent to which the study operations like data collection and analysis can be repeated to provide consistent results (Yin, 2014). Ultimately, reliability should seek to minimize the errors and biases in any study. As Stake (1995) suggests, the case study researcher can play many roles including teacher, observer, advocate, evaluator, and interpreter, among others. Not acknowledging these roles can threaten the reliability of the findings you present. For instance, if you are playing an "advocate" role for the program you are studying and the report becomes more of a promotional piece, this causes major problems for the reader of the case to believe what you are saying. Instead, clearly stating your role and then discovering the best arguments against your assertions then providing data that either are supportive of or contrary to those assertions can be better in terms of reliability.

The case study report should adopt the following suggestions to improve reliability: Clearly acknowledging your role as a case study researcher, developing and using case study protocols, and using databases and keeping detailed fieldnotes and memos to track fidelity (Miles & Huberman, 1994; Schwandt, 2007; Stake, 1995; Yin, 2014). The most important thing to note is that you as a researcher cannot just go on-site somewhere and start collecting data to have adequate reliability in the study. Having plans for meta-analysis and review at the conclusion can also help in increasing the reliability of the findings (Yin, 2014).

Data Collection

As suggested earlier in this chapter, certain qualitative data collection approaches are often associated with case study research. However, approaches to data collection can range from fairly simple to more complex. Numerous textbooks and courses cover all of these data collection strategies, but the typical approaches used with case study outlined in Table 6.3 can include document review, interviews, observations, artifact review, and surveys (Berg, 2004; Stake, 1995; Yin, 2014).

Data Analysis and Interpretation

Obviously, certain data analysis approaches are better suited to answer certain types of research questions with the type of data that is collected, as "the aim of analysis is to convert

Table 6.3 Common Data Collection Strategies

Data Collection Strategy	Overview	Some Possible Sources
Document Review	Includes collecting documents previously produced by or about the case	Any documents current or past about the case produced by various stakeholders including letters, websites, articles, promotional materials, photography, video, social media, databases, personal correspondence, or administrative documents
Interviews	Incorporates question-and-answer direct conversations using structured and/or open prompts and questions	Targeted individuals or focus groups; interviewees might be directly or indirectly aware and involved in the case. These should seek to uncover in-depth data about expectations and reflections about the case.
Observations	Involves observing or watching the case in its typical setting or state	Direct observations of the entire case or subunits of the case
Artifact Review	Consists of collecting tools, objects, instruments generated by or used in the direct observations	Physical artifacts (like observed and unobserved work, assessments) generated by participants or used by stakeholders in the case
Surveys	Incorporates questions and answers in a questionnaire-type format using simple descriptive research for longitudinal purposes	Large-scale surveys from national and international governing bodies, topic-specific surveys commonly used in the field of study, customized questions directly created to study the case

a mass of raw data into a coherent account" (Weiss, 1998, p. 271). Analysis in developing an understanding of the case is an ongoing process. Stake (1995) asserts, "There is no particular moment when data analysis begins. Analysis is a matter of giving meaning to first impressions as well as to final compilations" (p. 71). Moreover, because the case can have so many different types of data collection, you need to have an idea about analysis from the onset to prevent becoming overwhelmed with the data. In my experience, it takes approximately three to five times as long to clean and analyze the data as it does to collect it. Meaning if you do a one-hour interview it will take approximately three to five hours to transcribe verbatim or summarize your notes, to put it into a format that you can use, and to analyze the actual interview data. While advances have been made in transcription services and software programs for analyzing qualitative and quantitative data, it still takes researcher time and effort to get to know your data. Some common analytic techniques in case study research include trend or pattern analysis, explanation or theory building, and time series analysis.

Trend or Pattern Analysis

The purpose of trend or pattern matching is to compare the theoretical patterns to empirical outcomes (Weiss, 1998). Pattern analysis is not always solely based on consistencies, as this type of analysis can be commonly categorized to summarize (a) convergence or similarity, (b) divergence or difference, (c) frequency, (d) order or sequence, (e) correspondence, or (f) causation (Hatch, 2002; Patton, 2015; Saldaña, 2015; Weiss, 1998). The goal of trend or pattern matching is to compare the pattern with the predicted one so that this does not simply become a quantitative exercise with qualitative data (Yin, 2014).

Explanation or Theory Building

It is more complicated than pattern matching, as it is used "to 'explain' a phenomenon to stipulate a presumed set of causal links about it, or 'how' or 'why' something happened" (Yin, 2014, p. 147). Yin (2014)stresses that this type of analysis should be an iterative, systematic process in which a theoretical framework is proposed, an initial case study is done, a revision is done to the original theoretical framework, additional case studies are done and compared to the original framework, and then final explanations and frameworks are proposed.

Time Series Analysis

The final analytic technique is the same for any time-series analysis conducted in experimental and quasi-experimental studies in which you compare data from one time period to data from other periods (see Bickman & Rog, 2009 and Cook & Campbell, 1979). These can range from simple to complex designs. When adequate numbers of data are appropriate and available about the case, simple to complex statistical analysis can be used if it adds to the richness of the case (Yin, 2014). For instance, in a simple pre–post design, Wester and associates (2016) wanted to explore the data they collected on non-suicidal self-injury (NSSI), where descriptive statistics and frequencies were generated from eight individuals to explore their NSSI frequency and methods from intake to termination in outpatient counseling. An example of more complex design is the case study done by Berson and Avolio (2004), in which they used hierarchical linear modeling (HLM) to do a case study of a large telecommunications organization in order to examine group-level effects and relationships between aggregates in their study about leadership style of top- and middle-level managers and their ability to convey organizational goals.

Reporting a Case Study

Depending on the data that are generated, case study affords you the opportunity to utilize many strategies for data presentation. Academic writers like Wolcott (1990) assert that "You cannot begin the writing process early enough" (p. 20) because of the potential large amount of data that you can collect with case study. Stake (1995) warns, "a 20-page case study is likely to run 50 if the researcher doesn't 'ruthlessly winnow and sift'" (p. 121). So decisions about audience and reporting formats are crucial in case study.

Traditionally, writing reports is what most case study researchers within academia discuss in the literature. However, giving thought to your case study audience as well as reporting formats "serves as a good starting point for composing your case study" (Yin, 2014, p. 179). The overarching goal of reporting case study research is

> to describe the study in a manner to enable the reader to feel as if they had been an active participant in the research and can determine whether or not the study findings could be applied to their own situation.
>
> (Baxter & Jack, 2008, p. 555)

Yin (2014) encourages case study researchers to consider that case study reporting might be received by multiple audiences, such as those who are academic colleagues as well as nonspecialists.

Most case study reporting is delivered via a traditional report structure of some sort. Stake (1995) talks about the importance of using story formats in case study reporting to engage the reader and illustrate what is happening with vignettes, which are short descriptions of an issue or episode to illustrate something about the case. He recommends a report structure of having an entry vignette, background and purpose discussion, issue development, narrative about data analysis and triangulation discussion, assertions, and then closing vignettes. Yin (2014) also talks about six different types of compositional structures for case study report, including the standard research reporting style he identifies, linear-analytic structure. This structure commonly used by journal articles would start with an introduction to the issue or problem being studied, a review of the literature, methods, data collection, data analysis and findings, and conclusions and implications.

While the traditional case study reporting approaches are great for certain audiences, sometimes additional pieces should be considered for nonspecialists. Adapting communication and reporting to think about potentially making them more interactive is important in getting different audiences to understand and use the research (Patton, 2015; Torres, Preskill, & Piontek, 2005; Yin, 2014). Looking at Figure 6.2, there are examples of traditional and non-traditional pieces to help discussion. For instance, in doing a larger case study research project on digital learning within an organization, we needed to produce a data visualization infographic (see Figure 6.3) in addition to the traditional report in order to help communicate about the interview results with a broader audience (see Evergreen, 2014).

Continuing to Apply

Evident from the discussion, case study research is more than conducting qualitative research on a single individual or situation. This approach can be simple or complex, encouraging the researcher to ask different types of questions in order to study phenomena in depth within their own contexts. For new researchers, case study can be very informative, as it provides a rich opportunity to do single- or multiple-case study designs to gain insight into the case

Least Interactive	Potentially Interactive	Most Interactive
Memos, emails, newsletters, bulletins, briefs, brochures, websites	Verbal presentations (visual slides and flipcharts)	Working discussion sessions (skits, group sense making)
Paper reports (interim and comprehensive)	Video and multimedia presentations	Interactive dashboards
Executive summaries	Data visualizations and posters (live or digitized)	Webinar presentations (i.e., chat rooms, interactive whiteboards, web conferences)

Figure 6.2 Communication and Reporting Formats by Level of Potential Interaction.

(adapted from Torres et al., 2005).

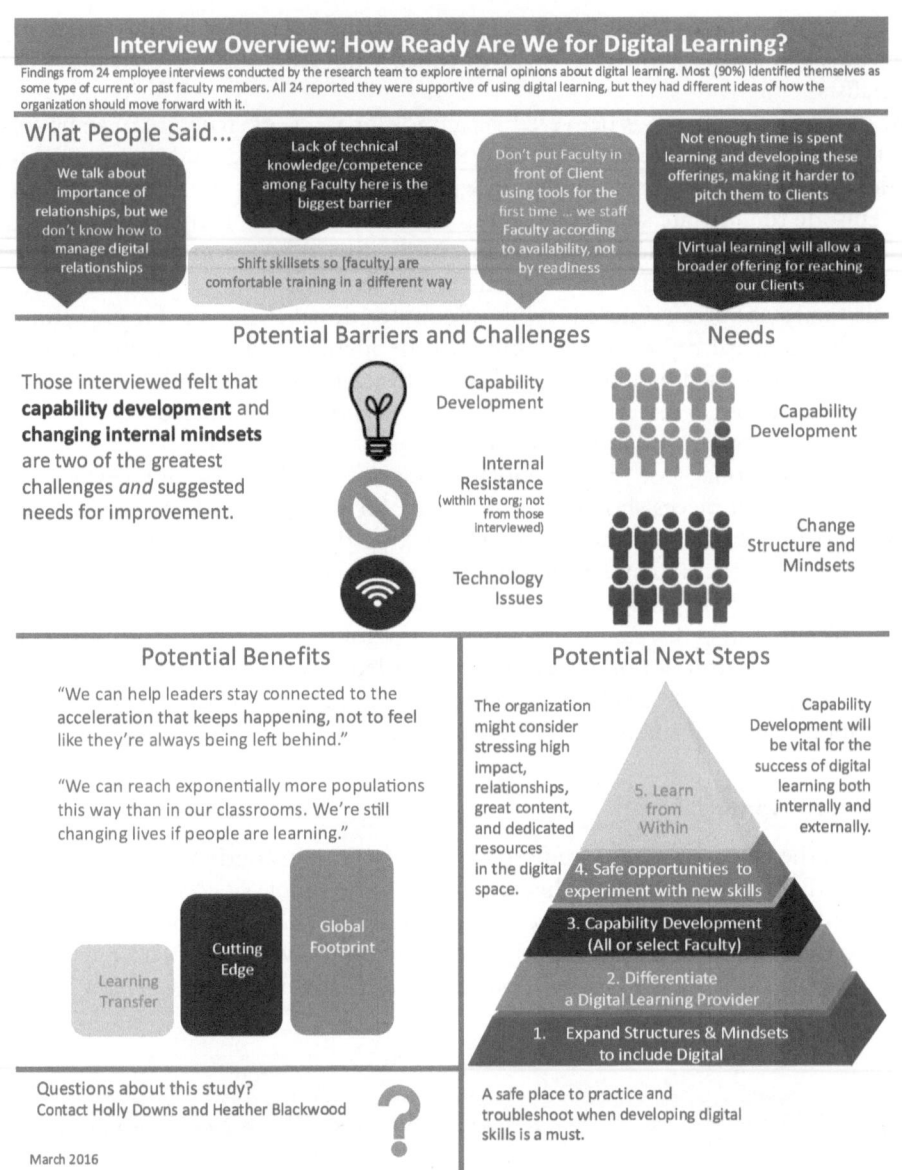

Figure 6.3 Example of an Infographic Displaying Interview Findings.

using myriad data sources and analyses to inform multiple audiences. The best way to get started is to review case studies from empirical journals within and outside your field of study. There is a great compilation of case studies from many different fields mentioned in this chapter and covered in Yin's book, *The Case Study Anthology* (2004).

Practice-Based Application

In Chapter 1, you were asked to consider a client and their presenting concern. You had jotted down a broad question, something that you had interest in knowing or gaining information or data on. Take a moment and consider the client, their presenting concern, and the broad question you had in Chapter 1. Consider the following questions:

- Is this client the "case" that you want to examine, or how would you define the "case" for this methodology? Understanding the case is needed in order to be able to answer or gain information and data on what you want to know.
- What type of case study would be appropriate to answer what you want to know?
- What data do you need to collect to gain a holistic, in-depth picture of this case? Consider whether this is multiple formats of data from just the client, or if you would be collecting data from other individuals or stakeholders as well.

Resources for More Information

Peer-Reviewed Journal Articles

Eisenhardt, K. M., & Graebner, M. E. (2007). Theory building from cases: Opportunities and challenges. *Academy of Management Journal, 50*(1), 25–32.

Flyvbjerg, B. (2006). Five misunderstandings of case-study research. *Qualitative Inquiry, 12*(2), 219–245.

Nespor, J. (2000). Anonymity and place in qualitative inquiry. *Qualitative Inquiry, 6,* 546–571.

Stringfield, S. C., & Yakimowski-Srebnick, M. E. (2005). Promise, progress, problems, and paradoxes of three phases of accountability: A longitudinal case study of the Baltimore City public schools. *American Educational Research Journal, 42*(1), 43–75.

Wells, A. S., Hirshberg, D., Lipton, M., & Oaks, J. (1995). Bounding the case within its context: A constructivist approach to studying detracking reform. *Educational Researcher, 24,* 18–24.

Books

Hancock, D. R., & Algozzine, B. (2015). *Doing case study research: A practical guide for beginning researchers.* Teachers College Press.

Stake, R. E. (1995). *The art of case study research.* Sage Publications.

Yin, R. K. (2004). *The case study anthology.* Sage Publications.

Yin, R. K. (2014). *Case study research: Design and methods* (5th ed.). Sage Publications.

Questions for Further Review on Case Study

1 Find a case study from your area of study. What was the purpose of this case study? What are the strengths of the case study you reviewed? What limitations do you see in this case study? What types of research questions (i.e., descriptive, process, issue questions) were presented?
2 What would you do differently if you were to undertake a case study on the same case?
3 If you were developing a case study, what design would you most likely use? Would you use a single- or multiple-case study approach? How would you justify this decision?
4 What are some common characteristics across all case studies that you have read or been exposed to? What can you apply to your own research?
5 Will you develop a theoretical framework for your case study? How will you justify your decision?
6 What are the data collection and analysis strategies being considered? What issues of validity and reliability will you need to attend to in order to strengthen the quality of your case study?
7 Identify the audiences you anticipate for your case study report. Do you think that one report would serve all the audiences adequately? Why or why not?

References

Baxter, P., & Jack, S. (2008). Qualitative case study methodology: Study design and implementation for novice researchers. *The Qualitative Report, 13*(4), 544–559.

Berg, B. L. (2004). *Qualitative research methods for the social sciences* (Vol. 5): Pearson.

Berson, Y., & Avolio, B. J. (2004). Transformational leadership and the dissemination of organizational goals: A case study of a telecommunication firm. *The Leadership Quarterly, 15*(5), 625–646. http://doi.org/10.1016/j.leaqua.2004.07.003

Bickman, L., & Rog, D. J. (2009). *The SAGE handbook of applied social research methods.* Sage Publications.

Cann, A. (2005). Extended matching sets questions for online numeracy assessments: A case study. *Assessment & Evaluation in Higher Education, 30*(6), 633.

Chmiliar, L. (2010). Multiple-case designs. *Encyclopedia of Case Study Research, 1,* 1–2.

Cho, J., & Trent, A. (2006). Validity in qualitative research revisited. *Qualitative Research, 6*(3), 319–340.

Cook, T. D., & Campbell, D. T. (1979). *Quasi-experimentation: Design & analysis issues for field settings.* Rand McNally & Co.

Cosmides, L., & Tooby, J. (1989). Evolutionary psychology and the generation of culture, part II: Case study: A computational theory of social exchange. *Ethology and Sociobiology, 10*(1–3), 51–97.

Creswell, J. W. (2009). *Research design: Qualitative, quantitative, and mixed method approaches* (3rd ed.). Sage Publications.

Denzin, N. K., & Lincoln, Y. S. (2011). *The Sage handbook of qualitative research.* Sage Publications.

Downs, H. A. (2014). Evaluation in STEM online graduate degree programs in agricultural sciences and engineering. *Journal of Case Studies in Education, 5*(1), 1–18.

Egel, A. L., & Barthold, C. H. (2010). Single subject design and analysis. *The Reviewer's Guide to Quantitative Methods in the Social Sciences.* Routledge. 357–370.

Eisenhardt, K. M., & Graebner, M. E. (2007). Theory building from cases: Opportunities and challenges. *Academy of Management Journal, 50*(1), 25–32.

Evergreen, S. D. (2014). *Presenting data effectively: Communicating your findings for maximum impact.* SAGE Publications.

Gall, M. D., Borg, W. R., & Gall, J. P. (1996). *Educational research: An introduction.* Longman Publishing.

Garrett, L. A., & Vogt, C. L. (2003). Meeting the needs of consumers: Lessons from business and industry. *New Directions for Adult and Continuing Education,* (100), 89–101.

Hatch, J. A. (2002). *Doing qualitative research in education settings.* SUNY Press.

Hill, C. E., Carter, J. A., & O'Farrell, M. K. (1983). A case study of the process and outcome of time-limited counseling. *Journal of Counseling Psychology, 30*(1), 3.

Korzilius, H. (2010). Quantitative analysis in case study. *Encyclopedia of Case Study Research, 2.*

Luo, W., & Wang, F. (2003). Measures of spatial accessibility to health care in a GIS environment: Synthesis and a case study in the Chicago region. *Environment and Planning B: Planning and Design, 30*(6), 865–884.

Maxwell, J. (1992). Understanding and validity in qualitative research. *Harvard Educational Review, 62*(3), 279–301.

Maxwell, J. (2013). *Qualitative research design: An interactive approach* (3rd ed.). Sage publications.

McAdams, D. R., Hess, G. A., & Viteritti, J. P. (1999). Lessons from Houston. *Brookings Papers on Education Policy,* (2), 129–183.

Merriam, S. B., & Tisdell, E. J. (2015). *Qualitative research: A guide to design and implementation.* John Wiley & Sons.

Mertens, D. M. (2010). *Research and evaluation in education and psychology* (3rd ed.). Sage Publications.

Messick, S. (1989). Meaning and values in test validation: The science and ethics of assessment. *Educational Researcher, 18*(2), 5–11. https://doi.org/10.3102/0013189x018002005

Miles, M. B., & Huberman, A. M. (1994). *Qualitative data analysis* (2nd ed.). Sage Publications.

Patton, M. Q. (2015). *Qualitative research and evaluation methods* (4th ed.). Sage Publications.

Perren, L., & Ram, M. (2004). Case-study method in small business and entrepreneurial research mapping boundaries and perspectives. *International Small Business Journal, 22*(1), 83–101.

Saldaña, J. (2015). *The coding manual for qualitative researchers.* Sage Publications.

Schwandt, T. A. (2007). *The Sage dictionary of qualitative inquiry* (3rd ed.). Sage Publications.

Shavelson, R., & Towne, L. (2002). *Scientific inquiry in education.* National Academy Press.

Stake, R. E. (1995). *The art of case study research.* Sage Publications.

Torres, R. T., Preskill, H., & Piontek, M. E. (2005). *Evaluation strategies for communicating and reporting: Enhancing learning in organizations* (2nd ed.). Sage Publications.

van Oort, L., Schröder, C., & French, D. P. (2011). What do people think about when they answer the brief illness perception questionnaire? A 'think-aloud' study. *British Journal of Health Psychology, 16*(2), 231–245. https://doi.org/10.1348/135910710x500819

Weiss, C. H. (1998). *Evaluation* (2nd ed.). Prentice Hall.

Wester, K. L., Downs, H. A., & Trepal, H. C. (2016). Factors linked with increases in nonsuicidal self-injury: A case study. *Counseling Outcome Research and Evaluation, 7*(1), 3–20.

Wieringa, R. J. (2014). Observational case studies. In *Design science methodology for information systems and software engineering* (pp. 225–245). Springer.

Wolcott, H. F. (1990). *Writing up qualitative research* (Vol. 20). Sage Publications.

Yin, R. K. (2004). *The case study anthology*. Sage Publications.

Yin, R. K. (2014). *Case study research: Design and methods* (5th ed.). Sage Publications.

7 Using Single-Case Research Designs to Evaluate Outcomes

A. Stephen Lenz

So far, you have reviewed some of the many important ways that researchers determine how efficacious interventions or programs are when looking at desired effects. In this chapter, we will review single-case research designs (SCRDs), one of two approaches that have been endorsed as supportive for making inferences about what works, for whom, how, and under what circumstances (Kratochwill et al., 2023; Tolin et al., 2015). The purpose of this chapter is to orient you to the general activities associated with SCRDs and get you started along the road to designing your own. Within this discussion, you will begin to understand how foundational concepts, design and analysis activities, and prudent interpretation of findings contribute to a defensible depiction of relationships between interventions and associated outcomes. Following, we have provided you with some resources that provide a more comprehensive discussion of these topics.

What Are SCRDs?

Single-case research designs (SCRDs) are a practical way to evaluate the efficacy of an intervention, establish preliminary support for novel practices, and assess applications of established programs with low incidence or understudied populations. Similar to the other experimental methods (e.g., randomized controlled trials, Chapter 10), well-designed SCRDs are suitable for demonstrating a cause-and-effect relationship between an intervention and dependent variables; unlike other experimental designs, in SCRDs, participants function as their unit for analysis, and progress is determined on an individual level instead of across groups (Cook et al., 2017; Lenz, 2015; What Works Clearinghouse, 2020). Within these designs, the *single case* of interest is not bound to an individual and instead can be representative of an individual client, family, classroom, group, or system (Morgan & Morgan, 2009; What Works Clearinghouse, 2020). Regardless of how your case is defined, your participants will always serve as their own comparison through the process of contrasting data collected during and after the intervention with those collected prior to the introduction of an independent variable (Egel et al., 2018; Rubin & Bellamy, 2012). As a result, SCRD analyses provide a wealth of information related to the unique magnitude and course of outcomes that individuals experience during an intervention. Although the data collected for a single participant's experience can be useful, the power of SCRDs lies in the accumulation of many cases whose data can be visually inspected and statistically aggregated to depict an overall effect (Brown et al., 2024; Lenz, 2013).

The beauty of using SCRDs to evaluate the outcome of interventions lies in their many practical advantages related to sample size, self as control, flexibility and responsiveness, ease of analysis, and type of data yielded. For example, the minimum sample size required for an

DOI: 10.4324/9781032706139-7

SCRD is one, but most will include between three and ten participants as a precaution against attrition. Also, being able to compare participant performance during and after an intervention with their experiences prior to it starting provides the basis for a functional relationship and thus causal inferences about outcomes. Within an SCRD, the repeated and consistent assessment of participant performance allows researchers to adjust their interventions so that people who may not respond to an intervention will have the chance to do so. Once an SCRD is completed, there are many statistically based approaches available to estimate intervention effect; however, the many trustworthy approaches require little more than a graph of your data, a straightedge, a pencil, and some basic arithmetic. As you will see in our discussion of situating SCRD results to participant context, the data yielded from these inquiries provides a depiction of the course of intervention effects and the amount of dosage that may be required to meet the intended criterion. What emerges from well-designed SCRDs is a body of empirical literature that can support practitioners in monitoring the progress of individual clients, completing larger program evaluations, maintaining evidence-based practice, and completing stakeholder reporting.

Situations Most Appropriate for SCRDs

Earlier in this chapter, we identified SCRDs as being a practical way to evaluate the efficacy of interventions and assess how programs are applied with underrepresented populations. One of the great things about using SCRDs is the ability to apply this design in a variety of settings such as inpatient, outpatient, partial hospitalization, private practice, community agencies, institutions of learning, and within your community. The results from SCRDs can be useful when reporting to stakeholders about treatment efficacy and the impact on the community. Kazdin (2020) also identified SCRDs as being applicable across several disciplines including education, psychology, social work, business, counseling, law enforcement, medicine, and corrections. SCRDs are appropriate when you have a low number of participants in your research, as the design is not likely to fail, because the minimum number of participants needed for SCRDs is one. In addition, researchers who desire to identify the course of treatment and observe for efficacy will find SCRDs an appropriate design (Barrio Minton & Lenz, 2019).

Types of Research Questions Best Suited for SCRDs

Although a number of case study approaches are suitable for answering myriad research questions, the quantitative SCRDs discussed in this chapter are particularly well-suited to answer two general types of research questions – those that estimate the degree of intervention effect and those related to exploring how individuals respond to an intervention. Research questions concerning degree of treatment effect should include language that establishes a causal relationship between a participant's experience with a dependent variable before your intervention and after it is introduced. Examples of these prompts include, "To what degree does an in-home reading intervention increase reading comprehension among school-aged children following a traumatic brain injury?", "How effective is a Graston treatment for increasing hip mobility among collegiate volleyball players?", and "How efficacious is a 12-week child-centered play therapy intervention for increasing on-task behavior in children with attention deficit hyperactivity disorder?" In each of these examples, the introduction of the interventions (i.e., in-home reading intervention, Graston treatment, and play therapy) is situated in a way that is intended to cause desired change among outcomes of interest (i.e., reading comprehension, hip mobility, and on-task behavior).

Research questions concerning how individuals respond to an intervention should include language related to important concepts such as immediacy of effect, course of response to intervention, and time until a desired criterion is met. Examples of these prompts include, "How many sessions are required to increase reading comprehension?", "What is the course of hip mobility gains during treatment?", and "How many sessions of play therapy are required for participants to no longer meet criteria for hyperactivity?" In each of these examples, the interest is associated with understanding the participant's personal response to the intervention. The answers to research questions related to intervention effect are best inferred from inspection of quantitative estimates of treatment effect and effect size, such as the nonoverlap and regression-based approaches discussed ahead. By contrast, the answers to questions related to how someone responds to an intervention are best inferred by using strategies for visual analysis of graphical data. We will address both approaches in our discussion of methodology, but first, let's consider an illustrative case example.

Case Example: Treating Trauma Symptoms Following Interpersonal Violence

To illustrate the application of methodological concepts, we present an example evaluating a 12-week, community-based, trauma-focused cognitive behavior therapy (Cohen et al., 2017; TF-CBT) program for adolescents who have been the victim of repeated interpersonal violence at school. The five participants range from ages 13 to 15, and all met the criteria for a diagnosis of posttraumatic stress disorder (PTSD) following a clinical interview and converging evidence from formal PTSD assessments. Participant symptoms were monitored weekly for three weeks ($N = 3$) and five weeks ($N = 2$) across participants. Once treatment began, participants completed the Child PTSD Scale one time a week while waiting for their scheduled appointment. As part of the TF-CBT treatment, all participants received a manualized series of coping skills training modules during the first seven weeks with the remaining five weeks oriented to completing a trauma narrative and safety planning for post-termination life.

SCRD Methodology

This section will discuss the characteristics and common designs used when implementing SCRDs. You will also learn about considerations for designs and what is involved in data analysis.

Characteristics Across All SCRDs

In SCRDs, inferences about the efficacy of interventions are made by comparing observations of an outcome across various phases of the study. A few key characteristics across all SCRDs are fundamental to their experimental nature. Among some of the most important to be familiar with are the concepts of baseline assessment, continuous assessment, performance stability, self as comparison, minimal sample size, and flexibility/responsiveness.

Baseline Assessment

In SCRDs, data is collected prior to any intervention during what is referred to as a *baseline phase*. Through baseline data, researchers can gather information about the level of particular behaviors before introducing an intervention. This initial period of observation serves two important functions. The first function, referred to as the *descriptive function*, describes the extent to which a participant engages in the behavior being studied. The second function is *prediction* of the immediate level of performance when intervention is not administered. This data serves as the comparison to all other data in an SCRD.

Continuous Assessment

One of the central requirements of an SCRD is the dependence on outcome variables being continually assessed over time. The researcher observes the participant's behavior across several occasions, occurring pre- and postintervention. Continuous assessment is a basic requirement of SCRDs, as this design examines the efficacy of interventions across time. Researchers can establish trends and patterns of behavior before implementing an intervention.

Performance Stability

Stability of performance can be explained by the absence of a slope in the data. The slope of data refers to the increase or decrease in performance over time. In addition, stability can be determined based on the level of variability of performance over time. Increased variability may adversely impact any conclusions about treatment efficacy.

Self as Comparison

Researchers utilizing an SCRD also can observe and evaluate the impact of interventions on overt behavior using visual inspection. Additionally, researchers are able to use the participant as their own control in an SCRD. This means the participant is their own comparison condition when comparing their scores during and after the implementation of an intervention. The researcher is then able to examine the data for a cause-and-effect relationship between the intervention and behavior being observed.

Minimal Sample Size

One characteristic central to SCRDs is the focus on one or a few participants. These designs are referred to as *small N research, single-case design*, or *N = 1 designs*. Since these designs are developed to study individual behavior over time, SCRDs can be implemented with one participant; however, to account for attrition, at least three to five participants are recommended.

Flexibility and Responsiveness

SCRDs can be implemented with diverse or unique populations in a variety of settings. SCRDs are not limited to a single set of standards or protocols; therefore, researchers can be flexible and adaptive in their approach to capture as many participants as needed. In addition, accommodation can be made for the amount of intervention needed across phases.

Common Designs

We have discussed the idea that SCRDs are used to evaluate the efficacy of an intervention over a period of time. SCRDs begin with repeated measurement of an outcome before introducing the intervention, but what happens afterward can take various forms in the effort to answer your research questions. Two general categories of SCRDs are those that are best suited for monitoring and those that are well-suited for garnering evidentiary support.

Designs Suitable for Monitoring

The most basic SCRD, the A-B design, can be used to document change in target behaviors at a single point and is the foundation of all SCRDs. In this design, the researcher collects baseline data (A) until stability is observed, then the intervention is implemented (B) while continuously observing the target outcome.

Researchers may make inferences from visual analysis of the graphed data while observing for any change in trends and patterns. Although important details about participants' experience can be observed using an A-B design, they are less defensible for demonstrating a cause-and-effect relationship between an intervention and the outcome of interest. To ease concerns about the threats to internal validity, researchers can implement another baseline (A) at the end, resulting in an A-B-A design. However, it should be noted that even with an A-B-A design, the threats-to-interval validity associated with an absence of replication persist.

Designs Suitable for Garnering Evidentiary Support

One of the characteristics of SCRDs is continuous assessment, in which the participant's behavior can be monitored across several occasions, as the intervention is repeated or replicated over time. Replication designs strengthen the conclusion that improvement can be attributed to the intervention. Examples of replication designs include A-B-A-B or A-B-A-B-A-B. Within these designs, the withdrawal of an intervention and reintroduction of it demonstrates a truer effect over time on participant experience, and thus, there is more internal validity as an effect is observed with every replication (Figures 7.1 and 7.2).

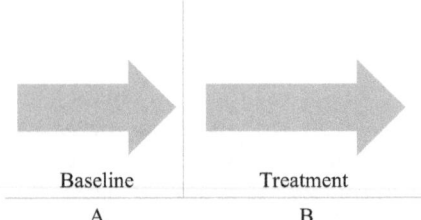

Figure 7.1 A-B Design.

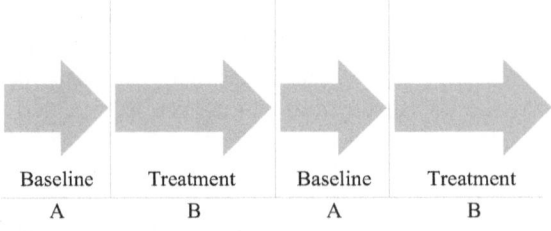

Figure 7.2 A-B-A-B Design.

Replication designs may be difficult to implement, or, in some settings, withdrawing an intervention may be unethical; therefore, using a multiple baseline design is a prudent alternative. Multiple-baseline designs comprise a series of A-B designs repeated in numerous ways: With the same individuals across various behaviors (multiple baselines across behaviors), the same behavior across various individuals (multiple baseline across subjects), or same individual across different settings (multiple baseline across settings). With multiple baselines, researchers collect baseline data at the same time across several participants, introducing the intervention only at systematic times when stability has been established. Baseline data can be collected on two or more behaviors, and the effect of an intervention is demonstrated by showing that the participant's behavior changes only when the intervention is applied. Multiple baselines do not require withdrawal or reversal of interventions; therefore, this is an appropriate design for establishing new behaviors.

Design Considerations

The best SCRDs clearly depict functional relationships between an intervention and the dependent variable of interest. When this relationship is clearly established through multiple baselines or replication designs, the design is thought to be more defensible to scrutiny than when those characteristics are present to a lesser degree. Within any design, some important considerations should be addressed, including those related to sample size, homogeneity of the sample, sensitivity of measurements, and fidelity of the intervention.

Sample Size

As mentioned, some useful information can be garnered from an SCRD with a sample size of one. However, heuristic guidelines for demonstrating evidentiary support require demonstration of treatment effect across a small series (3–9 participants) or large series (10 or more participants) to be regarded as modest or convincing support, respectively. In either scenario, evidence is most robust when findings converge across at least two different research teams residing at different sites. In the example of our illustrative case, there are five participants; therefore, even if the results depicted a clear picture of efficacy, the quality of support may yield only modest support. Therefore, the meta-analytic synthesis of samples across studies most likely provides the truest depiction of the relationships between intervention and outcomes (Tolin et al., 2015).

Homogeneity of the Sample

Because there is a small number of participants within an SCRD, those participants should be similar in some important ways. The amount of similarity across participants, referred to as the homogeneity of the sample, is directly related to the defensibility of inferences about the intervention effect. In our case example, the participants were all boys who were about the same age and experiencing the same response (PTSD symptoms) to a common problem (bullying). When making inferences, the findings from this sample are more trustworthy than an alternative sample of five participants from a wide range of ages (e.g., 8 to 17 years) and genders with different types of trauma and presenting symptoms (PTSD versus depression and self-injury).

Sensitivity of Measurements

The consistent, repeated nature of outcome measurement in SCRDs presents a unique consideration for researchers. Approaches to measuring outcomes should closely align with the phenomena intended to influence. In our case example, the change target was PTSD symptoms, and the associated measurement, the Child PTSD Symptom Scale (CPSS), was developed to reflect diagnostic criteria for PTSD. Several informal and formal assessments are available to facilitate this practice, but guidelines for use and adaptation-intended use should be considered in relationship to the frequency of your measurement interval. For example, the Direct Observation Form (Achenbach & Rescorla, 2001) is designed to rate observations of children's behavior and can be administered with some amount of regularity, whereas the Beck Anxiety Inventory (BAI; Beck & Steer, 1990; Beck et al., 1988) captures symptom expression over the last month and is not intended for multiple uses within the same week. In the case example, the instructions of the CPSS were modified from reporting changes in the previous two weeks to reflect progress in between sessions (1 week).

Fidelity of Intervention

Although flexibility is a prominent strength of SCRDs, the intervention should share some important commonalities across participants. Approaches to promote fidelity include demonstrating provider competence, using manualized approaches, and documenting adherence to essential intervention content and processes. In our case example, the providers were master's-level mental health counselors with at least five years of experience working with adolescents and advanced training in TF-CBT. Additionally, they were using a manualized approach to treating PTSD among adolescents (TF-CBT), and they were documenting completion of program modules weekly. It is important to remember that fidelity is not categorical (i.e., you have it or you do not); instead, it is an estimate of credibility upon which we can infer degrees of internal and external validity.

Taken together, when SCRDs have a sufficient sample that is homogeneous, features sensitive measurements, and accounts for fidelity of the intervention, the design is more likely to depict the actual intervention effect rather than influences from other extraneous influences.

Data Analysis and Interpretation

We suggested earlier in this chapter that certain data analysis approaches are best suited to answer certain types of SCRD research questions. We also mentioned that approaches to data analysis ranged from simple to more complex. In either case, important inferences can be made about the effectiveness of an intervention. Regardless, we submit that the data analysis used in an SCRD should be based on at least two things: (a) the nature of your research question and (b) the characteristics of your baseline data. Among the many available analysis options, most can be clustered within the general categories of visual analysis, measures of treatment effect, and estimates of effect size.

Visual Analysis

Visual analysis is the process of making determinations about intervention effects based on impressions derived from graphical representation of data, such as that represented in Figure 7.3. Brossart et al. (2006) suggested that depictions of data should include

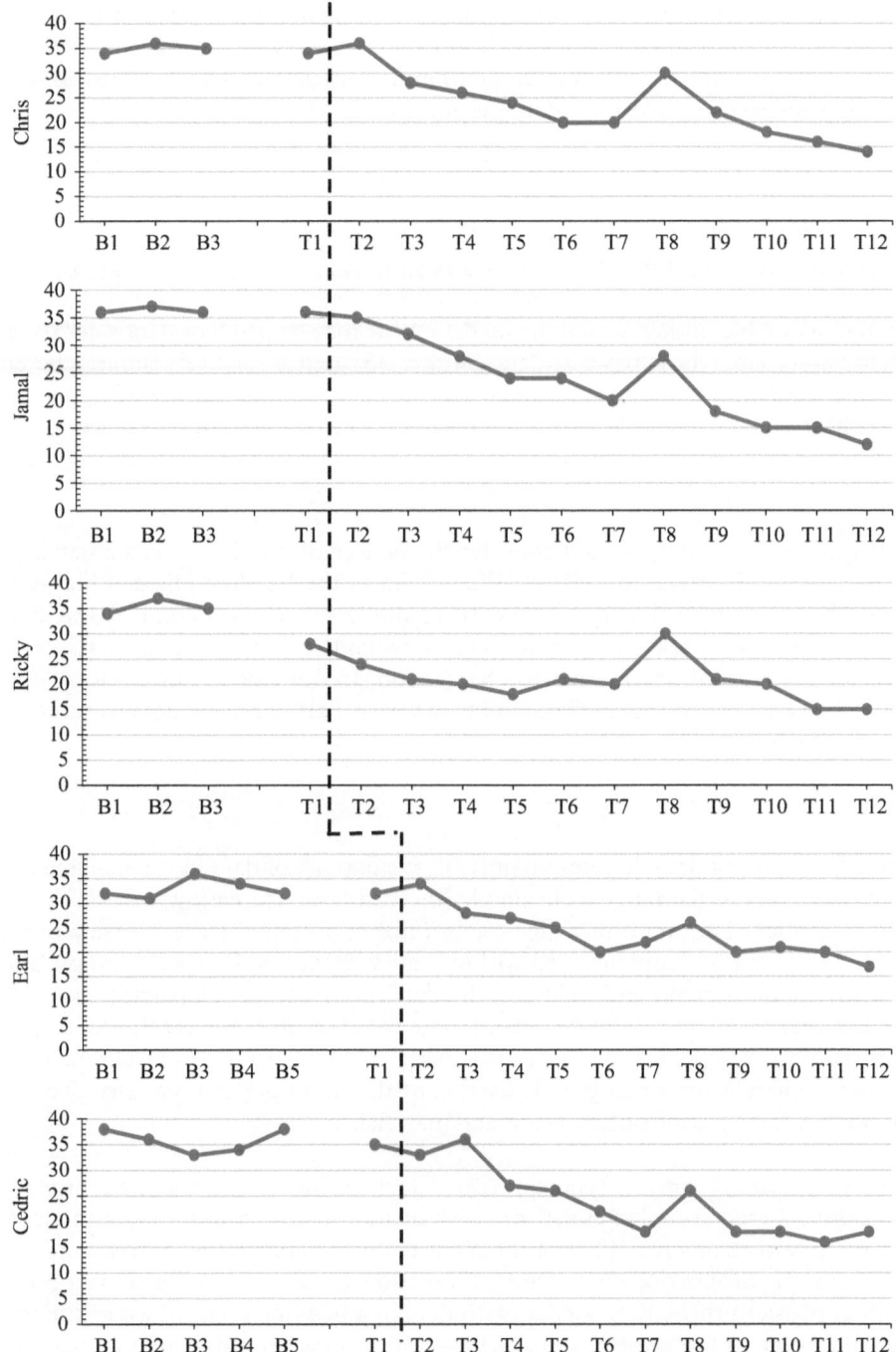

Figure 7.3 Scores on the Childhood PTSD Symptom Scale Across Baseline and Treatment Phases.

information to place findings in context (target behavior, time frame, instrument used), be considered in terms of practical effect, lead to impressions about degree of effect, and be accompanied by quantitative metrics. At a minimum, visual analysis takes into consideration characteristics referred to as level, variability, and trend.

LEVEL

Evaluation of the level refers to comparing general representations of data in each intervention phase, typically represented by either the mean or median. When baseline data are stable, the mean of data points across phases is indicated; however, in the presence of an unstable baseline data trend or a notable outlier, use of the median value may be prudent. Consider the example of Chris in Figure 7.3, whose baseline data (34, 36, 35) appear relatively stable. Therefore, we can compare the range of distance between average scores in the baseline (35) and intervention (24) phases and estimate the practical usefulness of this 11-point difference.

VARIABILITY

Interpretations of visual data should consider the degree of variability versus stability of data within baseline and intervention phases. When data in the baseline phase is highly variable, inferences about the way that the intervention influences the outcome is less defensible. Similarly, intervention-phase data is more reliable when the desired change is stable and does not vacillate greatly from observation to observation. In our case example data (Figure 7.3), Chris's baseline data shows distinctive stability, whereas Earl's baseline data features comparatively more variability.

TREND

Evaluating the trend of data denotes identifying the pattern of data in the baseline and intervention phases in ways that range from simple (increasing or decreasing) to complex (cyclical, curvilinear, erratic). The trend provides useful information about the course and nature of treatment, which can be supplemented with narrative accounts to explain complexities, such as apparently spurious peaks and valleys in the data. For example, all participants in our case example had seemingly linear and decreasing data trends with the exception of a peak in T8. Accounts from the researcher can share that this is the phase of TF-CBT at which the focus moves from coping skills training and practice to developing a trauma narrative and more directly and concretely confronting traumatic material.

Measures of Treatment Effect   Whereas visual analysis has a longstanding history within SCRD traditions, their complementary use with quantitative measures of treatment effect has become a standard of practice. One of the most enduring approaches is to compute an estimate based on the proportion that results when comparing the number of data points in an intervention phase to those that overlap with data in a baseline phase. Two of the more predominate and easy to use are the percentage of nonoverlapping data (PND; Scruggs et al., 1987) and the percentage of data points exceeding the median (PEM; Ma, 2006). In PND and PEM, the number of data points in the intervention phase that do not overlap with an identified point in the baseline phase is divided by the total number of observations in the intervention phase. For PND, the identified datum point is the most therapeutic value, and for PEM, that value is the median among scores. In either case, the resulting values are interpreted using a handy rubric suggested by Scruggs and Mastropieri (2001), wherein scores greater than 90% represent very effective treatments, scores ranging from 70 to 90% represent effective treatments, scores from 50 to 70% are debatable, and scores below 50% are regarded as ineffective.

Estimates of Effect Size   In contrast to providing estimates of treatment effect that are based on proportions of overlap, more true estimates of effect size are available such as those based in linear regression of scores, standardization of mean gain (Hedges et al., 2012), and statistically combining nonoverlap with trend analysis (Parker et al., 2011). Although all of these can be computed by hand, use of Excel or a related program is recommended. Each of these choices provides valuable information that explains the amount and direction of change between baseline and intervention phases.

Putting It All Together

SCRDs are a wonderful addition to the researcher's toolbox because they allow for the evaluation of outcomes in a way that requires small samples yet still yields causal data. Just like any other approach to research, there are strengths and limitations, and some designs are more robust than others. When done well, SCRDs can give voice to the experience of low-incidence populations, depict the utility of novel interventions, and support evaluation of existing programs that may not have access to large numbers of participants needed for a between-groups comparison. The body of literature related to SCRDs is growing month to month, and we have included some resources in what follows that may support your curiosity and application within your setting.

Practice-Based Applications

- Consider your responses that you identified in Chapter 1. What are some interventions and measures that would be suitable for inclusion in a related SCRD project?
- Now that you have walked through the possibilities of SCRD, more specifically A-B and A-B-A designs, how might either of these designs fit into your clinical experiences or practice setting? Is there an intervention or program that would be helpful for you to evaluate using an SCRD?
- Think about the characteristics of your current or future practice setting. How could you address the issue of participant homogeneity while also assuring equitable, fair, and ethical access to evidence-supported intervention during the SCRD development process?

Resources for More Information

Online

Computing measures of treatment effect and effect size. www.singlecaseresearch.org/
List of resources and seminal references. http://ethics.iit.edu/projects/single-subject-research

Peer-Reviewed Journal Articles

Brown, C. L., Peltier, C., Lee, D. Y., Webster, F. R., & Shabibi, A. A. (2024). A systematic review of single case research design graph construction in counseling. *Measurement and Evaluation in Counseling and Development, 57*(1), 72–88. https://doi.org/10.1080/07481756.2023.2189123

Cook, A., Codding, R., Silva, M., & Hayden, L. (2017). Enhancing school counselor research and practice in data-based assessment through single-case research design. *Counseling Outcome Research and Evaluation, 8*, 48–62. https://doi.org/10.1080/21501378.2017.1327746

Foster, L. H. (2010). A best kept secret: Single-subject research design in counseling. *Counseling Outcome Research and Evaluation, 1*, 30–39. doi:10.1177/2150137810387130

Kratochwill, T. R., Horner, R. H., Levin, J. R., Machalicek, W., Ferron, J., & Johnson, A. (2023). Single-case intervention research design standards: Additional proposed upgrades and future directions. *Journal of School Psychology, 97*, 192–216.

Lenz, A. S. (2015). Single-case research: Using single-case research designs demonstrate evidence for counseling practices. *Journal of Counseling & Development, 93*, 387–393. https://doi.org/10.1002/jcad.12036

Ray, D. (2015). Single-case research design and analysis: Counseling applications. *Journal of Counseling & Development, 93*, 394–402. https://doi.org/10.1002/jcad.12037

Books

Barlow, D. H., Nock, M. K., & Hersen, M. (2009). *Single case experimental designs: Strategies for studying behavior change* (3rd ed.). Pearson.

Kazdin, A. E. (2020). *Single-case research designs: Methods for clinical and applied settings.* (3rd ed.). Oxford University Press.

Morgan, D. L., & Morgan, R. K. (2009). *Single-case research methods for the behavioral and health sciences.* Sage Publications.

Vannest, K. J., Davis, J. L., & Parker, R. I. (2013). *Single case research in schools: Practical guidelines for school-based professionals.* Routledge.

Questions for Further Review and Application

1 SCRDs are useful for answering two categories of research questions. What are the two categories? Develop a research question for each one based on your interests.
2 SCRDs are helpful for evaluating the effect of an intervention across a single individual. If you were developing a study, what design would you use? What would your outcome variable be? How long would you collect data at baseline? How long would your intervention phase be?
3 What are some common characteristics across all SCRDs? How do they each support cause-and-effect inferences?
4 What are some design considerations for all SCRDs? How do they each support cause-and-effect inferences?
5 What are the three approaches to visual analysis, and what are some aspects of those analysis that are important to consider?

References

Achenbach, T. M., & Rescorla, L. A. (2001). *Manual for the ASEBA school-age forms & profiles.* Burlington, VT: Achenbach Research Center for Children, Youth, and Families.

Barrio Minton, C. A., & Lenz, A. S. (2019). *Applied research and program evaluation for helping professionals.* Routledge.

Beck, A. T., Epstein, N., Brown, G., & Steer, R. A. (1988). An inventory for measuring clinical anxiety: Psychometric properties. *Journal of Consulting and Clinical Psychology, 56*, 893–897.

Beck, A. T., & Steer, R. A. (1990). *Manual for the Beck Anxiety Inventory.* Psychological Corporation.

Brossart, D. F., Parker, R. I., Olson, E. A., & Mahadevan, L. (2006). The relationship between visual analysis and five statistical analyses in a simple AB single-case research design. *Behavior Modification, 30*, 531–563.

Brown, C. L., Peltier, C., Lee, D. Y., Webster, F. R., & Shabibi, A. A. (2024). A systematic review of single case research design graph construction in counseling. *Measurement and Evaluation in Counseling and Development, 57*(1), 72–88. https://doi.org/10.1080/07481756.2023.2189123

Cohen, J. A., Mannarino, A. P., & Deblinger, E. (2017). *Treating trauma and traumatic grief in children and adolescents.* Guilford Press.

Cook, A., Codding, R., Silva, M., & Hayden, L. (2017). Enhancing school counselor research and practice in data-based assessment through single-case research design. *Counseling Outcome Research and Evaluation, 8*, 48–62. https://doi.org/10.1080/21501378.2017.1327746

Egel, A. L., Barthold, C. H., Kouo, J. L., Maajeeny, F. S. (2018). Single-subject design and analysis. In G. R. Hancock, L. M. Stapleton, and R. O. Mueller (Eds.) *Quantitative Methods in the Social Sciences* (2nd ed.). Routledge.

Hedges, L. V., Pustejovsky, J. E., & Shadish, W. R. (2012). A standardized mean difference effect size for single case designs. *Research Synthesis Methods, 3*, 224–239.

Kazdin, A. E. (2020). *Single-case research designs: Methods for clinical and applied settings.* (3rd ed.). Oxford University Press.

Kratochwill, T. R., Horner, R. H., Levin, J. R., Machalicek, W., Ferron, J., & Johnson, A. (2023). Single-case intervention research design standards: Additional proposed upgrades and future directions. *Journal of School Psychology, 97*, 192–216.

Lenz, A. S. (2013). Calculating effect size in single-case research: A comparison of nonoverlap methods. *Measurement and Evaluation in Counseling and Development, 46*, 64–73. https://doi.org/10.1177/0748175612456401

Lenz, A. S. (2015). Single-case research: Using single-case research designs to demonstrate evidence for counseling practices. *Journal of Counseling & Development, 93*, 387–393. https://doi.org/10.1002/jcad.12036

Ma, H. H. (2006). An alternative method for quantitative synthesis of single-subject research: Percentage of data points exceeding the median. *Behavior Modification, 30*, 598–617.

Morgan, D. L., & Morgan, R. K. (2009). *Single-case research methods for the behavioral and health sciences.* Sage Publications.

Parker, R. I., Vannest, K. J., Davis, J. L., & Sauber, S. B. (2011). Combining nonoverlap and trend for single case research: Tau-U. *Behavior Therapy, 42*, 284–299.

Rubin, A., & Bellamy, J. (2012). *Practitioner's guide to using research for evidence-based practice* (2nd ed.). John Wiley & Sons, Inc.

Scruggs, T. E., & Mastropieri, M. A. (2001). How to summarize single-participant research: Ideas and applications. *Exceptionality, 9*, 227–244. https://doi.org/10.1207/S15327035EX0904_5

Scruggs, T. E., Mastropieri, M. A., & Casto, G. (1987). The quantitative synthesis of single subject research: Methodology and validation. *Remedial and Special Education, 8*, 24–33.

Tolin, D. F., McKay, D., Forman, E. M., Klonsky, E. D., & Thombs, B. D. (2015). Empirically supported treatment: Recommendations for a new model. *Clinical Psychology, 22*(4), 317–338. https://doi.org/10.1111/cpsp.12122

What Works Clearinghouse. (2020). *What Works Clearinghouse Standards Handbook, Version 4.1.* Washington, DC: U.S. Department of Education, Institute of Education Sciences, National Center for Education Evaluation and Regional Assistance. https://ies.ed.gov/ncee/wwc/handbooks.cpsp.12122

8 Using Correlational and Causal-Comparative Research Designs in Practice

Exploring Relations Among Client Variables

Lindsey K. Umstead and Heather Delgado

As practitioners, we typically have questions about our services or clients. These may include questions such as why does some classroom guidance impact students more than others, why do female clients self-injure more than male clients, or why do children who attend counseling with their parents fare better than those who do not? Different research methodologies are used to answer different questions. In this chapter, we provide an overview of both correlational and causal-comparative research methods, which are used when you want to examine the relationship between two or more variables without any manipulation. Put simply, these research designs involve looking at two or more variables, as they currently exist, to determine if they are related in some way. In other words, manipulation is when you change something, such as an intervention, educational guidance, or medication, to see if that change works better or differently than what was done previously (as you read about in Chapters 7, 9, and 10 with single-case research, quasi-experimental, and randomized controlled trials). While this manipulation is important to answer some research questions, through correlational and causal comparative designs, you would not manipulate or change anything that you are currently doing with your students or clients; you would simply be examining how things relate or how groups differ based on how they currently exist. The purpose of this chapter is to expose you to each design in order to help you understand and practically apply this in your own clinical setting. By the end of the chapter, you will have a foundational understanding of both correlational and causal-comparative research designs with regard to their methodologies, data analyses, specific types of research questions, and interpretation of your findings in addition to an understanding of the similarities and differences between the two methods. Additionally, you will learn how to design your own correlational and/or causal-comparative design, interpret the results, and determine if there is a relationship that exists between two or more different variables of interest.

Introduction to Correlational and Causal-Comparative Research Designs

Correlational and causal-comparative research designs are two types of quantitative descriptive methods that seek to define the existence and characteristics of various phenomena (Heppner, Wampold, & Kivlighan, 2008). Specifically, these two particular research designs aim to explore and identify associations, or relationships, between and among variables. While they are similar in what they are seeking to do, they also differ. Let's take a moment and start first with correlational research designs. With correlational designs, you are seeking to determine whether two variables are connected in such a way that as one increases, the other one either increases or decreases, or whether these two variables are not connected at all, thus unrelated. For example, you might notice that as clients spend more hours in counseling, they

DOI: 10.4324/9781032706139-8

begin to acquire more healthy coping skills. Here, you would use a correlational research design to see if there is a positive relationship between the number of hours in therapy and the number of healthy coping skills acquired. This works similarly to exploring whether a negative relationship would exist between the number of hours spent in group counseling and behavioral disruptions in the classroom for students in a school; thus, as the number of hours spent in group counseling increases, the frequency of behavioral disruption decreases.

Causal-comparative research, on the other hand, would be used to examine whether individuals in one group are different on one or more variables than individuals in at least one other group. For example, you might observe in your practice that clients who use substances use more maladaptive coping strategies than individuals who do not use substances. To see if a difference between these groups actually exists, you could use a causal-comparative design to see if clients who abuse substances use a significantly higher number of maladaptive coping strategies than clients who do not abuse substances.

A key difference between correlational and causal-comparative research involves the number of variables and the number of groups being studied (Gay & Airasian, 2000). Correlational research involves examining relationships among two or more independent and dependent variables for a single group in order to describe how these variables are related. Whatever variable you believe causes or leads to a change in another variable (i.e., dependent variable), is the independent variable(s) (refer back to Chapter 5 for a more thorough discussion on independent and dependent variables). Alternatively, causal-comparative research seeks to compare two or more groups on one or more dependent variables of interest. For causal-comparative research, the groups you choose to examine serve as your independent variable. By using causal-comparative designs, a researcher aims to determine whether the independent variable(s) (i.e., the group status or assignment one is in) causes the difference in the dependent variable(s) – or the outcome variable you are interested in. In general, correlational research aims to describe the relationship among variables, whereas causal-comparative research aims to identify whether an independent variable of a group (i.e., demographic variables, identities, group categories) acts as the cause or reason for differences in one or more dependent variable of interest. Table 8.1 outlines the differences between these research designs.

On the other hand, there are some important similarities between correlational and causal-comparative research designs. First, both of these designs are considered *ex post facto*, or "after-the-fact," research designs. This means that the relationships between and among the variables you are studying are thought to have been present prior to the research being

Table 8.1 Similarities and Differences Between Correlational and Causal-Comparative Research

Similarities	*Differences*	
	Correlational	**Causal Comparative**
• Descriptive quantitative designs • Examine relationships between and among variables • Lack of control over variables – neither is experimental • Cannot infer direct causality from results • Results may lead to experimental research to test a hypothesis	• Aims to understand relation between dependent variables • Does not attempt to understand cause and effect • One group • Two or more dependent variables • Requires a numerical score for each variable of interest for every person	• Aims to begin understanding a causal relation between independent and dependent variables • Two or more groups (independent variable) • One or more dependent variables • Involves at least one categorical variable (e.g., gender, race, ethnicity)

conducted and not due to any manipulation of the variables by the researchers. Consequently, correlational research would be considered *ex post facto* because you are investigating a relationship between variables in a group that existed prior to the research being conducted. Similarly, causal-comparative research is also a type of *ex post facto* research due to the fact that the groups being looked at are predetermined, or already existing (e.g., gender, race, ethnicity, classrooms), as opposed to having been determined by the researcher (Heppner et al., 2008); thus, in both correlational and causal-comparative research designs, you are studying relationships that are between or among variables for groups that were present before your study began rather than being manipulated during your study (as you would in the experimental or quasi-experimental designs).

Another important similarity shared by correlational and causal-comparative research is that neither design allows you to infer direct causality from the results. With regard to correlational research, although you may find results showing a positive relationship between x and y variables, you cannot say that x causes y, and you also cannot say that y causes x. In other words, correlational research does not allow you to establish the *direction of causality*, or the path of a causal effect, between two variables (Aron, Aron, & Coups, 2008). For example, you may find that as clients' anxiety levels increase, their happiness levels decrease; however, from this, you do not know whether increased anxiety directly leads to decreased happiness or if decreased happiness directly leads to increased anxiety. Here, you cannot establish a direct causal relationship between increased anxiety and decreased happiness because there may be other factors influencing anxiety and happiness levels. Similarly, if you find in a correlational research study that a positive relationship exists between clients' stress levels and the number of positive coping skills they use, you would not be able to say that stress causes an increase in the number of positive coping skills they use, nor would you be able to say that the number of positive coping skills they use causes an increase in stress level. Instead, you simply understand that as one of these variables increases, the other one also increases.

Likewise, although the goal of causal-comparative research is to determine a causal relationship between an independent variable and a dependent variable, you cannot establish a true cause-and-effect relationship between these variables. That is, even though you may observe a difference between groups on a variable of interest, you cannot say that the groups themselves directly cause this difference. For example, in your practice, you may find that female clients report lower levels of workplace satisfaction than male clients; however, you would not be able to infer that being a female causes lower levels of workplace satisfaction. It may be that there are other factors contributing to lower levels of workplace satisfaction, such as more sexual harassment experienced in the workplace or receiving lower salaries than male coworkers. Additionally, because the groups you examine in causal-comparative research are preexisting before your study, you cannot say that a group status directly created or caused the difference in the dependent variable. In fact, for both correlational and causal-comparative research designs, you collect data on groups that were determined before your study instead of collecting data as groups are being manipulated or determined by you during the study. Due to this limitation, you would not be able to say that one variable truly causes the other because you did not manipulate or change anything or control other variables that might have influenced your results (Mitchell & Jolly, 2010).

When to Use Correlational and Causal-Comparative Methods

As we discussed earlier in this chapter, correlational and causal-comparative research are useful quantitative descriptive designs when you are interested in increasing your understanding of phenomena that you may observe in your clinical practice (Heppner et al., 2008). Specifically, these designs allow you to identify whether one thing relates to another, such as how hours spent in classroom guidance relates to student academic achievement. For counseling practitioners, these research designs may be used in multiple settings to explore client variables (e.g., race, gender), treatment variables (e.g., type of intervention used), and client outcomes (e.g., anxiety level), ultimately providing us with answers as to how these variables are related. While you may want to know if time in counseling *causes* decreases in depression, it may seem silly to use these research designs that will not provide you the degree to which that is true; however, research using these particular designs can serve as the foundation for experimental research or more exploration of cause and effect without needing the same levels of control or time and effort needed to manipulate how counseling is offered, or the length and time spent in counseling, yet allows you to explore what currently exists among all of your clients at the same time. While limitations to these designs exist, correlational and causal-comparative research can be used to increase the effectiveness of counseling interventions used in your practice or school. Another way to think about the utility of correlational and causal-comparative research is to consider the bigger picture for your results. That is, what might be the implications for the results you find using a correlational or causal-comparative design? Subsequently, this may lead to better outcomes for the clients you serve in your practice. Even though cause and effect cannot be determined with these designs, relationships can, and this information about these relationships can apply to what you do with the clients you serve.

While earlier it was noted that similarities and differences exist between these designs, the question becomes when you would select correlational versus causal-comparative. Reflecting, if you have a question that is asking about the differences between two or more groups – such as what the difference is in disciplinary referrals from students in Ms. Smith's class versus Mr. Martin's class – you would select a causal-comparative design. But if you were interested in knowing how food insecurity related to disciplinary referrals, thus the relationship between two or more variables within groups as a whole, you would select correlational design.

Finally, these research designs may be used in any setting to answer important research questions. When considering where to use these research designs, consider settings such as community agencies, schools, colleges and universities, and inpatient or outpatient settings where you can gather data from several clients or students to answer correlational or causal-comparative questions. Later in this chapter, we will discuss the importance of your sample size, or how many clients you observe in your study, when conducting correlational and causal-comparative research.

Research Questions Answered by Correlational and Causal-Comparative Designs

When developing research questions, you should first observe or identify your dependent variable(s), or the variable(s) you want to measure. The next step involves hypothesizing that your dependent variable is related to either another variable (in the case of a correlational research design) or a group status (in the case of a causal-comparative research design). For example, if you are interested in the depression level of adolescent females, this would be considered your dependent variable, which you may measure using a depression inventory, such as the Beck Depression Scale. Subsequently, you may hypothesize that social support (measured by counts of the number of friends and family members who provide support) has an influence on depression levels; therefore, this would be your independent variable.

It is important to note that how you measure any of the variables you are interested in will determine how you can answer your questions. This provides a specific way to define, or operationalize, your variable so that you are able to measure it according to that definition. It is important to note that in the case of both correlational and causal-comparative research, you need to use appropriate ways of measuring or assessing your variables of interest; however, that discussion is outside of the scope of this chapter and can be found more specifically in Chapter 4, "Evaluating and Designing Surveys."

When you are simply asking whether a relationship between two or more variables exists, you are asking a research question that would fit nicely within correlational research design. When developing a correlational research question, it is important to use language that establishes a relationship between the different variables you are studying. Here are some examples of research questions for correlational research:

- Is the number of hours spent practicing yoga related to counselor burnout?
- Is there a positive association between positive client outcomes and social support among African American women?
- Are there relationships among the hours of classroom guidance received, hours spent doing homework, and academic achievement in middle school students?

On the other hand, for a causal-comparative research design, you would be asking about differences between two or more different groups on one or more dependent variables. When developing this type of research question, it is important to use language that establishes an intent to compare two or more groups for differences. Example questions might include:

- Is there a difference between females' and males' depression scores after receiving outpatient therapy?
- Does the number of incidents per week of self-harm differ among Caucasian clients, African American clients, and Latino clients who present with depression?
- Are there differences in standardized test scores and number of days absent among high school students who report low, moderate, and high parental involvement?

Case Example: Is Social Support Related to Anxiety? Exploring Differences Between Male and Female Clients

The following case study will illustrate the application of both correlational and causal-comparative research methods. Imagine that you are a practitioner at a community mental health agency. Recently, you have noticed some differences between male and female clients with regard to the amount of social support they have and their levels of anxiety. You want to compare a sample of the agency's male clients to a sample of female clients on their social support and anxiety. Specifically, you are interested in (1) whether social support is related to anxiety levels across all clients (i.e., including both men and women) and (2) if there are differences between men and women in the amount of social support they have and in their anxiety levels. You will select similar-sized groups of men and women from your community agency, and you will collect their social support and anxiety scores.

For this study, you need to operationally define each variable. This means you need to determine the scope of what you want to know and how to measure it. For the sake of this case example, social support will be defined as the number of friends and family that provide some form of support to the individual each week, and this construct will be measured informally using the intake form clients complete before beginning mental health services. Anxiety will operationally be defined and measured according to the Beck Anxiety Inventory (BAI; Beck & Steer, 1993). Each client selected by you to participate in this study, to answer your research questions, will complete the BAI in addition to the information they provided originally at intake about their social support. To answer your research questions, you will use a correlational research design to see if there is a relationship between social support and anxiety for both men and women combined as one group. If you were interested in exploring the differences between men and women, then you will use a causal-comparative research design to determine whether men and women differ in both social support and anxiety. For the purposes of this chapter, we are staying with simpler designs, but these can also be used to explore more complex practice-oriented questions. For example, you could explore how social support impacts the differences in anxiety between men and women. Answering this question involves mediating and moderating relationships, which you can learn to use once you master the basics of research design. Just know that this ability to combine relationships and group differences does exist.

Methodology

Now that you have your research question outlining what you want to know, and you have your samples of men and women and understand how you are collecting this information through various measures, let's walk through the methodology of both of these designs.

Research Questions

It is important to determine your research questions before setting out to conduct your study, because the questions will determine the methodology you use.

Box 8.1   Research Questions

Correlational Research Questions

1 Is there a relationship between social support and anxiety in male clients?
2 Is there a relationship between social support and anxiety in female clients?

Causal-Comparative Research Questions

1 Is there a difference in the amount of social support between male and female clients?
2 Is there a difference in anxiety level between male and female clients?

As you can see in Box 8.1, the language used in these research questions indicates the type of research design you will use. Specifically, research questions 1 and 2 use a correlational design, and research questions 3 and 4 use a causal-comparative design.

Hypotheses

For each of these designs, it is important that you establish *hypotheses,* or predictions about what you expect to find in your results. The hypotheses can be directional, where you are predicting that there is a positive or negative relationship between two variables. Alternatively, your hypotheses can be nondirectional, where you are predicting that there is a relationship between the two variables, but you are not certain what kind of relationship. For example, a directional hypothesis would imply that there is a positive relationship between social support and anxiety, whereas a nondirectional hypothesis would imply that there is a relationship between social support and anxiety, but you are not clear on the direction. Notice that there is one hypothesis for each research question originally noted (Box 8.2).

Box 8.2   Hypotheses

1 There is a relationship between social support and anxiety in male clients (nondirectional).
2 There is a positive linear relationship between social support and anxiety in female clients (directional).
3 Female clients have more social support than male clients (directional).
4 There is a difference in the level of anxiety between male and female clients (nondirectional).

Sample Size

There are many different ways to sample, including random sampling (selecting randomly from your clients) or convenience sampling (selecting specific clients, or the first few clients who walk into your office to complete the BAI). You may even use volunteer sampling (posting an advertisement or flier in your agency asking clients if they would like to participate). While there are pros and cons of each of these sampling methods, for this case example, your sample will consist of 35 males and 35 females from your community agency. While you could randomly sample, in this case you decide to simply use convenience sampling, and you sample the first males and females who come to your agency this month *and* agree to participate. It is important to note the impact of sample size, as the number of people you get to participate in a study influences what you may find and is influenced by a combination of factors including the statistic needed to answer your question, your measurement of the variables, the number of groups, and the number of variables, among many others. However, your sample may also be bound by the number of clients you have or who decides to participate. If you are running the statistical analysis to answer your question, know that in quantitative designs such as correlational and causal-comparative, it is important to determine your sample size through determining your statistical power. We are not going to spend time talking about that in this chapter, but know that it is important to determining final sample size.

Confounding Variables

In addition to determining the independent and dependent variables, you should consider if there is anything other than the independent variable (social support in this case) that might be influencing the dependent variable (anxiety). For example, while you believe social support may be one of the main reasons why anxiety is increasing or decreasing, you also believe that the number of sessions your clients have attended with you is also important to control, as it may confound (or change/alter) the relationship between social support and anxiety. In order to prevent this from happening, you would want to either control for these irrelevant variables (such as selecting only clients who have attended 30 counseling sessions with you, a homogenous sample) or randomly select clients from your practice, which controls for the possible effect through the sampling method or you could control for the confounding nature of number of counseling sessions by collecting this information and including it in your analysis.

Statistical Significance

In order to say that a relationship exists between two variables, you need to achieve statistical significance. Achieving statistical significance means that the relationship you observe in your results is likely not due to chance alone (Mitchell & Jolly, 2010). To determine this, you will refer to the appropriate test statistic for the statistical analysis you use. For both correlational and causal-comparative research, you will typically set an alpha level of 0.05 or lower to determine whether your results are statistically significant. Once you get your results, you compare the p-value determined by the statistical analysis you use to your preestablished alpha value in order to know whether your results are significant.

Data Analysis: Correlational Research Design

Many different analyses are appropriate for a correlational research design. These include but are not limited to correlations, regressions, and path analysis. We will not go in depth into all of these analyses, but know that they are all used for different reasons and ultimately may depend on how many variables you are comparing. What underlies each of these analyses is the correlation, so we are going to focus solely on the Pearson correlation coefficient (but note that there are many other correlation coefficients available as well).

Pearson Correlation Coefficient (r)

This is a measure of the strength of the relationship between two variables. The r-value will consist of (1) a numerical value ranging from -1 to 1 and (2) a positive or negative sign. These values correspond to the strength and the direction of the relationship. More specifically, a positive or negative sign indicates the *direction* of the association, and the r-value itself indicates the *strength* of the association; thus, the higher the absolute numerical value the stronger the relationship, with an r-value of (0.00) representing no relationship, an r-value of (± 0.50) representing a moderate relationship, and an r-value of (± 0.90) representing a strong relationship.

Visual Expression of Your Data

Providing your data in a scatterplot will allow for a visual understanding of the strength and direction of the relationship. The scatterplot graph can be created by plotting both values of social support and anxiety for each individual. There is no specific requirement for which variable goes on which axis. After the data have been plotted, the best-fit line will be drawn to visually see the linear relationship between the two variables more clearly (see Figure 8.1).

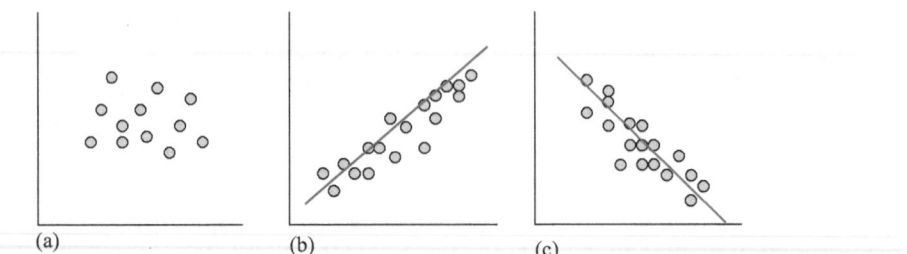

Figure 8.1 Examples of Correlations.

Note: (a) no correlation, (b) strong positive correlation, (c) strong negative correlation.

Interpreting Your Results

The interpretation of the results is structured based on the strength and direction of the relationship of the correlation. For a positive relationship, as one variable increases, the other variable increases as well. For a negative relationship, as one variable increases, the other variable decreases. The results of a correlational design can only inform the researcher about the relationship, but the results do not infer causality of the relationship. In other words, a correlation would not imply that one variable causes another variable but rather would describe the relationship between the two.

Data Analysis: Causal-Comparative Research Design

Descriptive Statistics

Descriptive statistics are used to describe your data. Typically, these statistics include the mean, mode, and median for your groups. For example, when conducting a causal-comparative study, you are testing whether there is a difference in the *mean* scores of each of your groups. In the case of the present example, you would test whether there is a difference in the mean scores of social support and anxiety between male and female clients. Descriptive statistics do not typically allow you to draw inferences or conclusions based on the mean scores but simply provide you a visual of whether one group is, on average, greater or less than another group.

Inferential Statistics

Inferential statistics are used in a causal-comparative research to demonstrate a relation between your independent and dependent variables (Brewer & Kubn, 2012). Unlike descriptive statistics, inferential statistics allow you to make inferences, or conclusions, about your results. There are several types of statistical analyses that may be used when conducting causal-comparative research; however, the three most commonly used statistical tests for causal-comparative research designs include the chi-square test, paired-samples and independent *t*-tests, and a statistical test from the analysis of variance (ANOVA) family (e.g., ANOVA, multiple ANOVA [MANOVA], or analysis of covariance [ANCOVA]). The analysis you use depends on the number and type of independent and dependent variables you observe in your study and the number of groups you are comparing.

Visual Expression of Your Data

When you use a causal-comparative design, there are various means by which to display your data and the results of your analysis. While most researchers may report the data simply using the statistics provided by the inferential analysis, another common way to present your data is through the use of bar or line graphs. These charts allow you to visually depict the descriptive statistics that show that a difference exists between your two groups (see Figure 8.2).

Interpreting Your Results

How you interpret your results will vary depending on the type of statistical analysis you use to answer your research question. Generally speaking, however, your results will inform you as to whether your groups are significantly different from each other and how your variables are related to one another. Specifically, for causal-comparative research designs, you will be able to determine from your results whether there is a difference between the groups you observe on your variable(s) of interest in order to infer that the difference you find is a result of an effect of the group.

Threats to Validity

In both correlational and causal-comparative designs, validity means that your data are accurate and that your findings reflect what they are intended to reflect. In causal-comparative research, there are various threats to the validity of your results. Because you are unable to randomly assign your clients to groups, the external validity of your results is limited. External validity refers to whether you can generalize your findings to those not included in your actual study or to clients that you did not collect data from. When your external validity is limited, this means that you cannot generalize, or apply, your results to all clients because your sample might not accurately represent your group of interest. Internal validity is also a consideration when it comes to these designs. Internal validity is the degree to which your results are actually true. As an example, if you found a difference in anxiety between males and females from your practice, to have internal validity would mean that you are confident that this difference found is truly due to being a male or a female. However, it may also be possible

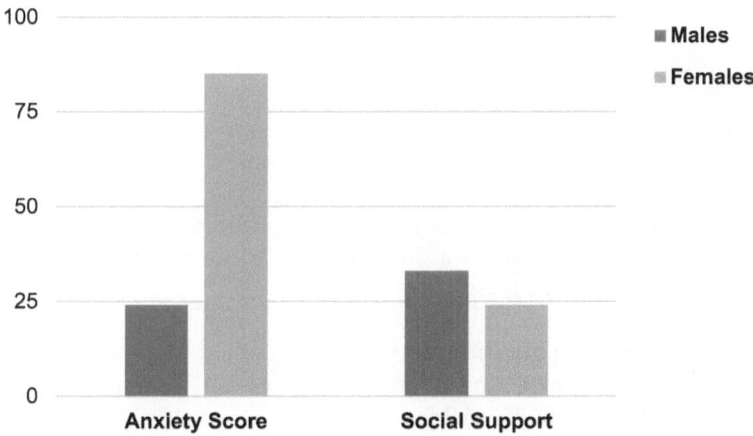

Figure 8.2 Bar Graph of Anxiety and Social Support Scores.

that some other innate difference may exist between groups, such as females attended more counseling sessions than males, which brings into question the internal validity of your study. This is why determining confounding variables is important.

Putting It All Together

Correlational and causal-comparative research designs both belong under the large umbrella of descriptive research studies and can be applied in any mental health setting to understand the relationship between two variables. Whether to use one design over the other depends on the specific research questions that are to be addressed. Despite the similarities and differences between these two specific designs, attempting to conduct this type of descriptive research has the potential to provide practitioners with valuable information concerning their clients, clients' outcomes, and clients' presenting concerns. In addition, correlational and causal-comparative research designs can provide the foundational step toward experimental designs that provide answers to causality of variables; therefore, these designs not only offer answers to your research questions, but they also provide insight into the bigger picture such as the effectiveness of treatment based on outcomes you observe. Looking beyond the possible benefits for clients, utilizing research methods allows practitioners to develop their own research skills and integrate their roles as both practitioners and researchers.

Continuing to Apply What You Have Learned

In this chapter, you have learned about correlational and causal-comparative designs, the types of research questions you can answer using these designs, and specific methodological considerations for each design. You have read through a case example illustrating how these research designs might be used in a counseling setting. Now it is your turn to think about applications for these research designs using your own experiences and interests as a counselor. First, consider how you might use one or both of these designs in your counseling setting. Are there two or more groups of clients that appear to show differences on a presenting issue that interests you (e.g., depression, anxiety, substance use)? Are you curious about whether a variable relates in some way to a certain issue for one group of your clients? As you work in your setting, begin to notice possible relationships between client groups, treatments, and outcomes.

Practice-Based Application

Think about the client-presenting concern, symptom, or situation that you identified in Chapter 1, and use that to answer the following questions:

- Describe what would it look like to examine your topic of interest from a *correlational* lens versus a *causal-comparative* lens? Consider the similarities and differences between these approaches with regards to your topic.
- Identify at least one correlation-based research question and at least one causal-comparative–based research question for your topic.
- For each of your research questions identified in Question 2, identify the following:
  - Independent and dependent variables
  - A directional hypothesis
  - A non-directional hypothesis

Resources for More Information

Online

Correlation sample size calculator. (n.d.). Retrieved from www.sample-size.net/correlation-sample-size/

Fraenkel, J. R., & Wallen, N. E. (2017). *How to design and evaluate research in education.* Retrieved from http://highered.mheducation.com/sites/0072981369/student_view0/index.html

Peer-Reviewed Journal Articles

Moinester, M., & Gottfried, R. (2014). Sample size estimation for correlations with pre-specified confidence interval. *The Quantitative Methods for Psychology, 10,* 124–130. doi:10.20982/tqmp.10.2.p124

Book Chapters

Brewer, E. W., & Kubn, J. (2012). Causal-comparative design. In *Encyclopedia of research design* (pp. 125–131). Thousand Oaks, CA: Sage Publications.

Questions for Further Review and Application

1 What are the similarities between correlational and causal-comparative research designs? What are the differences?
2 What are the design considerations for correlational research?
3 What are the design considerations for causal-comparative research?
4 Consider the setting in which you practice. How might you use correlational and/or causal-comparative research to understand two variables of interest to you?
5 What is an example of a correlational research question? What is an example of a causal-comparative research question?

References

Aron, A., Aron, E. N., & Coups, E. J. (2008). *Statistics for the behavioral and social sciences: A brief course* (4th ed.). Upper Saddle River, NJ: Pearson.

Beck, A. T., & Steer, R. A. (1993). *Beck anxiety inventory manual.* San Antonio, TX: Psychological Corporation.

Brewer, E. W., & Kubn, J. (2012). Causal-comparative design. In *Encyclopedia of research design* (pp. 125–131). Thousand Oaks, CA: Sage Publications.

Gay, L. R., & Airasian, P. W. (2000). *Educational research: Competencies for analysis and application* (6th ed.). Upper Saddle River, NJ: Pearson.

Heppner, P. P., Wampold, D. M., & Kivlighan, B. E. (2008). *Research design in counseling* (3rd ed.). Belmont, CA: Thomson Brooks-Cole.

Mitchell, M. L., & Jolly, J. L. (2010). *Research design explained* (7th ed.). Belmont, CA: Wadsworth.

9   Quasi-Experimental Methods

Casey A. Barrio Minton

As you are learning, there are many ways to investigate relationships in the helping professions. Quasi-experimental designs allow researchers to examine the impact of an event or intervention on groups of individuals, families, or organizations in a practical, feasible manner. The purpose of this chapter is to introduce you to quasi-experimental methods and their role in mental health and human services professions. This chapter begins with an overview of quasi-experimental methods, situations most appropriate for the design, and types of research questions researchers can address with quasi-experimental methods. After presenting a practice-based case study, we will turn attention to specific characteristics, design considerations, and data analysis procedures utilized within quasi-experimental methodology. The chapter concludes with additional research and questions for application or reflection.

What Are Quasi-Experimental Methods?

Before exploring quasi-experimental methods specifically, it is important to understand the broader continuum of experimental designs. Most simply, experimental designs involve making causal inferences regarding the impact of an experience or intervention on one or more groups. It may help to think of a group as a collection of units; for example, we may have groups of individuals, families, classrooms, schools, or organizations. In human services and mental health professions, we most often focus on individuals or families as the unit of study.

There are three broad types of experimental designs: preexperiments, quasi-experiments, and true experiments (Thyer, 2012). **Preexperiments** investigate the impact of an experience or intervention on just one group without comparison to other groups. For example, a researcher may provide a bullying intervention to a group of students, measuring students' likelihood to intervene as bystanders before and after the intervention. Although simple, preexperimental designs do not allow researchers to determine whether interventions caused changes. It is possible that participants in the preexperiment started thinking about their role as bystanders when they completed the initial assessment, there was a widely publicized community event between measurements, or participants naturally matured over time. Without careful comparison, it would be nearly impossible to determine what caused the observed changes.

True experiments, including **randomized control trials (RCTs) or randomized control designs** (see Chapter 10), involve manipulating treatment conditions or interventions *and* randomly assigning units of study to groups in ways that allow researchers to conclude that the interventions caused changes among groups (Miller et al., 2020). For example, researchers may identify a group of individuals eligible for a bullying intervention, assess likelihood to intervene as bystanders before the intervention, randomly assign so half of

DOI: 10.4324/9781032706139-9

participants engage in the intervention while the other half does treatment as usual through the school counseling curriculum, and compare changes in scores between groups. The controls taken in assessing pre- and postchanges and assigning groups helps researchers be relatively certain that the intervention is responsible for the changes observed.

As you will learn in this chapter, **quasi-experiments**

"involve comparing outcomes of one group receiving a treatment that is the focus of evaluation to one or more groups of clients who receive either nothing or an alternative real treatment, or to a group receiving a placebo-type treatment."

(Thyer, 2012, p. 9)

In contrast to true experiments, quasi-experiments do not feature random assignment, most often due to practical or ethical constraints (Miller et al.,. 2020). Rather, researchers create comparison groups based on self-selection (e.g., participants sign up to attend a certain group or at a certain setting), administrator selection, or self- and administrator selection (White & Sabarwal, 2014). Some quasi-experimental methodologists also find opportunities to investigate the impact of naturally occurring phenomena in ways that do not involve researcher-controlled manipulation of the intervention or experience. For example, I was working with a team on a broad-scale project related to older adults' mental health just before the onset of the COVID-19 pandemic. We had collected pre-test data in preparation for an RCT. Although we could not implement the intervention as designed, we had a dataset that allowed us to track changes in mental health for this vulnerable population during this global event.

The task of the quasi-experimental researcher is to design studies in ways that demonstrate that the intervention or experience, not a plausible alternative explanation, is most likely responsible for changes observed (Miller et al., 2020). To continue the example, researchers may identify a group of students eligible for a bullying intervention, assess likelihood to intervene as bystanders, and then assign students on one schedule to the intervention group and students on another schedule to treatment as usual through the school counseling curriculum. This method may have a reasonable chance of providing valuable information given assignment to groups was done in a thoughtful manner; for example, that there were no meaningful preexisting differences in classroom composition or assignment based on schedules.

As we will explore later in this chapter, there are several unique quasi-experimental designs. These designs vary regarding (1) use of no-treatment, comparison, or alternative-treatment interventions, (2) use of posttest only or pretest-posttest data, and (3) timing of interventions and observations. In addition, quasi-experimental researchers can utilize a variety of procedures for enrolling participants and assigning them to groups. For now, I turn attention to situations most appropriate for quasi-experimental methods.

Situations Most Appropriate for Quasi-Experimental Methods

Although many researchers consider quasi-experimental methods to be less rigorous than true experimental designs, quasi-experimental designs tend to be more practical and feasible for real-world practice settings. In other words, wherein quasi-experimental designs may have less internal validity due to lack of random assignment and control, they gain external validity in terms of ability to be carried out and practiced in real-world settings that are rarely as controlled as laboratory settings.

Thyer (2012) outlined several situations in which quasi-experimental designs might be the most appropriate method available. These included initial screening or piloting of interventions before investing in more time- and cost-intensive RCTs, testing and advancing theory, developing generalizable knowledge in contexts where it is not possible to conduct true RCTs, and as a teaching tool for those first learning experimental methods.

Handley et al. (2018) argued convincingly that quasi-experimental designs can be viable, rigorous alternatives that account for impossibilities or ethical quandaries raised by random assignment and controlled manipulation in some situations, collaboration with field-based practitioners, and need for exploration of conflicting or inconsistent findings. For these reasons, quasi-experimental designs are particularly relevant to mental health and human services professionals and settings.

Types of Research Questions Best Suited for Quasi-Experimental Methods

In short, quasi-experimental designs are most appropriate when researchers want to understand the effect of an experience or event, including a mental health intervention, on two or more groups. As will be explored later in this chapter, the effect must be able to be assessed quantitatively, and the researcher must have a large enough sample to compare groups in a way that allows for detection of changes over time.

To understand construction of research questions best suited for quasi-experimental methods, it is important to understand a few general concepts as applied to this design. The **independent variable** is the treatment, event, or experience being investigated in the study. In quasi-experimental design, the independent variable is comprised of two or more groups (e.g., treatment group, no-treatment control group, or comparison group). The **dependent variable** is the outcome the researcher believes will change as a result of exposure to the independent variable.

Quasi-experimental methods help researchers answer the general question *Do those who experience [independent variable/experimental condition] report changes in [dependent variable] compared to those who [independent variable control/comparison condition]?* In the bullying example, the research question might read, "To what degree do students who engaged in a bullying intervention report changes in likeliness to intervene as bystanders compared to students who participated in treatment as usual through the district's school counseling curriculum?" In this case, the research question makes clear both the independent variable (bullying intervention vs. treatment as usual) and the dependent variable (likelihood to intervene as a bystander).

Quasi-experimental research questions may be simple or complex. For example, quasi-experimental designs can assess effectiveness of multiple treatment conditions on multiple dependent variables. In the case study that follows, a sexual violence response center decides to evaluate impact of a mindfulness-based stress reduction (MBSR) group for waitlist clients (independent variable) on symptoms of posttraumatic stress disorder and overall outcome (two dependent variables). The overall outcome assesses three separate variables: Symptom distress, interpersonal relations, and social functioning. Their research question was: **"To what degree do survivors who participate in an MBSR group demonstrate improvements in PTSD, symptom distress, interpersonal relations, and social functioning compared to waitlist clients who have access to a peer support group only?"**

Case Study: Sexual Violence Recovery

The Sexual Violence Recovery Center is a nonprofit organization that serves adolescents and adults who self-report as having survived sexual assault. The center employs five full-time clinicians and two part-time interns and uses a trauma-informed approach to care. Historically, the center has offered individual counseling services to clients, and the average time on wait-list is two months. To provide initial support for clients on the waitlist, the center offers unstructured, weekly peer support groups facilitated by volunteer advocates.

Recently, the staff has been exploring evidence-based approaches to trauma and decided to implement an MBSR group in which participants would learn skills for noticing, accepting, and managing symptoms of traumatic stress (see (Boyd et al., 2018). The center director is exploring new sources of grant funding and wonders whether they can develop a rationale for state funding to fully implement the intervention as part of their treatment menu.

Center staff contact a local university researcher who has interest in trauma-based services to develop a study that would provide preliminary evidence for effectiveness of the services offered. The research team identifies symptoms of posttraumatic stress as assessed by the PTSD Checklist 5 (PCL-5; Blevins et al., 2015) and overall outcome as assessed by the Outcome Questionnaire (OQ-45.2; Lambert et al., 1996) as dependent variables. Based on an a priori power analysis, discussed in what follows, the researchers determine they need complete data for at least 14 people in each group.

Given the number of individuals needed for the MBSR groups, the staff decides to invite all new clients to participate in the MBSR group on Tuesday nights, and they continue this practice until the new group is full and ready to begin. On the first and last night of the six-week group, clients complete the PCL-5 and the OQ-45.2. If new clients are not available on Tuesday nights, the staff invites them to join one of two ongoing peer-support groups instead; they complete instruments the first day of group and again after six weeks. Once the MBSR group is filled, the staff invites all new clients to the peer support groups; they complete the instruments as described.

Quasi-Experimental Methods

This section delineates technical characteristics and design considerations for quasi-experimental research designs. This includes attention to nomenclature, development of experimental conditions, observations of dependent variable(s), and strategies to rule out plausible alternative explanations. The section ends with attention to data analysis in quasi-experimental methods.

Nomenclature

It is important to understand common nomenclature and symptoms used when writing about various experimental methods. The following nomenclature and symbols are adapted from Thyer (2012).

- **X** is used to refer to the independent variable of focus and most often refers to the **novel treatment or experimental group** in which the researcher is most interested.
- **Y** (and sometimes **Z)** is also used to refer to the independent variable; in this case, it most often refers to **comparison situations or conditions**.
- **O** stands for **observation** and refers to measurement of the dependent or outcome variable of interest. Quasi-experimental designs vary in the number of observations utilized, so a subscript is used to denote the order of observations. For example, O_1 refers to the first time a researcher measures the dependent variable. O_2 refers to the second time a researcher measures the dependent variable. O_3 refers to the third time a researcher measures the dependent variable, and so forth.

- N refers to the size of the **population** from which the sample was obtained.
- n refers to the size of a group or a **sample**, for example, the number of individuals in condition **X**, **Y**, or **Z**.

Researchers often use these symbols to denote specific types of quasi-experimental designs. For now, refer to Table 9.1 to see the various design configurations possible with quasi-experimental methods (see Thyer, 2012, for a complete discussion). For simplicity, each example in the table includes just two levels of the independent variable (X and Y). Note that any of the interventions could compare more than two levels of the independent variable (X, Y, and Z). Additionally, any of the designs could have additional measures of the dependent variable during or after treatment.

Treatment or Experimental Conditions

As discussed previously, all quasi-experimental studies feature an independent variable comprised of at least two different treatment or experimental conditions. Quasi-experimental designs are unique in that they use nonrandom assignment to experimental conditions. The types of conditions to which participants may be assigned include novel/experimental group, no-treatment control group, treatment-as-usual or placebo group, and competing or dismantled interventions group.

Novel or Experimental Group

Most often, researchers are interested in one approach or experience, that which is represented by X in the nomenclature from earlier. The literature most often refers to this as the **novel or experimental group**. In this chapter, the bullying bystander intervention and MBSR groups are two specific examples of possible treatments of focus.

Table 9.1 Quasi-Experimental Design Considerations

Notation	Name	Brief Description
$X\ O_1$ $Y\ O_1$	Posttest-only comparison/control design	Compares whether individuals in two conditions have different scores after an intervention or experience
$O_1\ X\ O_2$ $O_1\ Y\ O_2$	Pretest-posttest comparison/control design	Compares degree of change experienced before and after two or more interventions or experiences
$O_1\ X\ O_2\ O_3$ $O_1\ O_2\ X\ O_3$	Switching-replications design (also known as delayed treatment, lagged-groups, or stepped wedge design)	Provides the same intervention to different groups at different points in time; allows researchers two chances to show change based on a single intervention; introduces the ability to assess for maintenance of change over time
$O_1\ X\ O_2$ $O_1\ X_{-1}\ O_2$	Dismantling study	Creates comparison condition in which the same intervention, minus one component, is delivered to groups; allows researchers to determine the importance of different parts of treatment

No-Treatment Control Group

Quasi-experiments differ from preexperiments because they include some type of comparison or control group to help rule out other plausible explanations for change. Researchers can choose from several possible configurations for this level of the independent variable. The simplest option is to use a **no-treatment control group** in which those receiving an intervention are compared to those who do not receive any intervention or treatment, perhaps those on a waitlist for services. In helping professions, withholding treatment for those in emotional distress or with worsening conditions may go against fundamental ethical principles to do no harm. Although the use of a no treatment control group may help answer the question *Is this treatment better than nothing at all?*, it cannot answer whether the intervention is better than current practices.

Treatment-as-Usual or Placebo Group

For reasons noted already, researchers may prefer to compare those in the novel or experimental group with those who are having some other sort of experience. There are several options for comparison groups. One option would be to compare the novel or experimental group with effectiveness of **treatment as usual**. In the examples within this chapter, researchers compared a novel bullying program to curricula already provided to school counselors. Similarly, counselors at the sexual assault violence center realized that long waitlists for their clients were problematic, so they had already implemented the peer-support group. In the proposed design, researchers compared the MBSR intervention to treatment as usual. Alternately, researchers could decide to compare the novel treatment with a **placebo** experience designed to elicit hope for change and provide a degree of attention to participants but not, in theory, assumed to facilitate change.

Competing or Dismantled Interventions Group

In more advanced quasi-experimental designs, researchers may compare the novel or experimental group with other carefully designed conditions. For example, you may design a competing intervention or intentionally manipulate an intervention to determine the degree to which specific elements of the treatment are important. Manipulation could involve adding a specific element to the intervention or taking away a different component of the intervention. For example, individuals researching a play therapy intervention for which parent/caregiver consultation is considered an important element may decide to compare outcomes of those in the traditional condition with those in a condition offering no parent consultation. Results of that study could confirm the importance of that element of treatment or, if not supported, indicate an opportunity to save time and resources by not offering an element of care that does not make a practical difference to client outcome.

Observations of Dependent Variables

All quasi-experimental designs involve observations of at least one dependent variable; however, they vary regarding the number of times dependent variables are assessed. At the most basic level, researchers may observe the dependent variable only at posttest or both pretest and posttest. As you will see in this section, there are many creative opportunities to observe dependent variables.

Posttest-Only Designs

Posttest-only designs involve observation of the dependent variable for two or more nonrandomly assigned groups only after the groups have experienced the independent variable. These studies can answer whether individuals in condition X have different outcomes than individuals in condition Y. A posttest-only design could be useful when assessing changes in naturally occurring, noncontrollable events. This might be particularly helpful in assessing impacts of crisis and disaster or taking a broader look at the impact of widespread educational policy or preventative programming.

There are several limitations to posttest-only designs. Because there is no pretest comparison, one can only compare *how different* groups are from each other after the event rather than comparing *the degree of change* each group experienced related to the intervention. This distinction becomes particularly important because researchers are responsible for making a strong case that preexisting, uncontrolled factors or differences between the groups did not account for differences observed (Thyer, 2012). This is particularly difficult to do in the absence of pretest data.

Pretest-Posttest Designs

Pretest-posttest designs involve assessing participants in all groups at least once before and at least once after experiencing the experimental condition. These studies allow you to compare *the degree of change* each group experienced related to the intervention. In addition, the studies allow you the opportunity to *explore possible preexisting differences* across groups that might impact response to the experimental condition.

Although researchers may assess each group just once pre- and postintervention, there are a few reasons to include more frequent observations of dependent variables. In longer interventions, you may be interested in identifying periods of time during which the most change occurs. For example, if the most change occurred during the first four weeks of the MBSR group, the agency might offer shorter groups to serve more clients; if the most change occurred between weeks four and six, they would have a data-based rationale for keeping the groups longer. Similarly, you may be interested in understanding whether participants maintain changes after the intervention. Thus, they may decide to integrate one or more follow-up posttests in the design. From a statistical perspective, having a greater number of observations means researchers need fewer participants to yield meaningful data. This may be important in settings in which access to participants or clients is limited.

Strategies to Eliminate Alternate Explanations

When researchers use random assignment in true experimental designs, they engage in a process that increases internal validity and, with it, the likelihood that any changes or differences observed between groups were due to the intervention. By definition, quasi-experimental designs do not involve random assignment. This means researchers have a special responsibility to take steps to eliminate alternate causal explanations to the extent possible (Hadley et al., 2018). In this section, I explore several strategies and considerations researchers may use to rule out alternative explanations. These include treatment fidelity, assignment to groups, demonstrating equivalence of groups, measurement sensitivity, and statistical sensitivity.

Treatment Fidelity

Treatment fidelity refers to the degree to which treatments or conditions in the independent variable are designed and delivered in an intentional, replicable manner. When treatments are designed and delivered with fidelity, researchers are better able to conclude the degree to which the interventions were responsible for changes. If researchers do not provide interventions as they were intended, they may contaminate the design in such a way that one cannot determine what actually happened and contributed to change or lack of change. The most common treatment fidelity strategies used in helping professions include use of standardized manuals or curricula and video monitoring of interventions for compliance with the manual.

The National Institute of Health Behavior Change Consortium (Bellg et al., 2004) delineated a number of treatment fidelity goals and strategies that are still in strong use today. Many focused on ensuring equivalence of designs (e.g., length of contact, number of sessions) within and between conditions, standardizing treatment protocols, monitoring provider implementation, and ensuring designs were appropriate to the participant population. The report provides an excellent, in-depth exploration regarding steps researchers can take to improve treatment fidelity. Intentional work toward fidelity is especially important in research that focuses on behavior change (Toomey et al., 2020).

In the case study presented earlier, fidelity steps related to MBSR may include ensuring adequate provider training, using published MBSR curricula, and utilizing an outside observer to ensure the curricula are delivered as planned. In addition, the center may monitor the peer support group so a well-intentioned volunteer does not hear about the new MBSR material and find ways to bring in little doses or exercises for the groups, thus altering their experiences.

Assignment to Groups

As noted previously, there are a number of options for assigning participants to groups. These may include allowing participants to self-select into groups, assigning to groups by an administrator, or using a combination of self- and administrator selection (White & Sabarwal, 2014). You should consider potential benefits and drawbacks of each design carefully. If using self-selection, for example, it is possible that participants will self-select into a condition because of a characteristic, belief, or preference that might influence their experience and, ultimately, their outcomes. Similarly, those who engage in administrative assignment should consider whether there may be meaningful differences as they make their assignments. For example, if conducting the treatment condition at one center and the control condition at another center, one should ask whether the centers vary on basis of provider experience or populations served. Similarly, if using intact classrooms for an intervention, you will want to make sure there was not an outside factor guiding student assignment to classes (e.g., student achievement or special needs).

When creating groups, you must also decide whether to hold initial data collection until all groups are established and then implement concurrently, stagger implementation so data collection within groups begins at one time but data collection between groups begins at another time, or engage in rolling enrollment wherein each individual starts as they are ready and completes instruments on a set schedule. As with all design considerations, there are positives and negatives to each decision. Although engaging in simultaneous implementation might be strongest from a design perspective, it might not be practical given the number of participants available at any given time and the nature of the phenomenon being addressed. For example, it might take the sexual violence center three months to collect enough people for the group design; by then, potential participants will be enrolled in counseling services, have sought treatment elsewhere, or perhaps have experienced a degree of healing on their own. Thus, the staff decided to use a modified rolling enrollment design for their study.

When you choose to collect data at different points in time, you should also consider how outside, seemingly unrelated events might influence the groups differently (Thyer, 2012). Sometimes these influences may be as simple as the natural ebbs and flows of academic semesters or seasonal change. Imagine that researchers were implementing a stress-management program in a school. They collected data for the group in the fall, and they implemented the experimental condition in the weeks leading up to standardized testing in the spring. Although groups looked equivalent at pretest, timing of examinations may have influenced students' stress in ways that made it appear the intervention was not effective.

Other times, communities may experience disasters, unrest, turmoil, or significant changes that influence participants. Imagine, for example, that the sexual violence center was collecting data when news broke that a major political figurehead had been accused of sexual violence *and* was planning to defund a number of grant-funded organizations like the one they were attending. Participants may have found themselves reliving elements of their assaults through incessant media reports and wondering where they could go for support and safety. As a result of these confounds, the interventions may have appeared ineffective (or not as effective). If data collection for the comparison and intervention group was occurring on different schedules, the impact of these outside events on study findings could be even more profound.

Demonstrating Equivalence of Groups

How researchers create groups may have a profound impact on quasi-experimental designs, and researchers are responsible for presenting a strong case regarding the equivalence of groups. By showing that groups are as equivalent as possible before the intervention, researchers can be more certain that the intervention led to changes between groups at the end of the intervention.

The first step toward demonstrating equivalence of groups is being intentional regarding selection of data collection sites and participant profiles. If collecting data across centers or schools, you should take care to ensure that the experimental and control/comparison groups do not vary on important elements such as participant gender, age, race/ethnicity, socioeconomic status, resources, and general design. Similarly, if using intact classrooms within a school, you would not want to compare effectiveness of an intervention for students in a gifted and talented classroom with a control group of students in a self-contained classroom, as preexisting differences may influence the study outcome.

In some cases, researchers may decide to use nonrandom matching to assign participants or units to groups (Hadley et al., 2018). For example, researchers may gather demographic and pretest data and systematically assign individuals to conditions so the groups are as balanced as possible in terms of important characteristics. In the classroom example, researchers may examine classroom composition and divide up assignments so that each group contains one gifted and talented classroom, three general education classrooms, and one self-contained classroom.

Even if researchers do not intentionally match group assignments, they should provide evidence of group equivalence when conducting data analysis. For example, you might provide demographic descriptives and pretest profiles for each group, showing that they were roughly equivalent at pretest. Some researchers also engage in advanced methods to consider how to handle dropouts (e.g., efficacy subset analyses, intention-to-treat analyses; Thyer, 2012). White and Sabarwal (2014) presented advanced techniques such as regression discontinuity design and propensity score matching procedures to make the case for similarity of groups at baseline. Across all examples, you need to monitor and report characteristics of groups, design studies to ensure optimal equivalence, and interpret findings with attention to this fundamental consideration.

Measurement Sensitivity

Although not unique to quasi-experimental designs, the repeated-measures nature of most quasi-experimental designs makes measurement sensitivity particularly important. Researchers who are conducting pre–post designs should ensure that they are selecting instruments that are (1) related to the dependent variable, (2) appropriate for the population of focus, (3) designed to be used at intervals relevant to the study, and (4) sensitive to change. Measurements that assess experience over a long period of time (e.g., 6 months, 1 year, or a lifetime) or trait-like characteristics are not designed to be sensitive to change over time. In addition, you will want to select instruments that provide meaningful information for the group of participants under study.

For example, I once conducted a study regarding empathy in counselors-in-training; however, I selected an instrument on which my sample scored nearly two standard deviations above the normed mean. This created a ceiling effect in which the instrument was not able to detect changes in participants' already high levels of empathy. In our running example, researchers should carefully consider how the population tends to score on the PCL-5. If initial measures of client symptoms are below threshold at the beginning, it will be unlikely to discern meaningful change from the intervention. On the other hand, if participants score in clinical or higher ranges, the assessment tool is sensitive enough to detect change over the six-week intervention. In the sexual violence example, both the OQ-45.2 and PCL-5 were designed to detect clinically meaningful change of periods of weeks to one month, and their manuals included reliable change metrics and cut points that provided support for interpreting degree of meaningful change on the scales.

Statistical Sensitivity

Statistical sensitivity relates to the degree to which one can use statistical tests to detect changes between groups. Although it is a concept related to data analysis and interpretation, it is an important consideration when designing quasi-experimental studies. Those who design quasi-experimental research need to consider a unique interplay between number of participants, number of groups in the independent variable, number of measurements of the dependent variable(s), degree of change they wish to be able to observe, and amount of error they are willing to accept in their tests of statistical significance.

In order to do this, researchers will often use a program such as G*power (Faul et al., 2007) to conduct an a priori power analysis. The program calls for researchers to enter a variety of design factors (e.g., level of Type I error, level of Type II error, anticipated effect size, number of groups, number of measurements, correlations between measures, and statistical test to be used). In turn, the program generates an estimate regarding the number of participants needed to run the analysis. Researchers can use G*power to see how design decisions influence the number of individuals needed for different designs. Being intentional about number of participants during the design stage sets researchers up to be able to make accurate conclusions about the impact of their independent variable on the dependent variable(s) when it comes time for data analysis and interpretation. Certainly, you do not want to leave an intervention wondering whether the intervention really did not work or whether you simply did not have enough participants or use the right instruments to conclude whether it worked.

Data Analysis and Interpretation

There are a broad range of statistical procedures available to researchers, and intricacies of these decisions depend on level and nature of measurement, sample size, and overall sophistication of the design. In this section, I review the most common and typical data analysis considerations including exploration of descriptives, inferential tests of statistical significance, effect size, and clinical significance.

Exploration of Descriptives

Researchers should begin data analysis by exploring their entire dataset. This includes looking at score ranges, means, and standard deviations for groups as a whole and exploring the dataset for individual cases or outliers that might indicate errors in scoring, extreme cases, or other problems. Researchers may find it helpful to examine scatterplots for each group and time of measurement as well as graphics showing each group mean at each time of measurement. Exploration of distributions also helps researchers to determine whether certain assumptions are met for statistical tests.

Inferential Tests of Statistical Significance

Quasi-experimental researchers may use a variety of inferential statistics that test for changes between groups over time. The appropriate test depends on number of groups, number of independent variables, number of dependent variables, type of data (e.g., nominal, ordinal, or interval-ratio), and special characteristics of the data (e.g., normality). Most commonly, *t*-tests allow researchers to determine whether there are mean differences among two independent groups, including groups with pre–post data. **Analysis of variance (ANOVA)** is used to test for mean differences among two or more independent groups on one interval and can answer more complex questions including whether there are changes in mean differences by group, by time, and by group and time. **Multivariate analysis of variance (MANOVA)** is similar to ANOVA, but it has capacity to test for differences among multiple, theoretically related dependent variables at one point in time. Other statistical methods may include descriptive discriminant analysis, hierarchical linear modelling, and growth curve modeling (Watson et al., 2021). These are just a few of many available statistical procedures that are beyond the scope of this chapter. In all, these tests help researchers answer whether two or more groups are different in a way that is not likely due to chance.

Effect Size

While statistical tests answer the question if/whether a change is present, researchers need to use measures of effect size or practical significance to determine the degree or size of the changes observed (Balkin & Lenz, 2021; Watson et al., 2021). This consideration is particularly important because results of inferential statistical tests are heavily influenced by sample size. The specific type of effect size used depends on the statistical test of interest. Often, researchers will report effect sizes such as Cohen's d, eta^2, or Adjusted R^2, which they then determine to account for small, medium, or large degrees of change.

Clinical Significance

Finally, clinical significance refers to the idea that interventions should result in real-life changes for real-life people (Balkin & Lenz, 2021). Imagine, for example, that the MBSR intervention earlier in this chapter was tested and found to produce statistically significant changes compared to the peer-support group, and the effect size was decided to be moderate (both good things!). Now, imagine that participants started with severe levels of PTSD as assessed on the PCL-5. Although scores went down at posttest, participants still mostly fell in the severe range. We would have to ask whether the participants experienced meaningful change in their day-to-day experience. If, however, half of the group moved from severe to mild range on the PCL-5, one might conclude that the intervention had a very real impact on some clients' well-being. It might open up exploration regarding why some participants benefited when others did not. In short, researchers have a responsibility for exploring individual-level impacts even within group comparison designs.

Summary

You may use quasi-experimental designs to navigate a delicate balance between rigorous, laboratory-based research and the real, complex world of practice many helping professionals encounter. By building designs in ways that help rule out plausible alternative explanations, you may build an evidence base for practice that deepens both theoretical, academic understanding and practical, field-based implementation.

Practice-Based Application

Think about the client-presenting concern, symptom, or situation that you identified in Chapter 1. Imagine that you have decided to implement a quasi-experimental study to investigate the impact of an intervention in your setting.

- Write a research question and use standardized notation to indicate the type of design you selected. Be sure to name the independent and dependent variables.
- How will you assign participants to groups or conditions? What are the benefits and drawbacks of this approach?
- What strategies will you use to rule out plausible alternative explanations? What are the benefits and drawbacks of this approach?

Resources for More Information

Bellg, A. J., Borrelli, B., Resnick, B., Hecht, J., Minicucci, D. S., Ory, M., … Czajkowski, C. (2004). Enhancing treatment fidelity in health behavior change studies: Best practices and recommendations from the NIH behavior change consortium. *Health Psychology*, 23(5), 443–451. https://doi.org//10.1037/0278-6133.23.5.443

Handley, M. A., Lyles, C., McCulloch, C., & Cattamanchi, A. (2018). Selecting and improving quasi-experimental designs in effectiveness and implementation research. *Annual Review of Public Health*, 39, 5–25. https://doi.org/10.1146/annurev-publhealth-040617-014128

Miller, C. J., Smith, S. N., & Pugatch, M. (2020). Experimental and quasi-experimental designs in implementation research. *Psychiatry Research*, 283, 112452. https://doi.org/10.1016/j.psychres.2019.06.027

Thyer, B. A. (2012). *Pocket guide to social work research methods: Quasi-experimental research designs*. Oxford.

Trochim, W. M. K. (2023). Quasi-experimental design. In *Research methods knowledge base.* https://conjointly.com/kb/quasi-experimental-design/

White, H., & Sabarwal, S. (2014). Quasi-experimental design and methods. In *Methodological briefs: Impact evaluation No. 8.* Florence: UNICEF Office of Research. https://www.unicef-irc.org/publications/pdf/brief_8_quasi-experimental%20design_eng.pdf

Questions for Further Review and Application

1   Quasi-experimental design exists on a continuum from preexperiments to a true experimental design. What are the primary features distinguishing these three types of designs?
2   In which situations might a quasi-experimental design be favorable to a true experimental design?
3   What are the options for assigning participants to groups in quasi-experimental designs? What are the strengths and limitations of each option?

References

Balkin, R. S., & Lenz, A. S. (2021). Contemporary issues in reporting statistical, practical, and clinical significance in counseling research. *Journal of Counseling & Development, 99*(2), 227–237. https://doi.org/10.1002/jcad.12370

Bellg, A. J., Borrelli, B., Resnick, B., Hecht, J., Minicucci, D. S., Ory, M., … Czajkowski, C. (2004). Enhancing treatment fidelity in health behavior change studies: Best practices and recommendations from the NIH behavior change consortium. *Health Psychology, 23*(5), 443–451. https://doi.org/10.1037/0278-6133.23.5.443

Blevins, C. A., Weathers, F. W., Davis, M. T., Witte, T. K., & Domino, J. L. (2015). The posttraumatic stress disorder checklist for DSM-5 (PCL-5): Development and initial psychometric evaluation. *Journal of Traumatic Stress, 28*, 489–498. https://doi.org/10.1002/jts.22059

Boyd, J. E., Lanius, R. A., & McKinnon, M. C. (2018). Mindfulness-based treatments for posttraumatic stress disorder: A review of the treatment literature and neurobiological evidence. *Journal of Psychiatry and Neuroscience, 43*(1), 7–25. https://doi.org/10.1503/jpn.170021

Faul, F., Erdfelder, E., Lang, A. G., & Buchner, A. (2007). G*Power 3: A flexible statistical power analysis program for the social, behavioral, and biomedical sciences. *Behavior Research Methods, 39*, 175–191.

Handley, M. A., Lyles, C., McCulloch, C., & Cattamanchi, A. (2018). Selecting and improving quasi-experimental designs in effectiveness and implementation research. *Annual Review of Public Health, 39*, 5–25. https://doi.org/10.1146/annurev-publhealth-040617-014128

Lambert, M. J., Hansen, N. B., Umphress, V., Lumen, K., Okiishi, J., Burlingame, G. M., & Reisenger, C. W. (1996). *Administration and scoring manual for the OQ-45.2.* American Professional Credentialing Services.

Miller, C. J., Smith, S. N., & Pugatch, M. (2020). Experimental and quasi-experimental designs in implementation research. *Psychiatry Research, 283*, 112452. https://doi.org/10.1016/j.psychres.2019.06.027

Thyer, B. A. (2012). *Pocket guide to social work research methods: Quasi-experimental research designs.* Oxford University Press.

Toomey, E., Hardeman, W., Hankonen, N., Byrne, M., McSharry, J., Matvienko-Sikar, K., & Lorencatto, F. (2020). Focusing on fidelity: Narrative review and recommendations for improving intervention fidelity within trials of health behaviour change interventions. *Health Psychology and Behavioral Medicine, 8*(1), 132–151. https://doi.org/10.1080/21642850.2020.1738935

Watson, J. C., Ho, C., & Boham, M. (2021). Advancing the Counseling Profession Through Intervention Research. *Journal of Counseling & Development, 99*(2), 134–144. https://doi.org/10.1002/jcad.12361

White, H., & Sabarwal, S. (2014). Quasi-experimental design and methods. In *Methodological briefs: Impact evaluation No. 8.* Florence: UNICEF Office of Research. Retrieved from www.unicef-irc.org/publications/pdf/brief_8_quasi-experimental%20design_eng.pdf

10 Randomized Controlled Trials

Dee C. Ray

Randomized controlled trials (RCTs) are considered the "gold standard" of research designs for the purposes of evaluating effectiveness of intervention. As indicated by the design title, RCTs are characterized by the random assignment of a sample into comparison groups receiving or not receiving the tested intervention in the context of a controlled environment. Both random assignment and internal validity controls serve to allow the exploration and conclusion of effectiveness related to a given intervention. In this chapter, I will discuss the required components and methods involved in RCTs for research. Although the process of conducting an RCT may seem daunting to practitioners, this chapter presents clear steps for implementation of an RCT or possibly as criteria for reviewing published RCTs to determine evidence-based practices.

Public and government organizations typically emphasize RCTs as the highest level of evidence to support mental health interventions (e.g., American Psychological Association, 2006; California Evidence-Based Clearinghouse, 2023; Title IV-E Prevention Services Clearinghouse, 2023; What Works Clearinghouse, 2022). In order for interventions to be noted as evidence based, they must be supported by research studies in which effectiveness is proven. Effectiveness is determined by outcome studies in which variables that may interfere with results are controlled for and positive outcomes can reasonably be attributed to participation in treatment. For example, if a university counseling center wanted to test whether a specific type of orientation activity was more effective for building knowledge about mental health resources on campus, the staff could work with the orientation office to select students at random who will participate in that activity during the normal orientation period. Other students not selected might not receive anything during that time or might participate in an alternative activity. After the orientation, all students might fill out a survey that assesses their knowledge about mental health resources on campus.

Due to the random assignment, RCT designs offer the most control over variables that may interfere with outcomes (internal validity) in combination with the ability to generalize findings to the greater population (external validity). The rigor necessary to offer acceptable levels of internal and external validity is found within the well-designed RCT. Hence, RCT design is well-regarded, carefully scrutinized for thoroughness, and lauded as an exemplary design under which to test intervention. Although other intervention research designs such as single-case and quasi-experimental designs are considered contributory to evidence-based practice, the RCT is respected as the most appropriate design for determining effectiveness.

The well-designed RCT includes several components that contribute to rigor and to internal validity. Specifically, if you use RCT, you seek to isolate intervention as the most likely cause of change for participants through controlling for passage of time, client expectation of

DOI: 10.4324/9781032706139-10

change, therapist attention, repeated assessments, and regression to the mean (Kendall, Comer, & Chow, 2013). In other words, clients participating in a research study with few variable controls may demonstrate improvement for a wide range of reasons. It may have been due to getting older or time passing, or because they believe that they will get better, or just because a therapist spent time with them. Maybe they become more sophisticated about instruments that are provided and how to best answer items, or they moved away from the more severe ends of the symptom spectrum to a more middle ground. These are just a few factors that have been shown to interfere with credibility of results. In order to control for these possibilities, RCTs employ the use of random assignment of participants to treatment conditions and measure change over time. By randomly assigning participants, you most likely control the internal validity factors (e.g., for every participant assigned to the treatment group who improves by passage of time, there is a participant in the control group who improves simply through time passage who serves as a counterbalance). Internal validity controls such as random assignment and comparison conditions help to rule out factors that interfere with treatment outcome (Kazdin, 2021).

When an RCT's findings result in favorable outcomes related to the intervention and internal validity has been established, indicating that results can be considered credible, external validity should also be addressed. External validity refers to the ability to generalize findings across other people, units, outcomes, and settings (Heppner, Wampold, Owen, Wang, & Thompson, 2016). External validity for an individual RCT is likely accounted for by conclusions drawn by researchers regarding the applicability of their findings to other groups or populations. For example, if an RCT results in decreased depressive symptoms for participants in the treatment group and all participants were college-educated White American females, conclusions that treatment is broadly effective across gender and race would be inappropriate and a violation of external validity. However, researchers could offer implications that treatment appears effective for college-educated White American females whose situations are similar to those of study participants. As discussed, the concepts of internal and external validity are central to the RCT design, establishing the context for the detailed components necessary for an RCT to be considered for evidence-based decision making.

Appropriate Contexts for RCTs

The RCT design is used when you desire to explore the effectiveness of an intervention or program. The design and statistical analyses used in RCTs serve to compare the effects of receiving an intervention when compared with not receiving the specified intervention or receiving another form of intervention. The design determines cause and effect, thereby allowing for conclusions regarding the impact of the intervention on targeted outcomes. Typically, when you use RCT, you embark on research with a defined intervention and a specific outcome of interest. Simply put, you want to know if an intervention works, with whom it works, and with what problems or issues. The RCT is designed to answer these questions from a positivistic philosophical framework (Heppner et al., 2016) with a yes or no, an objective truth. For example, RCT design is used to determine if Intervention X is effective in reducing trauma symptoms with female adults who have been sexually abused. The RCT design is useful in clinical settings, as well as other institutions such as schools and workplaces, where subgroups can be defined and then assigned to different conditions.

Alternately, in some contexts, RCTs are inappropriate and possibly an ethical challenge to client service. When RCT designs employ experimental conditions that withhold or delay treatment, clients who have substantial needs may be negatively affected. In a community clinic, counselors may determine that it would be unethical to withhold services from a client in crisis who is randomly assigned to a control condition, especially if resources are available. In these settings, you must determine ethical practice, which may include the use of a non–RCT design or your willingness to accept higher attrition (dropout) rates when a person who is delayed service is determined to be in greater need and is terminated from the study in order to receive services. Institutions legally and morally committed to equitable services, such as schools, may also struggle with the concept of no-treatment control conditions. In these settings, the use of waitlist-control conditions and alternative services may help institutional administrators be more favorable to RCT conditions.

Types of Research Questions and Hypotheses Related to RCTs

Because the purpose of the RCT is to test the effectiveness of an intervention, research questions suitable for RCTs focus on determining the impact of the intervention on the targeted variable. The research question encompasses variables that are measurable and clearly interpretable regarding effectiveness. Additionally, RCT research questions include a "compared to what" feature in which the intervention will be compared to another condition (Solomon, Cavanaugh, & Draine, 2009, p. 87) in order to conclude effectiveness. Some examples of research questions include: "For parents of foster-care children, is ABC parent education more effective in teaching parenting skills than the current agency curriculum?" "For adult clients who are clinically depressed and seeking mental health services in a community-based clinic, does participation in XYZ counseling intervention result in reduced depressive symptoms when compared to symptoms of clients who do not participate in XYZ?"

In addition to stated research questions, RCT designs often generate testable hypotheses in order to drive the statistical analysis of data. Because of the positivistic nature of RCT design and goals, hypotheses are suitable to the discovery of an objective truth regarding the relationship between intervention and outcomes. RCT hypotheses consist of statements that correlate intervention delivery with measurable outcomes. Examples of testable RCT hypotheses generated from the previous research questions include: "Parents of foster-care children who participate in ABC parent education will demonstrate no significant difference in attainment of parenting skills when compared to parents of foster children who participate in current agency curriculum (null hypothesis)." "Adult clients who qualify as clinically depressed and participate in XYZ counseling will demonstrate a significant reduction in depressive symptoms when compared to adult clients who qualify as clinically depressed but do not participate in XYZ (directional hypothesis)." In these hypotheses, the relationship between the independent variable (intervention) and dependent variable (target outcome) is well-defined and measurable through data analysis.

Case Study

In order to highlight the detailed components involved in designing and implementing an RCT, I will present a case in which a researcher wants to explore the effectiveness of child-centered play therapy (CCPT) in reduction of aggressive behaviors among children who are enrolled in first through third grade in a public-school setting. The research question for this study is: Do young children identified as exhibiting clinical levels of aggressive behaviors who participate in 16 sessions of CCPT demonstrate a reduction in aggressive symptoms in comparison with children who do not participate in CCPT? In the following listed steps

Table 10.1 Steps to Conduct RCTs

Step 1	Define Intervention
Step 2	Target Outcomes
Step 3	Define Experimental Conditions
Step 4	Identify Valid and Reliable Measures
Step 5	Define Inclusion Criteria
Step 6	Implement Recruitment and Informed Consent Procedures
Step 7	Conduct Criterion and Baseline Testing
Step 8	Perform Random Assignment
Step 9	Monitor Intervention and Control Conditions
Step 10	Monitor Participant Flow
Step 11	Conduct Posttest and Follow-Up
Step 12	Explore Statistical, Practical, and Clinical Significance

(see Table 10.1), I will address issues related to the implementation step and present the specific procedures followed for this case study.

Step 1. Define Intervention

The first step in RCT design is to decide what intervention will be explored. In this case, the intervention is identified within the research question as CCPT. Because the intervention itself is what will be manipulated through delivery or nondelivery to participants, it is considered the independent variable in an RCT. In order for RCTs to be deemed credible evidence of an intervention, intervention must be specified in a manual or detailed protocol of procedures (Appelbaum et al., 2018). The length and format of intervention should also be specified. Although intervention manuals or rich description of treatment is required for a credible RCT, they may consist of guidelines to treatment and not necessarily detailed instruction of intervention delivery (Carroll & Rounsaville, 2008; Solomon et al., 2009). In this case study, CCPT will be delivered according to the published CCPT manual (Ray, 2011) and, as the research question specifies, over the course of 16 sessions (30 minutes each) delivered twice a week for eight weeks. Additionally, the qualifications and training of treatment providers should be detailed. For this case, the counselors are doctoral-level students who are state-licensed interns and have completed three courses in CCPT as well as a two-day training on the CCPT protocol.

Step 2. Target Outcomes

The second step in RCT is the identification of a target outcome or multiple outcomes, also referred to as the dependent variables. In this case, as in most RCTs, step 2 is conducted simultaneously with step 1. The example research question identifies the target outcome as reduction in aggressive symptoms. Because RCTs are conducted to test what intervention works with what types of issues, the identification of treatment and outcome variables occurs concurrently. Best practices in RCT encourage the limiting of outcome target variables to a minimal number of constructs (Kazdin, 2021). The tendency to cast a broad net by attempting to target multiple and diverse outcomes indicates that the researcher may have limited theoretical rationale for how the intervention works and is on a "fishing" expedition to find any possible positive outcome. RCTs are ideally grounded in the conceptual framework that defines the role of intervention in behavioral or emotional change (Solomon et al., 2009).

Step 3. Define Experimental Conditions

Once the intervention and target outcomes are well-defined, the researcher determines the control condition from which to compare the treatment condition. Kendall et al. (2013) identified four control conditions in treatment outcome research that include a no-treatment control, waitlist control, attention-placebo/nonspecific control, and standard treatment (treatment as usual) control. In the no-treatment control condition, participants assigned to this group receive assessments on repeated occasions at the same time as the treatment group, but they do not receive treatment. In the same procedures as the no-treatment control, the waitlist control does not receive treatment and participates in assessment, but they will be scheduled to receive treatment following final data collection. The attention-placebo control receives a treatment that involves attention or contact at the same time as the treatment group; however, the treatment is not intended to address the target outcome. In the standard treatment control, participants receive an intervention that is already in place but not the intervention being tested. For this case study, wherein the research was scheduled to take place in a school setting, the researchers selected a waitlist control condition as the experimental condition from which to compare the treatment group. Administrators at the school agreed to participation in the study with the stipulation that every child who qualified for the study would eventually receive treatment. The waitlist control group seemed most suitable to meet this requirement.

Step 4. Identify Valid and Reliable Measures

The fourth step involves the identification of valid and reliable measures in order to assess changes in the target outcomes. Prior to implementation of an RCT, researchers will select instruments with strong psychometric properties that capture the construct of the targeted outcomes. Although researchers may be tempted to create an assessment to more fully match their RCT design, this practice is discouraged. The development of reasonably valid and reliable assessments is a research agenda in and of itself (see Chapter 4) and should be embarked on with caution and care. For most outcomes, assessments with solid psychometric properties can be identified. Using inadequately supported instruments to measure dependent variables in an RCT results in credibility and interpretation limitations. Kazdin (2021) recommended the use of multiple measures in order to operationalize a construct. Limiting assessment of a key construct to one instrument may result in the inability to fully interpret change in the construct.

In the case study, researchers identified aggressive symptoms as the target dependent variable. In order to capture the construct of aggression fully, the RCT design included the use of the Children's Aggression Scale (CAS; Halperin & McKay, 2008) for both parents and teachers, as well as the Aggression Scale on the Child Behavior Checklist and Teacher Report Form (CBCL/TRF; Achenbach & Rescorla, 2001). Thereby, change in aggression was captured by two different reporters (parent and teacher) and two instruments, resulting in a fuller picture of how aggression was affected by participation in CCPT.

Measurement preference for RCTs is the utilization of objective raters to report and assess behavioral changes. RCTs often employ objective raters who are trained in an assessment protocol and establish interrater reliability prior to observation or participant interview.

This type of measurement is considered most objective and of highest credibility. However, RCTs more frequently utilize self-report and other-report on reasonably valid and reliable instruments due to the lack of availability of objective measurements, as well as the high interest in change of emotional status for mental health interventions, normally only captured through self-report.

Step 5. Define Inclusion Criteria

Once design features regarding independent variable (intervention), dependent variable (targeted outcomes), control conditions, and measures of change have been determined, the RCT researcher must establish criteria for participant inclusion and necessary sample size. RCT researchers seek participants that have a connection with the target outcome and favorable candidates for the intervention. In the case study, because CCPT is an intervention that is directed to younger children, sample children needed to be between first and third grade. Because the dependent variable of interest was aggression, a clinical score on the parent or teacher aggression scales was required for participant inclusion. In order to extend external validity, children of both genders and various ethnicities were recruited across three elementary schools. In all, inclusion criteria for the case study required that children were (1) enrolled in first through third grade at one of the recruiting schools, (2) scored by a parent or teacher in the clinical range on one aggression scale, and (3) not participating in any other mental health intervention over the course of the study.

Prior to recruitment for an RCT, researchers must determine the sample size necessary for results from statistical analysis to be credible. This procedure is referred to as a power analysis. In order to conduct a power analysis, the researcher determines the magnitude of the desired effect size, the alpha level at which the null hypothesis will be rejected, and the likelihood that you want to reject the null hypothesis if there is a relationship between intervention and outcome, known as power (Cooper, 2018). Traditionally, the alpha level is set at .05 and power is set at .80 or above. Desired effect sizes are ideally selected based on previous research, but researchers often default to a medium effect size (e.g., $d = .5$). Power analysis also requires that the researcher has decided the type of statistical analysis that will be used to test differences in treatment conditions. G*power is one online program to help run a power analysis (www.gpower.hhu.de/). The result of running a power analysis is the determination of how many participants a researcher will need to recruit for adequate power to run analyses and find credibility in results. Power analysis for a factorial analysis of variance based on .95 power, .05 alpha level, and medium effect size of $d = .5$ indicated that 36 participants were needed for the CCPT RCT example study.

Step 6. Implement Recruitment and Informed Consent Procedures

Up to this point, the RCT has been in the planning stages. Prior to making contact with potential participants, the researcher has organized a plan for intervention, targeted outcomes, determined a comparison design, selected reasonably valid and reliable measures, set criteria for participant inclusion, and analyzed the number of participants necessary to address the research question. The delineation of steps emphasizes the detailed planning and organization required prior to implementation of an RCT design. Now that the researcher has a plan of action, recruitment can begin. Because RCTs involve human subjects by virtue of the design, human subjects approval from an institutional review board is a prerequisite for research implementation. Human subjects approval involves the development of a recruitment plan and participant informed consent that notifies the potential participants of the nature of the study and extent of participation, and addresses confidentiality, benefits, and risks. Upon human subjects approval, the researcher can embark on participant recruitment.

When recruiting, the RCT researcher works within the context setting to inform potential participants of the upcoming RCT and criteria for participation. Often, researchers will design a simple statement of recruitment disseminated to staff or clients in order to identify participants. For this particular case study, the researchers sent out a notice to parents and teachers that play therapy services were being offered in their schools through a research study. If parents or teachers were concerned about a child being aggressive or defiant, the child might qualify for free services. Once the parent contacted the researcher, the researcher explained the use of the waitlist control group and that children may not immediately receive services but they would be guaranteed services immediately following posttest data collection. If parents were still interested, the researcher reviewed the informed consent with the parent and acquired signature for participation.

Step 7. Conduct Criterion and Baseline Testing (Pretest)

Participants have now been recruited, and it is time to determine whether they meet the qualification criteria stated necessary for the RCT. Recruitment procedures generally limit participants to those who meet some criteria. In the case study, only parents and teachers of children who were between first and third grade in the recruiting schools were notified of the study. Hence, most potential participants met some criteria at initiation of the study. However, criteria for qualification that require assessment may only be met through the potential participant's inclusion in preliminary procedures. For example, although potential child participants may have met age and referral criteria, it is unknown whether they would qualify as clinical on the selected instruments. Therefore, pretest instruments were administered to parents of all potential participants. Inclusion could not be determined until all pretest assessments were scored. Once scored, the researchers identified participants who met all inclusion criteria, as well as those who did not. According to RCT procedures and human subjects approval, it is common to dismiss potential participants who do not meet full criteria. However, RCT researchers should consider the demoralization possible for participants who become excited about participation and then are rejected for inclusion. In this circumstance, it is recommended that when RCT researchers recruit, there should be an alternate plan for how to serve potential participants who do not meet criteria.

Step 8. Perform Random Assignment

In this step, participants have been screened for inclusion, met criteria, and are now ready for assignment to an experimental condition. Random assignment is the crucial component of a credible RCT. Random assignment is the key distinguishing feature between conducting an experimental design and a quasi-experimental design. Ideally, random assignment would occur directly following the identification of all participants so that the sample is equally and simultaneously distributed, referred to as simple random assignment (Hsu, 2008). However, the identification of all participants is often not possible, and random assignment occurs in block assignments in which the researcher decides a priori how many participants will be blocked at a time before random assignment occurs, referred to as randomized blocks assignment (Kendall et al., 2013). In the case study example, upon the identification of 12 children who met inclusion criteria, those 12 were randomly assigned to the treatment or waitlist control groups. Hence, random assignment took place at three different points in order to reach the desired number of 36 participants. Further ideas regarding types of random assignment can be found in Hsu (2008).

Proper random assignment includes the use of a mathematical procedure to determine assignment to conditions (Solomon et al., 2009). Although some random assignment procedures are described informally, such as every other participant is assigned to a group or participants are assigned according to the first initial of their last name, these types of procedures are considered unacceptable in ensuring the equality of groups. Credible procedures include the use of a table of random numbers or computerized random number generator. For the case study, once 12 participants had met inclusion criteria, the research team employed the website Research Randomizer (randomizer.org) to generate assignment to groups.

The purpose of random assignment is to ensure that participants in experimental conditions are comparable. Using credible procedures for random assignment allows the researcher to assume that groups are similar, start approximately in the same place, and can be compared to one another. However, even with random assignment, there are likely to be slight differences among groups such as small non–statistically significant variances in pretest data. Even though researchers may be encouraged to demonstrate equivalence of groups through pretest analyses, this type of analysis is considered superfluous and unnecessary (De Boer, Waterlander, Kuijper, Steenhuis, & Twisk, 2015) when proper assignment procedures have been used. Exceptions to this guideline may occur when attrition rates are high throughout the study, and pretest analysis would ensure comparability of the intact groups at follow-up testing.

Step 9. Monitor Intervention and Control Conditions

Once participants have been assigned to an experimental condition, treatment intervention is implemented. For participants who are assigned to the treatment group, they will begin intervention for the set amount of time as designated by the researcher prior to design implementation. As previously discussed, intervention is delivered according to protocol or manualized procedures by qualified and trained facilitators. Adherence to treatment is a critical piece of conducting solid research, and it has been shown that without monitoring, researchers will drift from manualized treatments (Nathan, Stuart, & Dolan, 2003). Monitoring of treatment goes beyond the general supervision and training of treatment providers in a given study. RCTs require the use of fidelity checks to confirm that intervention is being delivered as intended in the RCT design. Fidelity checks include objective evaluation that intervention is facilitated as designed such as employing objective raters to visually inspect and rate intervention delivery. For the example RCT case study, researchers enlisted two raters unaffiliated with the study to use the Play Therapy Skills Checklist (Ray, 2011) to rate the therapist responses in video-recorded sessions for adherence to protocol, resulting in a percentage adherence. The researchers had previously cited an acceptable adherence percentage at 80%, meaning that 80% of the therapist's responses in the evaluated session must match with protocol response categories to be considered as meeting fidelity standards.

In addition to monitoring the treatment condition, the RCT researcher also monitors the comparison or control condition. Comparison groups are typically subjected to the same types of fidelity checks used for the experimental group. For example, if the comparison group is supposed to be receiving a reading intervention, the RCT researcher ensures that the reader is not initiating discussions or engaging in therapeutic techniques with participants assigned to that condition. For no-intervention control conditions, the RCT researcher ensures that there is no cross-contamination of treatment to the control participants and that participants in that condition are not receiving other mental health services during the course of the experiment. For the case study, the researcher checked in with the school administrators, counselors, and teachers to monitor that the waitlist control group participants received no additional mental health services.

Step 10. Monitor Participant Flow

Throughout recruitment, inclusion, data collection, and treatment delivery, RCTs report an account of participant flow. Participant flow indicates how many participants were initially involved in the study, assigned to experimental conditions, dismissed or dropped out of the study, failed to provide usable data, and completed the study. A visual flowchart is recommended for publication to diagram the specifics of participant flow (Cooper, 2018). Transparency related to participant flow lends credibility to final results through the acknowledgment of limitations in participant completion. For the case study, the following description is an example of monitoring participant flow: Thirty-eight participants were recruited for the study who appeared to meet criteria. At pretest, two participants did not qualify due to lack of clinical ratings on the assessments. Thirty-six participants were randomly assigned to the CCPT treatment group ($n = 18$) and waitlist control group ($n = 18$). Over the course of the treatment period, two children from the treatment group moved from the area, and one child from the waitlist control group dropped out of the study due to substantial absences, resulting in 16 children in the treatment group and 17 children in the waitlist control group. The 16 children in the treatment group participated in 16 sessions of CCPT within ten weeks. All 33 children completed posttest data at the end of ten weeks.

Step 11. Conduct Posttest and Follow-Up

RCTs are characterized by evaluating the dependent variable(s) over the course of the study. Pretests serve as baseline assessments from which to measure change on the target outcome. Follow-up assessment may occur during, directly following, and/or substantially later after treatment. At minimum, RCT researchers provide a posttest assessment using the same measures from pretest directly following the treatment period. However, repeated measures over time improve the credibility of results for interpretation, as well as improving power in data analysis. Although follow-up assessment after a lengthy period is rare in RCTs, Kendall et al. (2013) advocate for follow-up data collection as a "signpost of methodological rigor" (p. 44). However, follow-up assessments delay treatment for the control condition participants due to the inability to start treatment prior to the last data collection point, a particularly salient challenge for RCT researchers who use waitlist control groups. For the case study, parents and teachers were administered the CAS and the CBCL/TRF at the end of the ten-week treatment period. Although the original design called for treatment to occur over eight weeks, the treatment period was extended to ten weeks due to absences and school holidays. All participants were administered posttesting in the same week.

The administration of posttest assessments appears to be a straightforward step in the RCT design. Yet experience reveals that the posttesting step of RCT design can be challenging. When subjective raters are used such as parents and teachers, or other reporters who have a relationship with the participant, it is often difficult to motivate them to complete assessments. Some challenges include avoiding contact with the researcher, hastily filling out assessments without thoughtfulness, or passive refusal to complete assessments. The RCT researcher is likely more successful at this stage if planning for these challenges has occurred. Strategies such as offering incentives, visiting homes, and providing a quiet space for assessments (e.g., volunteering to substitute or babysit while assessments are being completed) may address these normal challenges. Additionally, use of objective raters and measures circumvents the need for subjective raters. In the case study, researchers offered a "pizza day" after school for parent reporters to complete assessments. During the pizza day, researchers provided pizza and babysitting while parents filled out instruments. For teacher assessments, researchers served as substitutes in the classroom for 30-minute time periods while teachers went to another room to complete assessments.

Step 12. Explore Statistical, Practical, and Clinical Significance

The answers to RCT research questions are developed through analysis of statistically, practically, and clinically significant outcomes (Thompson, 2002). Statistical significance refers to the probability estimate regarding the null hypothesis that the intervention group will not differ from the comparison/control group at a predetermined probability threshold (i.e., $\alpha = .05$). If the treatment group performs in the desired direction at a probability difference below the set alpha level ($p < .05$), the result is determined to be statistically significant and the intervention is interpreted as effective. Yet statistical significance is artificially impacted by sample size; there must be substantial difference in outcomes between experimental conditions to detect significance when the sample size is small, but large samples often yield statistically significant results with small differences between groups. Statistical significance is seen by many as the traditional indicator of effectiveness but is limited in its scope.

Practical significance refers to the importance of the findings and is generally reported through effect sizes. Effect sizes quantify the difference between groups or the relationship between variables. In RCTs, effect sizes allow the researcher to understand the magnitude of difference or relationship between the groups, as well as between intervention and group assignment (Ellis, 2010). Clinical significance refers to the realistic value of intervention when applied to everyday life of a client (Kazdin, 2021). Although statistical and practical significance may be reached through a two-point mean decrease in assessed symptoms, clinical significance addresses whether this two-point difference means that the participants in the treatment group have a better quality of life following intervention. Clinical significance is often determined through comparison of participant groups to normative samples, which can be assessed through statistical methods (Kendall et al., 2013).

RCT researchers seek to answer their research questions through addressing the three types of significance. What is the probability that the treatment group would improve over another experimental condition group (statistical significance)? How much of the detected change can be attributed to intervention? Or, How different are the experimental groups from each other at posttesting (practical significance)? Did the intervention make a difference for the participants in real life (clinical significance)? All types of significance are addressed through analysis of collected data over the course of the RCT. Brown, Costigan, and Kendziora (2008) suggested three major approaches to data analysis for RCTs including analysis of variance (ANOVA) models, latent growth models, and hierarchical linear models. In these approaches, RCT researchers seek to explore the impact of intervention through analysis of patterns within subjects over time, between subjects, and within different contexts (Brown et al., 2008). A full description and investigation of these methods is beyond the scope of this chapter. Notably, RCT researchers necessarily are well-versed in complex statistical methods to understand how to determine the impact of intervention over time and between groups in the context of probability, magnitude, and realistic outcomes. If you find that you are unsure of your ability to perform some of these analyses, there are often individuals in your community who may be able to lend their expertise. Don't be afraid to ask for support!

In the case study, researchers conducted four factorial ANOVAs using the pre- and post-test CBCL Aggression scale score, TRF Aggression scale score, CAS-Parent, and CAS-Teacher Total Scores as the dependent variables and the experimental group as the independent variable. Statistically significant differences between the means across time were tested at the .05 alpha level for the dependent variable scores. Practical significance was calculated through Cohen's *d* (Cohen, 1988), a group difference effect size used to compare standard deviations between the two groups. Clinical significance was explored through the Reliable Change Index analysis calculating the number of participants moving from clinical range to normative sample range (Jacobson & Truax, 1991; Kendall et al., 2013).

All the Steps Together

The steps for implementation of RCTs emphasize the level of detail and planning required for findings to be considered credible. Conducting RCTs is not for the faint of heart. RCTs require that you have considerable knowledge regarding the intervention, experience with outcomes of interest and statistical analysis, resources to implement data collection and experimental conditions, and time dedicated to intense monitoring of procedures. However, RCTs can also be exciting endeavors into exploration of different interventions. Although practitioners may experience certain interventions to be effective, it is encouraging to show through rigorous methods that the intervention can be proven effective. Alternately, outcomes from RCTs may indicate that intervention is ineffective, which can be discouraging but also helps practitioners to understand conditions that may contribute to or limit treatment effectiveness. Researchers who employ RCT designs contribute directly to client services through production of outcomes related to intervention effectiveness.

Resources for More Information

Resources for Conducting RCTs

Nezu, A., & Nezu, C. (2008). *Evidence-based outcome research: A practical guide to conducting randomized controlled trials for psychosocial interventions*. New York, NY: Oxford University Press.

Solomon, P., Cavanaugh, M., & Draine, J. (2009). *Randomized controlled trials: Design and implementation for community-based psychosocial interventions*. New York, NY: Oxford University Press.

Resources for Reporting RCTs

Butcher, N., Monsour, A., Mew, E., Chan, A., Moher, D., Mayo-Wilson, E., Terwee, C., Chee-A-Tow, A., Baba, A., Gavin, F., Grimshaw, J., Kelly, L., Saeed, L., Thabane, L., Askie, L., Smith, M., Farid-Kapadia, M., Williamson, P., Szatmari, P., Tugwell, P., Golub, P., Monga, S., Vohra, S., Marlin, S., Ungar, W., & Offringa, M. (2022). Guidelines for reporting outcomes in trial reports: The CONSORT-Outcomes 2022 extension. *JAMA*. 328(22), 2252–2264.

Cooper, H. (2018). *Reporting research in psychology: How to meet journal article reporting standards* (2nd ed.). Washington, DC: American Psychological Association.

Hancock, G., Stapleton, L., & Mueller, R. (Eds.). (2018). *The reviewer's guide to quantitative methods in the social sciences* (2nd ed.). New York, NY: Routledge.

Resources for Power Analysis and Random Assignment

G*power. Retrieved from www.gpower.hhu.de/
QuickCalcs. Retrieved from www.graphpad.com/quickcalcs/randomize1.cfm
Research Randomizer. Retrieved from Randomizer.org

Resources for Finding Assessment Instruments

Mental Measurements Yearbook/Tests in print via EBSCOhost
PsycTESTS via EBSCOhost

Questions for Further Review and Application

1   In reviewing chapters from this book, what features of RCT design distinguish it from other designs?
2   In one column, create a list of obstacles that you might encounter in planning and conducting an RCT. In a second column, list strategies to address those obstacles.
3   Think of an intervention to which you are favorable. Search the internet to explore if RCTs have been conducted on this intervention. If so, what outcomes have been explored in these RCTs?
4   For one of your favorite interventions, develop a theoretical model that links the components of that intervention with an outcome of interest. Evaluate the possibility of testing your model. Develop a research question addressed through an RCT.
5   You are interested in the effectiveness of ABC intervention. You have already conducted a power analysis and know that you need 46 participants to run statistical analysis to compare two experimental groups. Go to the website for Research Randomizer. Follow directions to randomly assign your 46 participants.
6   Think of an outcome of interest to you. Search for instruments that measure aspects of this outcome. Use internet and academic sources such as Mental Measurements Yearbook or PsycTESTS (see Resources section in this chapter) to locate assessments. Find the reliability and validity support for the instruments.

Practice-Based Application

Think about the client-presenting concern, symptom, or situation that you identified in Chapter 1, and use that to answer the following questions:

• If you wanted to conduct an RCT in your setting, how would you explain the process to clients who are randomized into a control or treatment-as-usual group? How do you help clients who are randomized into a comparison group maintain hope?
• How would you ensure that the counselors in your setting are following treatment protocol? What would be reasonable methods to monitor counselors' fidelity to the protocol within the context of your setting?
• How would an RCT in your setting benefit the setting and the clients within the setting? What would be the obstacles to conducting an RCT in your setting?

References

Achenbach, T. M., & Rescorla, L. A. (2001). *Manual for the ASEBA school-age forms and profiles; Child behavior checklist for ages 6–18, teacher's report form, youth self report: An integrated system of multi-informant assessment.* Burlington, VT: ASEBA.
American Psychological Association Presidential Task Force on Evidence-Based Practice. (2006). Evidence-based practice in psychology. *American Psychologist, 61*, 271–285.
Appelbaum, M., Cooper, H., Kline, R., Mayo-Wilson, E., Nezu, A., & Rao, S. (2018). Journal article reporting standards for quantitative research in psychology: The APA Publications and Communications Board Task Force Report. *American Psychologist, 73*, 3–25.

Brown, C., Costigan, T., & Kendziora, K. (2008). Data analytic frameworks: Analysis of variance, latent growth, and hierarchical models. In Nezu & Nezu (Eds.), *Evidence-based outcome research* (pp. 285–314). New York: Oxford University Press.

California Evidence-Based Clearinghouse for Child Welfare. (2023). Retrieved from www.cebc4cw.org/ratings/scientific-rating-scale/

Carroll, K., & Rounsaville, B. (2008). Efficacy and effectiveness in developing treatment manuals. In A. Nezu & C. Nezu (Eds.), *Evidence-based outcome research: A practical guide to conducting randomized controlled trials for psychosocial interventions* (pp. 219–243). New York, NY: Oxford University Press.

Cohen, J. (1988). *Statistical power analysis for the behavioral sciences* (2nd ed.). Hillsdale, NJ: Erlbaum.

Cooper, H. (2018). *Reporting research in psychology: How to meet journal article reporting standards* (2nd ed.). Washington, DC: American Psychological Association.

De Boer, M., Waterlander, W., Kuijper, L., Steenhuis, I., & Twisk, J. (2015). Testing for baseline differences in randomized controlled trials: An unhealthy research behavior that is hard to eradicate. *International Journal of Behavioral Nutrition and Physical Activity*. Online publication. Retrieved from http://dx.doi.org/10.1186/s12966-015-0162-z

Ellis, P. D. (2010). *The essential guide to effect sizes: Statistical power, meta-analysis, and the interpretation of research results*. New York, NY: Cambridge University Press.

Halperin, J. M., & McKay, K. E. (2008). *Manual for the children's aggression scale*. Odessa, FL: Psychological Assessment Resources, Inc.

Heppner, P., Wampold, B., Owen, J., Wang, K., & Thompson, M. (2016). *Research design in counseling* (4th ed.). Boston, MA: Cengage.

Hsu, L. (2008). Random assignment procedures. In A. Nezu & C. Nezu (Eds.), *Evidence-based outcome research: A practical guide to conducting randomized controlled trials for psychosocial interventions* (pp. 179–200). New York, NY: Oxford University Press.

Jacobson, N. S., & Truax, P. (1991). Clinical significance: A statistical approach to defining meaningful change in psychotherapy research. *Journal of Consulting and Clinical Psychology, 59*, 12–19.

Kazdin, A. (2021). *Research design in clinical psychology* (5th ed.). Cambridge.

Kendall, P., Comer, J., & Chow, C. (2013). The randomized controlled trial: Basics and beyond. In J. Comer & P. Kendall's (Eds.), *The Oxford handbook of research strategies for clinical psychology* (pp. 40–61). New York, NY: Oxford University Press.

Nathan, P., Stuart, S., & Dolan, S. (2003). Research on psychotherapy efficacy and effectiveness: Between Scylla and Charybdis? In A. Kazdin (Ed.), *Methodological issues and strategies in clinical research* (3rd ed., pp. 505–546). Washington, DC: APA.

Ray, D. (2011). *Advanced play therapy: Essential conditions, knowledge, and skills for child practice*. New York, NY: Routledge.

Solomon, P., Cavanaugh, M., & Draine, J. (2009). *Randomized controlled trials: Design and implementation for community-based psychosocial interventions*. New York, NY: Oxford University Press.

Thompson, B. (2002). "Statistical," "practical," and "clinical": How many kinds of significance do counselors need to consider? *Journal of Counseling & Development, 80*, 64–71.

Title IV-E Prevention Services Clearinghouse. (2023). Retrieved from https://preventionservices.acf.hhs.gov/review-process/sesp

What Works Clearinghouse. (2022). What Works Clearinghouse procedures and standards handbook, version 5.0. U.S. Department of Education, Institute of Education Sciences, National Center for Education Evaluation and Regional Assistance (NCEE). https://ies.ed.gov/ncee/wwc/Handbooks

11 Content Analysis

Edward Wahesh

Content analysis (CA) is the systematic and replicable examination of texts. In CA, text is understood in the broadest sense, encompassing oral and verbal communication as well as images. While not an exhaustive example, you may consider texts to include things like client journals, or poetry, song lyrics, or case notes. Content analysts systematically categorize and assign numerical values to written text for the purpose of describing patterns within the communication or to make inferences about the meaning or context (Riffe et al., 2014). This process of systematic recording and assigning numerical values to text distinguishes CA from other research methods that seek to describe and explain symbols of communication, such as thematic analysis (Braun & Clarke, 2006). Researchers can use CA to examine research questions or test hypotheses that contribute to empirical literature or advance theory. This approach can also be used by practitioners in applied, pragmatic ways to help with program evaluation efforts or solve problems that arise in counseling practice. Let us now look at the unique features of CA as a research method.

Overview of Content Analysis

CA is systematic in that it follows the standards of the scientific method (Neuendorf, 2017), which includes asking a question, making a prediction or a theory of what you think is going to happen, gathering data to examine the question, analyzing the data gathered, and drawing conclusions. Researcher assumptions about the features of the texts are subject to a rigorous system of critical observation and empirical verification, meaning that hypotheses (or predictions you have about what you may find) are determined before the coding of texts begins. Additionally, the scope and framework of CA studies are determined in advance, which includes defining each variable, establishing coding procedures, and deciding what qualifies as evidence to support study hypotheses (Riffe et al., 2014). This process involves generating hypotheses to be tested and creating a standardized codebook containing definitions and measurement rules for each variable. Each of these processes of CA will be discussed later in a case study. Despite CA having an a priori design in which hypotheses are derived and tested deductively, there is room for the use of an inductive approach to identify variables and formulate hypotheses as well. Neuendorf (2017) argues that before the initial coding procedures are finalized, content analysts should examine a representative sample of texts to identify additional variables and ascertain whether changes need to be made to the coding process before actual coding of the texts begin. This type of exploratory work can help establish a more complete representation of the concepts being studied by addressing the limitations of existent theory and past research.

DOI: 10.4324/9781032706139-11

Another key feature of CA research is that it is replicable, meaning that the research pro-cedures should be objective and reproducible. Concepts are operationalized into discrete variables each with a definition and set rules of measurement. All procedures, from the selec-tion of texts to the final analysis, are reported in enough depth that they can be replicated by other researchers. This includes providing reliability data as evidence that the coding process was replicable within the study itself (Neuendorf, 2017). Reliability data includes calculating inter-coder agreement, which measures differences in coding among two or more raters and can be particularly helpful in determining the extent to which content analysts followed an objective process and that the coding procedures are reproducible.

Reliability of measurement procedures is necessary though not sufficient in establishing validity, which is another important consideration in CA research. In CA, validity refers to the extent to which the coding process adequately measures the underlying constructs being studied. Hence, semantic validity, which is the degree to which there is agreement about the meaning and categorization of a concept (Insch et al., 1997) and ecological validity, other-wise known as generalizability (Potter & Levine-Donnerstein, 1999), are important consid-erations when establishing standardized and replicable coding rules.

Content analysts summarize characteristics across texts and make inferences based on the aggregate of these observations (i.e., nomothetic), instead of documenting and present-ing each individual observation within a set of texts (i.e., idiographic). CA is a nomothetic approach because of its focus on producing findings that are generalizable and can be applied to other contexts. When presenting results, providing examples of specific observations can offer evidence of validity of the findings; however, a full accounting of all observations found within a dataset of texts is unnecessary and beyond the scope of CA. Think of this as supply-ing quotes as examples from one or two journals that a client provided in counseling rather than supplying a quote from every single journal entry. Part of the process of summarizing includes quantifying texts by assigning numerical values to each observation. Depending on the scales of measurement used to code the variables, content analysts could use descriptive statistics as well as parametric or non-parametric statistical analyses to gather evidence in sup-port of their hypotheses. For example, content analysts can examine relationships among variables coded within texts using bivariate correlations (e.g., how related were the concepts of sadness and the behavior of drinking for a client after coding their case notes), or test group differences among variables based on specific characteristics of the texts (e.g., what were the coping behavior differences among clients who experienced major depression, mild depression, and no depression after coding information you provided in their case notes). This process of systematically quantifying and analyzing texts highlights the unique nature of CA as a research methodology and points to a diverse array of possible research questions that can be explored using this approach.

When to Use Content Analysis Methodology

Researchers can use CA to quantify and explore patterns, trends, or differences within texts. And remember, texts can include anything such as books, case notes, journals, responses to open-ended questions, transcripts of counseling sessions, poetry, or anything else that you or a client may have written. As a result, CA can be useful when you have access to a large amount of textual data to analyze. How many texts do you need to conduct a CA? Well, that depends. Krippendorff (2018) suggests that decisions about sample size (i.e., the number of texts you should have) should be based on the frequency of the variables that are under examination. When variables necessary to answer the research questions are rare, the sample size should be larger than when these variables are common (Krippendorff, 2018). Having a larger sample of texts increases the likelihood that you will end up observing enough of these rare variables to answer your research questions. If you plan to use inferential statistics (i.e., correlations, regressions, Analysis of Variance) to test your hypotheses, the concept of statistical power applies; therefore, it is necessary to conduct a power analysis before collecting data to determine the minimum number of texts that you need to conduct your analyses. For more information on statistical power, refer to Chapter 5, "Quantitative Data Analysis and Interpretation".

CA is a concept-driven approach that uses existent theory and empirical literature to formulate research questions and develop coding procedures. If little is known about the phenomenon that you are studying, it is likely that exploratory and inductive approaches to data analysis are more suitable. CA is appropriate to use when studying manifest constructs, which are textual elements that can be readily observed and taken at face value. CA is less appropriate to use when the goal of the research is to examine constructs that cannot be observed directly but must be inferred through a more nuanced interpretation of the texts and their context (Riffe et al., 2014). For example, a client may say they are sad – which is directly observable and stated and thus can be an appropriate observable variable for content analysis. However, if you are interested in the subjective experience of client emotions (i.e., good or bad), then CA is more difficult and potentially not the correct methodology. When coding involves searching for latent meaning (like what the emotion means to a client), researchers should use qualitative methods that consider contextual factors and do not require high levels of inter-coder reliability (Schreier, 2012), such as phenomenology in the next chapter. The line between manifest and latent characteristics is impossible to draw; that said, if a great deal of context is needed, such as considering when the text was collected or who provided it, researchers should use a qualitative approach to data analysis.

Finally, given the emphasis placed on the concept of replicability, CA must be done with a minimum of two coders to calculate intercoder reliability. It is possible to calculate the reliability of a single coder using intra-coder reliability (i.e., a coder applies the coding procedures to the same textual content at two points in time); however, intra-coder agreement has been characterized as the weakest form of reliability (Neuendorf, 2017) and on its own is not considered acceptable evidence of replicability (Riffe et al., 2014). Intra-coder reliability can be used in addition to inter-coder reliability in CA studies when coding occurs over a prolonged period of time and the stability of coder adherence to coding procedures is a threat.

Types of Research Questions Best Suited for CA

CA has a long history of use in the social sciences (Neuendorf, 2017). Presently, the most common application of CA in counseling literature is to explore characteristics of articles published in counseling-affiliated scholarly journals (e.g., topics published, methods used, demographics of authors). In addition to coding journal articles, researchers can also use CA to examine other textual formats, such as websites, social media posts, course syllabi, clinical documentation, client artwork, and client-counselor exchanges. Analyzing texts can help researchers identify aspects of an experience or social interaction that might not be fully captured using traditional quantitative self-report measures. Another way that researchers can use CA is to summarize and quantify narrative responses to open-ended questions embedded within a survey also containing questions with numerical response options; in this scenario, researchers could conduct statistical analyses that involve a combination of data derived through the CA and numerical responses to the quantitative instruments. See Table 11.1 for examples of possible research questions.

Table 11.1 Examples of Texts and Research Questions

Text	Research Question
Social media posts that contain the hashtags sobriety and sober living.	What intersectional identities are represented in social media posts of people who are in recovery from substance use disorder?
Clinical documentation	To what extent do client demographics explain *DSM*-5 diagnoses assigned to clients?
Audio recordings of motivational interviewing sessions	How do clients respond to counselor use of simple and complex reflections?
Audio recordings of group supervision sessions	What types of peer feedback are exchanged during a group supervision session?
Counseling program websites	To what extent does CACREP–accreditation influence the discussion of counselor identity in counseling program mission statements?
Responses to the open-ended question: "Describe the constructive feedback you received from your supervisor."	Are there differences in supervisee scores on the Supervision Working Alliance Inventory-trainee (Efstation et al., 1990) version based on the feedback content discussed during supervision?

In addition to being used for research purposes, professional counselors can use CA to inform their work with clients. For instance, professional counselors who are interested in learning more about the typical characteristics of people who enter counseling can analyze narrative data gathered from intake questionnaires. Examining patterns in client homework can complement quantitative data collected via routine outcoming monitoring tools in determining counselor effectiveness. Further, analyzing clinical progress notes can identify the kinds of interventions and theoretical approaches used in session across client presenting concerns and demographics. On a broader level, CA can be used by counseling supervisors and agency leadership to evaluate programming and client services. By conducting a CA of treatment plans, agencies can identify the frequency and patterns in how particular referrals or resources are provided to clients, for example. Agencies can also analyze responses to post-termination client satisfaction surveys to identify meaningful experiences associated with treatment and gather feedback to improve existing policies, procedures, and staff expectations.

Case Study

The staff at a university counseling center provide mandatory counseling to undergraduate students who have been sanctioned for alcohol policy violations. During these sessions, the staff use motivational interviewing (MI; Miller & Rollnick, 2013) and cognitive behavioral therapy (CBT; Liese & Beck, 2022) to increase client motivation and capacity to change problematic alcohol use behaviors. To evaluate the efficacy of these interventions, the staff has students complete a questionnaire before their first session and again six weeks after their final session. The questionnaire uses the Brief Young Adult Alcohol Consequences Questionnaire (B-YAACQ; Kahler et al., 2008) to measure reported alcohol-related negative consequences during the past 30 days. After a year of data collection, the staff found that on average there were no changes in reported alcohol problems six weeks after clients had finished counseling. After calculating a reliable change index (Jacobson & Truax, 1992) for the B-YAACQ, inspection of individual client results revealed that only 62 out of the 143 clients reported clinically significant reductions in alcohol problems at follow-up. These results were surprising, given the evidence underlying their approach (Fachini et al., 2012) and because all staff received training as well as regular feedback and coaching on their use of MI and CBT.

To identify possible reasons for why these interventions did not result in reductions in alcohol problems among some clients, the staff immersed themselves in the literature to understand what makes these kinds of interventions effective. A meta-analytic study of CBT in the treatment of substance use disorder by Magill et al. (2020) showed that changes in self-regulatory coping skills led to improved outcomes. In a study of MI sessions with college student drinkers, Apodaca et al. (2014) found that client speech in session predicted drinking outcomes, suggesting that the way in which clients articulate their drinking plans can help explain their future behavior. Given these findings, the staff decided to content analyze student responses to questions in the Change Planning Form, which is a worksheet that clients fill out at termination that includes questions about how clients will change their alcohol consumption using strategies learned in counseling. See Table 11.2 for a list of questions in the Change Planning Form. Exploring client responses to these questions can help the staff understand why some clients were unsuccessful in their efforts to change their alcohol use behaviors and provide input on how to enhance the efficiency of these counseling interventions in the future.

Steps in Conducting a Content Analysis

Neuendorf (2017) describes a process for CA research involving nine steps:

1. Theory and rationale of study
2. Conceptualization of variables
3. Operationalization of measures and textual units
4. Developing a codebook
5. Sampling texts
6. Training coders and assessing pilot reliability
7. Final coding
8. Final assessment of reliability
9. Analyses and reportage

In the following section, I will describe each step and apply it to the case study.

Theory and Rationale of CA Study

The first step of a CA involves determining what texts to examine and why examining these texts is important (Neuendorf, 2017). Content analysts rely on theory and past research to

Table 11.2 Change Planning Form

Questions
1. I plan on making the following changes:
2. I will make these changes by taking the following steps:
3. I am making these changes because:
4. The people in my life who support and can help me with these changes are:
5. I will know that I am successful in making these changes if:
6. If my plan is not working, I will:

Note: Questions are based on the change plan worksheet in Miller and Rollnick (2013).

justify their selection of particular texts and to develop research questions and hypotheses. They also consider ways to link their CA with other data sources to gain a better understanding of the source of the texts. To examine why some clients changed their drinking behaviors while others did not, the staff looked to two theories of behavior change, the transtheoretical model of change (TTM; Prochaska & DiClemente, 1982) and self-determination theory (SDT; Ryan & Deci, 2020).

According to Prochaska and DiClemente (1982), when people change a behavior they progress through six stages of change. To move through these stages, they apply a number of different experiential and behavioral processes. Experiential processes, such as emotional arousal and consciousness raising, can help people move from not thinking about changing (i.e., precontemplation stage) to getting ready to act (i.e., preparation stage), whereas behavioral processes move people from thinking about change (i.e., contemplation stage) into action (i.e., action stage) through maintaining that change over time (i.e., maintenance stage). Because engaging in behavioral processes can move people into initiating change and maintaining change over time, the staff decide to content analyze client responses to questions two, three, and four of the Change Planning Form to identify evidence of the TTM behavioral processes – stimulus control, counterconditioning, reinforcement management, self-liberation, and helping relationships – believing that perhaps the number of processes reported by a client is related to their alcohol use behaviors following counseling.

Whereas the TTM explains the "how" of the behavior change process, SDT helps us understand "why" people decide to change a behavior. In SDT, motivation is understood as existing along a continuum ranging from amotivation (i.e., not being motivated at all) to intrinsic motivation, which involves engaging in a behavior for its own sake. Between these two poles is extrinsic motivation, which is when one engages in a behavior for some other outcome, separate from the behavior itself. Importantly, SDT describes four different types of extrinsic motivation, each reflecting a different degree of internalization including external regulation, introjection, identification, and integration. Based on the SDT principle that people who are internally motivated to change are more likely to be successful at change, the staff decide to content analyze Change Planning Form questions three and five to determine the degree to which clients were intrinsically motivated to change their alcohol use behaviors. See Table 11.3 for research questions and hypotheses as well as other important considerations in planning a CA study.

Conceptualization of Variables

In step 2, researchers define the variables that they will use in the study. To answer the first research question, the counseling center staff name and describe each of the TTM behavioral processes based on definitions from Marden Velasquez et al. (2015). Using this particular source for the definitions was intentional; Marden Velasquez and colleagues (2015) developed definitions of each process in relation to changing substance use behaviors. Using well-known definitions drawn from the literature helps with the semantic validity of the results (i.e., people who read the study will likely define the variables in the same way the researchers did). For the second research question, the staff uses the taxonomy of motivation by Ryan and Deci (2020) to create one variable with multiple levels for each type of motivation.

Neuendorf (2017) suggests that during step 2 researchers screen the texts they plan to analyze to ensure that all important variables are addressed. After reviewing approximately 20% of the Change Planning Forms ($n = 28$), the staff notice that some responses to questions two through four include examples of the TTM experiential processes of change. They decided to add these because, though they do not represent behavior-change strategies,

Table 11.3 Planning a CA Study

Research question	Hypothesis	Content	Theory	Linking data	Statistical analyses
RQ1: Are there differences in the number of reported TTM change processes based on whether clients reduced their alcohol use behaviors following counseling?	Clients who reported a reduction in alcohol problems will have reported more processes than clients who did not change their alcohol use or showed deterioration following counseling.	Responses to Change Planning Form questions 2, 3, and 4	TTM	Client data on alcohol use behaviors collected six weeks following counseling	Mann Whitney *U* test
RQ2: To what extent does a client's level of motivation explain changes in their reported alcohol problems following counseling?	There will be an inverse relationship between level of motivation and alcohol problems such that clients who described more intrinsically oriented reasons for change will report fewer alcohol problems following counseling.	Responses to Change Planning Form questions 3 and 5	SDT	Client data on alcohol use behaviors collected six weeks following counseling	Spearman's rank-order correlation

coding experiential processes can potentially shed light on client motivation and commitment to change. All variables have a definition and represent constructs that do not overlap, making it impossible for one messaging unit to have more than one code. Having variables that are mutually exclusive helps improve inter-coder reliability as it can reduce the number of disagreements among coders.

Operationalization of Measures and Textual Units

Step 3 involves determining how to measure each variable. For research question 1 there are ten separate variables, or one variable for each of the ten TTM experiential and behavioral change processes. To record these variables in the Change Planning Forms, the staff will use a nominal level of measurement: "Present" (1) or "Not Present" (0). The option "Unsure" will be available if coders are unable to determine if a variable is present. A composite variable representing the total number of processes of change described by each client will be included in the statistical analysis for research question 1. To answer the first research question, the staff will conduct a Mann Whitney *U* test comparing the total number of change processes between clients who reported a clinically significant reduction in alcohol problems six weeks following counseling ($n = 62$) compared to those who reported either no change or more alcohol problems ($n = 81$), hypothesizing that clients who reported fewer alcohol problems would have more total experiential and behavioral processes. They selected a non-parametric test because the dependent variable, processes of change total, is comprised of count data (i.e., counting the number of times a component of the TTM is "present" in their answers) and is not continuous (see Chapter 5 for more information on types of variables).

Research question 2 uses one variable, level of motivation, with six levels for the different types of motivation described in Ryan and Deci's (2020) taxonomy of motivation. Because these levels are ordered along a continuum the staff will use an ordinal measurement scale (see Box 11.1 for coding examples). The staff will use Spearman's rank-order correlation, which is a variation of Pearson's product moment correlation coefficient for ordinal variables, to examine the relationship between level of motivation with number of alcohol problems reported following counseling. The staff believe that the Spearman's rank-order correlation will reveal a negative relationship between level of motivation and reported alcohol problems such that more internally regulated motivation will be associated with lower levels of problems.

Another important consideration when operationalizing variables is determining how the variables will be captured within the texts – this requires the process of unitizing. The process of unitizing (Krippendorff, 2018) involves deciding how messaging units are coded. The staff could code each sentence or response to the questions on the Change Planning Form; however, because it is possible for there to be multiple change processes represented within one response, the staff chooses to code each discrete idea represented within the Change Planning Form questions two, three, and four for research question 1. This will result in more than one code, or idea, per client – which is something unique to CA.

Reading the texts to determine the number of ideas (i.e., number of codable messaging units for research question 1) is more time consuming than simply coding each word or sentence, but it will provide a more meaningful and accurate representation of the TTM change processes. The actual process of unitizing the dataset occurs during step 5 (sampling texts) before coding begins. Although no standards exist for assessing the reliability of the unitizing process and evidence of agreement in identifying codable units is rarely reported in CA research (Neuendorf, 2017), content analysts should take steps to ensure that the process of determining the number of message units is valid and replicable. This includes having a clear definition of what a unit is and using multiple coders to identify these units within the texts.

For research question 2, the staff decide to rate client motivation using responses to questions three and five on the Change Planning Form. The message unit was defined as client responses to questions three and five because this research question contains one CA variable representing a client's level of motivation. So, in this case, the messaging unit is the client, or in other words, the coders will provide one rating of motivation per client using responses to questions three and five. Making coding decisions based on multiple responses can potentially result in poor inter-coder reliability. For example, it is possible that a client might include examples of multiple types of motivation within their responses to question three and five, or a coder might interpret a combination of responses from one client differently than other coders. These challenges highlight the importance of codebook development and coder training. If disagreements occur during the initial reliability pilot test, revising the definition and operationalization of this variable, or revisiting the unitizing process, might be necessary.

Developing a Codebook

With each variable now defined and operationalized, the next step is to create a codebook and coding form. The codebook should contain enough detail for there to be little ambiguity regarding the coding protocol. Additionally, codebooks should include definitions of each variable and measurement unit. Although providing examples of the variables and levels of measurement can help improve inter-coder reliability, including examples can have an impact on the validity of the results. According to Neuendorf (2017), providing examples of each variable limits how coders perceive the text and makes them less likely to observe and code textual elements that were not similar to the examples in the codebook. The coding form can simply be a spreadsheet with each messaging unit that coders use to record their observations as they review the texts. Box 11.1 contains an excerpt from the counseling center staff's codebook.

Box 11.1   Excerpts from Codebook

Research Question 1

Coding units: Unique and discrete ideas presented in client responses to Change Planning Form questions 2–4 (e.g., if a client lists three different steps in response to question 2, code each of those steps separately).

Instructions: Provide a code (Yes or No) in the coding form for each variable across all message units. In the coding form, rows are messaging units, and the 10 change process variables are columns.

Definitions:

Behavioral processes of change: Efforts made by clients to change their alcohol use.

Helping relationships: Seeking or fostering interpersonal relationships that offer support and reinforcement of alcohol-related behavior changes.

   Present: Messaging unit contains an example of the helping relationships process.

   Not Present: Messaging unit does not contain evidence of this process.

   Unsure: Coder is not certain if a messaging unit contains evidence of this variable.

Environmental reevaluation: Recognizing the impact that one's current alcohol use behavior has on others (e.g., friends, family) and the community as a whole.

   Present: Messaging unit contains an example of environmental reevaluation.

   Not Present: Messaging unit does not contain evidence of this process.

   Unsure: Coder is not certain if a messaging unit contains evidence of this variable.

Research Question 2:

Coding units: Client responses to questions 3 and 5.

Instructions: After reading questions 3 and 5, select one categorical rating that best represents the client's level of motivation to change. In the coding form, each row is a client. Provide a numerical rating (using the levels below) in column 1.

Variable: Taxonomy of human motivation

Levels/Categories:

1. Amotivation
2. External regulation
3. Introjected regulation
4. Identified regulation
5. Integrated regulation
6. Intrinsic motivation

Definitions:

External regulation: Engaging in behavior change for extrinsic reward or to avoid negative contingencies (i.e., punishment).

Sampling Texts

In step 5, content analysts determine how much data are needed to answer their research questions (Riffe et al., 2014). If all relevant content is available and you have the time and resources to code every text, you can use a census of every messaging unit within that population of texts. However, if coding all textual content is impossible or impractical, you need to decide how to draw a sample that is an accurate representation of the entire population of texts. Neuendorf (2017) describes a number of ways to draw a representative sample from a population of texts, including random sampling, systematic sampling, and stratified sampling. With random sampling, researchers list all relevant text and randomly select the number of texts they wish to use in their study. Systematic sampling involves selecting every *k*th text after selecting a random starting point in the list of texts. Stratified sampling is when researchers divide the population of texts into smaller groups and randomly select from within those groups. If the full population or census of texts is unknown or it is more practical to use a sample of available texts, you can use convenience sampling; though, this approach has its limitations. Texts drawn through convenience sampling might not represent the full population of texts, which can impact the generalizability of findings.

As mentioned earlier, you should consider the frequency of the variables that are under study as well as the statistical power of your analyses when determining your sample size. There are no previous CA studies using TTM or SDT to code client post-treatment change plans; therefore, the probability of observing each variable within the texts is unknown. Given that there are ten variables for research question 1 and the variable for research question 2 has six levels, the staff decide to code all Change Planning Forms ($N = 143$). This increases the likelihood that there will be multiple observations of each variable and level of measurement within the dataset. Finally, to confirm that they will have enough units to achieve acceptable statistical power in their planned analyses, the staff conduct a power analysis using G*Power (Faul et al., 2007) for each research question. Using a medium effect size, alpha of .05, and power level of .80, the staff determined that the minimum sample sizes needed for research questions 1 and 2 are 102 and 67, respectively.

Knowing that they have a large enough sample to proceed (as they have a total sample size of 143 clients), the staff take steps to begin the coding process. First, they delete identifying information from the Change Planning Forms and ensure that coders do not code forms completed by their own clients during the final coding process (step 7). They take these steps to reduce bias and keep coders from considering any context beyond the Change Planning Form when coding client responses. Second, they unitize the forms to determine the number of unique ideas present in the sample. For research question 1, two of the three coders each independently review all 143 Change Planning Forms of clients, meeting periodically to reconcile disagreements in the number of units identified in each form. Coders underline each unique idea and assign a numerical code representing the client and number of ideas present on the form. Remember that each unique idea within questions two, three, and four for each client is one unit. Coders identified a total of 498 units within the 143 Change Planning Forms. See Box 11.2 for an example of the unitizing process for research question 1. Unitizing for research question 2 is simple as each client's responses to questions three and five is a single messaging unit, resulting in 143 total units to analyze. The coding team place the Change Planning Forms in a location they can access during the coding process. This entire process of determining the number of units occurs prior to actual coding (which occurs in Step 7).

Box 11.2   *Unitizing Client #12's Change Planning Form*

1. **I will make these changes by taking the following steps**:

   Pregaming less [Unit 139.12], eating a full meal before drinking [Unit 140.12], telling my friends my plans [Unit 141.12], delaying, or waiting 30 minutes between each drink [Unit 142.12], and not using cocaine at parties [Unit 143.12].

2. **I am making these changes because**:

   I don't want to end up in the hospital again. [Unit 144.12] Most people do not drink as much as I do [Unit 145.12], and I can use the money that I save on new clothes [Unit 146.12].

3. **The people in my life who support and can help me with these changes are**:

   My roommate, Julie. [Unit 145.12] I can ask for help from my sister, [Unit 146.12] too.

Training Coders and Assessing Pilot Reliability

Step 6 begins with having coders familiarize themselves with the content and coding procedures. To facilitate this process, I suggest holding a meeting in which coders read aloud and react to each variable and measurement definition in the codebook. Even if all the coders had been involved in developing the codebook, these conversations can sometimes shed new light on how to conceptualize and measure the constructs. After coders have reviewed the definitions and levels of measurement, the coding team then codes a small number of messaging units. Ideally, these units are not drawn from the sample used in the study; if that is not possible, content analysts can select at random a small percentage of messaging units (e.g., 3–5%) from their sample to review together. Once training is finished, these units are then returned to the sample to be used in the final coding process (step 7; Neuendorf, 2017).

During this process, coders apply their knowledge and communicate any questions they have about the codebook and coding form. Members of the coding team should discuss their rationale for selecting a particular level of measurement for each coded unit. This helps increase consensus among coders and can identify aspects of the codebook that need to be refined. Training also involves some discussion of the study timeline and coding procedures, such as what steps coders should take when coding (e.g., to prevent drift in how the variables are interpreted over time, all coders should read the entire codebook before each coding session), and how many messaging units coders should review at a time (e.g., to avoid decay, or reduced reliability in how units are interpreted over time, coders should not exceed 30 units per session).

Following training, the coding team conducts a pilot test of the coding scheme using a randomly selected subset of the texts. Using a random sample increases the likelihood that the texts used in the pilot test represent the characteristics of the full sample of texts. According to Neuendorf (2017), content analysts should conduct a pilot test to identify issues with the codebook as well as to spot problematic coders. Thus, pilot test coding is done independently, and the coding team gathers evidence to evaluate inter-coder reliability. Two important considerations when conducting a pilot test are selecting content for testing and strategies for evaluating coder agreement.

There are several strategies you can use to determine the size of your pilot test sample. Krippendorff (2018) provides a formula for determining sample size based on the probability of the least-frequent value observed within the texts. Riffe et al. (2014) offer their own formula based on the assumed level of inter-coder agreement within the full population of texts. Based on the logic of these formulas, Neuendorf (2017) provides a general recommendation for determining sample size, "the reliability subsample should be at least 10% of the full sample, probably never be smaller than 50, and should rarely need to be larger than about 300" (p. 187). Content analysts should consider drawing a sample closer to 300 when the population, or full sample of texts being used in the study, is large or when there is an assumption that there will be a lower level of coder agreement when coding the population of texts (Neuendorf, 2017).

Following the pilot test, it is time to evaluate the level of agreement among the coders. The simplest reliability coefficient is percentage of agreement, which is the number of agreements divided by total number of units coded. Percentage of agreement provides a straightforward way of determining concordance; however, it overestimates reliability because it does not consider chance agreements, or times when agreement among coders occurs accidentally and not because coders were carefully following the coding scheme (Riffe et al., 2014). Cohen's kappa (κ) and Krippendorff's alpha (α) are two commonly used reliability coefficients that account for chance agreement. κ measures reliability between two raters under the assumption that the data are a nominal level of measurement; whereas α assesses chance-corrected agreement among multiple raters with data measured as nominal, ordinal, interval, or ratio. Both κ and α have a range from .00 (no agreement) to 1.0 (complete agreement) with coefficients closer to 1.0 indicating higher levels of agreement among coders. Krippendorff's alpha coefficients at or above .80 indicate acceptable reliability; different benchmarks exist for interpreting Cohen's kappa. One common approach is to consider coefficients above .75 as indicating excellent agreement (Krippendorff, 2018). When perfect agreement is unlikely, such as when content analysts use ordinal, interval, or ratio levels of measurement, it can be more useful to examine covariation among coders using Spearman's rho (ρ) for ordinal variables or intraclass correlation coefficients (ICCs) for interval and ratio data. Higher Spearman's rho coefficients or ICCs on a scale of .00 to 1.0 indicate greater levels of agreement among coders.

Riffe et al. (2014) suggest calculating multiple measures of reliability, such as percentage of agreement and Krippendorff's alpha, for each variable in the study as they argue that the true level of reliability will likely fall somewhere between these two coefficients. It is important to examine the reliability coefficients of each variable rather than reviewing the average value of all inter-coder reliability coefficients because reviewing each coefficient can provide greater clarity as to what specific variables or levels of measurement are causing disagreements among the coders. When a study includes more than two coders, inter-coder reliability coefficients should be calculated for every possible combination of coders (e.g., if a team has three coders, you will calculate inter-coder reliability for coder 1 and coder 2, coder 1 and coder 3, and coder 2 and coder 3). Examining pairwise comparisons can reveal possible inconsistencies in coding decisions and identify coders who need more training. Finally, you have to decide how to manage coding disagreements. Two ways that disagreements can be resolved are using majority rule or having the coding team meet to discuss and try to resolve the disagreements. Making final decisions based solely on how the majority of coders interpreted a messaging unit is less time consuming; however, taking time to discuss disagreements and come to consensus during the pilot test can improve consistency among coders during the final coding process (step 7).

As part of their coder training, the counseling center staff met to review the codebook and practice coding using 15 Change Planning Forms from the previous academic year and before they began collecting data on client alcohol problems. Next, they independently coded a random sample of 50 messaging units for the pilot test. The coding form that they use is an Excel spreadsheet containing two tabs, one for each research question. There are multiple messaging units per Change Planning Form for research question 1, so the group coded units from 16 forms. For research question 2, they coded 50 Change Planning Forms. Despite this number being over a third of the total sample size, the staff decided to code 50 participants because it is the minimum number recommended by Neuendorf (2017) and because they anticipated challenges in agreeing on a single rating of motivation for each client in the full sample given that they were using responses to two questions on the Change Planning Form to make that determination. The pilot was conducted in two rounds with coders reviewing 25 units over two weeks, then meeting to reconcile differences and review the codebook before coding the remaining 25 units over another two-week time period. Using the KALPHA macro for SPSS (Hayes & Krippendorff, 2007), the staff calculated the percentage of agreement and Krippendorff's alpha reliability estimates for each combination of the three coders across all variables following each round. If you do not have access to SPSS, there are free online web applications that you can upload your data into to calculate Krippendorff's alpha and other reliability statistics (e.g., K-Alpha Calculator; Marzi et al., 2023). See Table 11.4 for final reliability estimates from the pilot test.

The pilot test improved the coding scheme in a number of ways. When coding the first batch of 25 messaging units, coders struggled with distinguishing between several of the TTM processes of change. Following discussion, the coding team revised the codebook to clarify the differences between counterconditioning and stimulus control (i.e., that stimulus control represented altering ones environment, not applying new behavioral or cognitive strategies), as well as consciousness raising and self-revaluation (i.e., consciousness-raising examples reflected learning new facts or information in support of change, whereas self-reevaluation represents self-reflection about the impact that drinking has had on the client's values or identity). When they completed the pilot test, the range of agreement coefficients for each combination of coders across the ten processes of change variables exceeded .80.

After coding 50 messaging units for research question 2, the coding team did not observe any examples of the level of measurement amotivation. Clients fill out the Change Planning Form as part of an intervention designed to increase their motivation; therefore, it was not surprising to the team that they did not observe client responses that reflected no motivation at all to change. Analysis of Krippendorff's alpha also revealed coder disagreement in assigning three levels of the taxonomy of motivation: Identified regulation, integrated regulation,

Table 11.4 Pilot Test Reliability Coefficients

Pairwise Comparisons	Percentage of Agreement	Krippendorff's Alpha
Research question 1		
Coders 1 and 2	85%–97%	.81–.97
Coders 1 and 3	86%–90%	.83–.87
Coders 2 and 3	82%–93%	.81–.90
Research question 2		
Coders 1 and 2	90%	.85
Coders 1 and 3	91%	.87
Coders 2 and 3	87%	.84

Note: Ranges reported in research question 1 include all ten processes of change. Coefficients were calculated following pilot test of 50 messaging units for each research question..

and intrinsic motivation. Recognizing that differentiating between these types of motivation in client responses was difficult, the coding team collapsed their scale into three levels: (1) amotivation and external; (2) introjected; and (3) identified, integrated, and intrinsic motivation. Whereas this change in scale impacts the semantic validity of the results, the coders believed that it was justified due to the subtle differences in how each type of motivation is defined and the type of data they were using in the study. They also believed that their revised scale was still a valid representation of the construct as it reflected increasingly internalized motives. After re-coding pilot test data using the revised scale, all Krippendorff alpha coefficients for coder pairwise comparisons exceeded .80.

Final Coding

In step 7, the coding team separately code the remaining messaging units. The number of messaging units left for research questions 1 and 2 are 448 and 93. To make a final assessment of reliability (step 8), a random sample of 50 messaging units are coded by all three coders. The remaining 398 messaging units for research question 1 are divided evenly among the coding team and coders are assigned an additional 132 messaging units each to code separately. For research question 2, coders are assigned an additional 14 messaging units. If coder agreement does not reach adequate levels during the pilot test, the coding team can conduct a second reliability assessment using a new random subset of messaging units from the full sample. Another option is to assign all units to multiple coders to estimate inter-coder reliability for the entire sample. The last option can yield robust evidence of replicability but is more feasible when there are fewer messaging units (Riffe et al., 2014).

If the coding process takes an extended period of time, content analysts should monitor intra-coder reliability. This can be done by having each member of the coding team code a small percentage of messaging units twice to calculate intra-coder percentage of agreement. This type of reliability is generally regarded as supplemental to inter-coder reliability (Neuendorf, 2017) and there are few guidelines available for determining when and how to measure intra-coder reliability in CA. Riffe et al. (2014) suggest assessing intra-coder reliability using a random sample of approximately 40 messaging units if the coding process exceeds a month. If there are concerns of possible coder drift because of the complexity of the coding scheme or length of time coders have to finish coding all messaging units, it can be advantageous to monitor the stability of the coding team's application of the codebook. Observing disagreements in how particular messaging units are coded might indicate that additional training or further refinement of the coding scheme are necessary. Because the counseling center staff planned to finish all coding within one month, they did not assess intra-coder reliability.

Final Assessment of Reliability

Inter-coder reliability is assessed once the final coding process is finished. Coders should not know which messaging units are used in the reliability sample; that way, the estimates of reliability will better reflect the level of coder agreement in the full sample (Riffe et al., 2014). Similar to the pilot test, multiple reliability coefficients should be calculated for each variable. Further, pairwise comparisons of each coder combination should be estimated to provide a more precise representation of agreement among coders. Once reliability is evaluated, the coding team settles any final coding disagreements and examines messaging units that they had trouble coding (i.e., messaging units coded as "uncertain"). As with the pilot test, content analysts can meet to discuss and reach a consensus about what codes to assign to these messaging units. Another way to manage disagreements is to use majority rule to determine the final codes that will be used in the analyses (Step 9).

In the final assessment of reliability, coefficients for all study variables exceeded Krippendorff's α = .80. Pairwise comparisons of all possible codes showed excellent concordance among coders. Because inter-coder reliability was acceptable, the staff decided to use a majority rule system to manage disagreements in coding messaging units. More specifically, the level of measurement assigned by two of the three coders would become the final coding decision. The coding team met to address messaging units that they were unable to code and decide on units in which all three coders provided a different level of measurement. Eight units for research question 1 were left coded as "uncertain" because they were either so vague or illegible that the coding team was unable to interpret what was written. All units were coded using the level of motivation variable for research question 2.

Analyses and Reportage

We have finally reached the last step of conducting a CA. In step 9, content analysts aggregate the messaging units based on the coding results and conduct statistical analyses to answer your research questions. Depending on the nature of the study, it may be useful to report descriptive statistics or create a table or bar graph of the frequency distribution of the variables. Because replicability is such a critical aspect of CA, it is important to provide a step-by-step description of the procedures used in the study (Krippendorff, 2018) along with evidence of inter-coder reliability for the pilot test and final coding stage in the final report.

The counseling center staff tabulated the coded messaging units for research question 1 into a table listing each TTM process of change. Next, they created a composite variable for clients with the total number of TTM processes of change found in their Change Planning Form. This was the dependent variable used in the Mann Whitney U test. The staff compared client total TTM processes between two independent groups, clients who had a clinically significant reduction in alcohol problems at follow-up ($n = 62$) and clients who either reported no reliable change or had reported a significant increase in alcohol problems at follow-up ($n = 81$).

After confirming that the data met the assumptions of a Mann Whitney U test, the counseling center staff conducted the analysis using SPSS version 29. Results indicated that there was a significant difference ($U = 113, p = .001$) with clients in the clinically significant change group reporting more TTM process ($M = 5.34, SD = 1.81$) than clients whose reported number of alcohol problems did not change or had increased at follow up ($M = 3.43, SD = 2.13$). The magnitude of this difference was meaningful, with Cohen's $d = 0.97$ signifying a large effect size (Cohen, 1992). Based on these findings, the staff can consider how they can provide clients with more exposure to the various processes that propel behavior change. They also can conduct exploratory post hoc analyses to determine if particular TTM processes of change (e.g., experiential compared to behavioral processes of change) vary based on reported change in alcohol problems at follow-up.

For research question 2, the staff computed descriptive statistics for the variable, level of motivation, as well as client scores on the B-YAACQ. Before conducting the analysis, they confirmed that the data met all the assumptions of Spearman's rank-order correlation. Results indicated that there was a negative correlation between level of motivation and alcohol problems, $r_s (141) = -.25$, $p = .022$. According to Cohen (1988), the strength of this relationship reflects a small to medium effect size. This relationship suggests that the way in which clients articulate their motives at termination can help predict future alcohol use behaviors. These findings can inform the way that the staff address extrinsic and intrinsic motivators during counseling and also can contribute to the development of novel approaches to checking in with clients who have low levels of internalized motivation post termination. Further, the staff could conduct an exploratory post hoc analysis examining the extent to which each TTM process of change accounts for variance in the taxonomy of motivation variable. Potentially, this kind of analysis (using ordinal regression) can identify what processes of change best explain levels of internally regulated behavior change.

Practice-Based Application

Think about the client-presenting concern, symptom, or situation that you identified in Chapter 1. Brainstorm possible hypotheses or assumptions that you have about these ideas.
Develop a CA study to investigate those hypotheses. Consider the following questions:

- What are some examples of possible texts (e.g., client homework, intake documentation, recorded sessions, etc.) that you can analyze to help test your hypotheses, and consider how you might unitize these texts.
- Consider how you will operationalize and measure the constructs you want to test.
- Who can you ask for help in coding the texts so you can gather evidence of reliability in your pilot test and final coding process?

Resources for More Information

Peer-Reviewed Journal Articles

McKibben, W. B., Cade, R., Purgason, L. L., & Wahesh, E. (2020). How to conduct a deductive content analysis in counseling research. *Counseling Outcome Research and Evaluation*, *13*(2), 156–168. https://doi.org/10.1080/21501378.2020.1846992
Nice, M. L., Brubaker, M. D., Gibson, D. M., McMullen, J. W., Asempapa, B., Kennedy, S. D., ... Moore, C. M. (2023). Wellness and well-being in counseling research: A 31-year content analysis. *Journal of Counseling & Development*, *101*(3), 251–263. https://doi.org/10.1002/jcad.12467

Books

Neuendorf, K. A. (2017). *The content analysis guidebook* (2nd ed.). SAGE Publications.
Krippendorff, K. (2018). *Content analysis: An introduction to its methodology*. SAGE Publications.

Questions for Further Review and Application

1 In what ways does CA differ from traditional qualitative methods of textual analysis?
2 What types of coefficients are used to evaluate reliability in CA?
3 How are reliability and validity evaluated in CA research?
4 What are the two approaches content analysts can use to manage coder differences? Describe the strengths and weaknesses of each approach.
5 Develop a research question suitable for CA. Follow steps 1–4 to establish a conceptual basis for your study, define and operationalize the levels of measurement for your variables, and consider possible texts that you can code to answer your research question.

References

Apodaca, T. R., Borsari, B., Jackson, K. M., Magill, M., Longabaugh, R., Mastroleo, N. R., & Barnett, N. P. (2014). Sustain talk predicts poorer outcomes among mandated college student drinkers receiving a brief motivational intervention. *Psychology of Addictive Behaviors, 28*(3), 631–638. https://psycnet.apa.org/doi/10.1037/a0037296

Braun, V., & Clarke, V. (2006). Using thematic analysis in psychology. *Qualitative Research in Psychology, 3*(2), 77–101. https://doi.org/10.1191/1478088706qp063oa

Cohen, J. (1988). *Statistical power analysis for the behavioral sciences* (2nd ed.). Lawrence Erlbaum Associates.

Cohen, J. (1992). Statistical power analysis. *Current Directions in Psychological Science, 1*(3), 98–101. https://doi.org/10.1111/1467-8721.ep10768783

Fachini, A., Aliane, P. P., Martinez, E. Z., & Furtado, E. F. (2012). Efficacy of brief alcohol screening intervention for college students (BASICS): A meta-analysis of randomized controlled trials. *Substance Abuse Treatment, Prevention, and Policy, 7*(1), 1–10.

Faul, F., Erdfelder, E., Lang, A.-G., & Buchner, A. (2007). G*Power 3: A flexible statistical power analysis for the social, behavioral, and biomedical sciences. *Behavior Research Methods, 39*, 175–191.

Hayes, A. F., & Krippendorff, K. (2007). Answering the call for a standard reliability measure for coding data. *Communication Methods and Measures, 1*(1), 77–89. https://doi.org/10.1080/19312450709336664

Insch, G. S., Moore, J. E., & Murphy, L. D. (1997). Content analysis in leadership research: Examples, procedures, and suggestions for future use. *The Leadership Quarterly, 8*(1), 1–25. https://doi.org/10.1016/S1048-9843(97)90028-X

Jacobson, N. S., & Truax, P. (1992). Clinical significance: A statistical approach to defining meaningful change in psychotherapy research. In A. E. Kazdin (Ed.), *Methodological issues & strategies in clinical research* (pp. 631–648). American Psychological Association. https://doi.org/10.1037/10109-042

Kahler, C. W., Hustad, J., Barnett, N. P., Strong, D. R., & Borsari, B. (2008). Validation of the 30-day version of the Brief Young Adult Alcohol Consequences Questionnaire for use in longitudinal studies. *Journal of Studies on Alcohol and Drugs, 69*(4), 611–615. https://doi.org/10.15288/jsad.2008.69.611

Krippendorff, K. (2018). *Content analysis: An introduction to its methodology.* SAGE Publications.

Velasquez, M. M., Crouch, C., Stephens, N. S., DiClemente, C. C. (2015). *Group treatment for substance abuse: A stages-of-change therapy manual* (2nd ed.). Guilford Publications.

Liese, B. S., Beck, A. T. (2022). *Cognitive-behavioral therapy of addictive disorders* (2nd ed.). Guilford Publications.

Magill, M., Tonigan, J. S., Kiluk, B., Ray, L., Walthers, J., & Carroll, K. (2020). The search for mechanisms of cognitive behavioral therapy for alcohol or other drug use disorders: A systematic review. *Behaviour Research and Therapy, 131*, 103648. https://doi.org/10.1016/j.brat.2020.103648

Marzi, G., Balzano, M., & Marchiori, D. (2023). K-Alpha Calculator - Krippendorff's Alpha Calculator. Retrieved [December 12, 2023], from https://www.k-alpha.org/

Miller, W. R., & Rollnick, S. (2013). *Motivational interviewing: Helping people change* (3rd ed.). Guilford Press.

Neuendorf, K. A. (2017). *The content analysis guidebook* (2nd ed.). SAGE Publications.

Potter, W. J., & Levine-Donnerstein, D. (1999). Rethinking validity and reliability in content analysis. *Journal of Applied Communication Research, 27*(3), 258–284. https://doi.org/10.1080/00909889909365539

Prochaska, J. O., & DiClemente, C. C. (1982). Transtheoretical therapy: Toward a more integrative model of change. *Psychotherapy: Theory, Research & Practice, 19*(3), 276–288. https://psycnet.apa.org/doi/10.1037/h0088437

Riffe, D., Lacy, S., Fico, F. (2014). *Analyzing media messages: Using quantitative content analysis in research* (3rd ed.). Taylor & Francis.

Ryan, R. M., & Deci, E. L. (2020). Intrinsic and extrinsic motivate ion from a self-determination theory perspective: Definitions, theory, practices, and future directions. *Contemporary Educational Psychology, 61*, 101860. https://doi.org/10.1016/j.cedpsych.2020.101860

Schreier, M. (2012). *Qualitative content analysis in practice.* SAGE Publications.

12 Phenomenological Methodology
Merging Research and Practice

Maribeth F. Jorgensen and Kathleen Brown-Rice

Carl Rogers stated, "So I have learned to ask myself, can I hear the sounds and sense the shape of this person's inner world? Can I resonate to what [they are] saying so deeply that I sense the meanings?" (Rogers, 1980, p. 8). Perhaps the most fundamental characteristic of an effective counselor is their ability to listen as a way to understand clients' lived experiences. The counseling process may be the most common platform practitioners think of for listening and gaining access to clients' view of the world; however, conducting research is another pathway. Previous literature has supported the idea that qualitative research may be especially suitable for counselors given the interpersonal connection with participants, and it uncovers and represents voices in different ways than through numbers and statistics (Jorgensen & Duncan, 2015; Kline, 2008).

Qualitative research is a broad term for different research methods such as grounded theory, narrative, case study, ethnography, and phenomenology (Creswell & Creswell, 2022). In this chapter, we will focus on phenomenological methodology. The goal of phenomenological research is to explore and describe the experiences of individuals related to a phenomenon (Creswell & Creswell, 2022). Counselor-researchers (i.e., you!) would aim to do this by collecting data from persons who experienced the phenomenon to extract and describe or give meaning to the what and the how (Moustakas, 1994). Phenomenological methodology guides counselor-researchers to approach their studies with an openness to multiple outcomes, seek and capture what emerges from participants, and continuously remain aware of their assumptions and biases (Husserl, 1931).

Haase and Johnston (2012) suggested phenomenological qualitative research serves to be the most similar to counseling, as it allows people to share their experiences and is most compatible with the process and practice of counseling. Further, phenomenological methodology encompasses philosophies and practices that align well with a counselor professional identity and ethical practices. For example, counselors are trained to acknowledge there are no absolute truths and that each client is an expert on themselves (American Counseling Association, 2014; Anderson & Goolishian, 1992; Bedi & Duff, 2014; Rogers, 1980). Phenomenological methodology also fits counseling ethics such as bracketing thoughts and biases (Kocet & Herlihy, 2014), being culturally competent, ensuring confidentiality, acquiring informed consent from participants, ethically storing documents, and having appropriate boundaries (American Counseling Association, 2014). Also, in phenomenological studies, the information-gathering process is typically done through interviews and asking participants questions, which is a skill counselors hone and use in sessions with clients. According to Jorgensen and Duncan (2015), introducing research methodologies that fit with the skill set of practitioners and goals of counseling best bridges the gap between research and practice.

DOI: 10.4324/9781032706139-12

This gives promise to the idea that counseling and research can easily overlap, and counselors can come to see themselves as counselor-researchers (i.e., develop their researcher identity).

Introduction to the Methodology

Qualitative phenomenological approaches can be traced back to the early 1900s when a German philosopher, Edmund Husserl, suggested people's realities and experiences of a phenomenon were the most valuable source of data (Husserl, 1931; Vagle, 2018). Since that time, many phenomenological research traditions have developed such as empirical/psychological, interpretive, hermeneutic, descriptive, existential, social, reflection/transcendental, and dialogue (Creswell & Creswell, 2022; Husserl, 1931; Merriam & Tisdell, 2015; Patton, 2014, Smith et al., 2022). Some of the differences between the listed phenomenological approaches relate to the researchers view of reality, how information is acquired and accessed (i.e., interview, letter, in-vivo experiences), how researchers engage with the participants and data, how data are analyzed (e.g., interpretive phenomenological analysis involves thorough analysis of each case before moving to the next [Smith et al., 2022]), and how data are conceptualized and shared (Creswell & Creswell, 2022; Smith et al., 2022). Giorgi (1994) indicated that regardless of the variations across the approaches, all seem to be similar in that they seek to honor what emerges from participants, are descriptive in nature, use phenomenological reduction, examine interactions between people and contexts, and capture essences of human lives.

In order to provide a concrete understanding of the phenomenological approach, we will discuss the key aspects such as beliefs about reality (i.e., research philosophy), design considerations (e.g., research questions, participants and sampling, data collection, research ethics), steps for ensuring credibility (i.e., trustworthiness procedures), and the ways to conceptualize information (i.e., data analysis).

Beliefs About Reality

Phenomenological research aligns with constructivism research philosophy. The constructivism research viewpoint honors that there is no absolute truth, and each person *constructs* their own reality around an experience (Smith et al., 2022). The research questions that come from a constructivism philosophy are open in nature and aimed at understanding the *how* and *what* in relation to the phenomenon. This particular philosophy suggests people are the experts on their own reality and, thus, the richest source of data is provided by understanding a specific phenomenon they have experienced (i.e., our lived experiences). This research philosophy parallels one that is widely held by counselors in that clients are the experts on their own lives. Additionally, given these ingredients of phenomenological research, this is a methodology that is particularly fitting to explore topics of diversity, equity, inclusion, and social justice (see Miller et al., 2018, for more detail).

When to Use Phenomenological Approach

Research questions drive the methodology; therefore, it is only appropriate to use phenomenological approaches if they connect *with* the research question(s) (Creswell & Creswell, 2022). Phenomenological approaches are driven by *how* and *what* research questions that are derived from curiosities and few assumptions about a topic and belief the best informants about a reality of a phenomenon are those who have experienced it (Creswell & Creswell, 2022).

Phenomenological research has a lot of utility and can be used in various settings and within multiple disciplines (Patton, 2014). Phenomenological approaches have been used to explore research questions in educational, counseling, nursing, and medical fields with clients, athletes, patients, educators, parents, and multiple other persons (Merriam & Tisdell, 2015). Phenomenological approach has also been used to conduct program evaluation (Patton, 2014). For more examples, see resources and references at the end of this chapter in which researchers utilized phenomenological approaches to explore their research questions.

Research Questions That Drive Phenomenological Approach

Researchers conducting phenomenological studies often have one or two main research questions and sometimes include more specific sub-questions (see Creswell & Creswell, 2022, for more detail). The main research question starts with *what* or *how*, as that allows researchers to get at the essence of experiences and approach a topic with openness to whatever emerges. Some examples of main research questions that start with *what* include: "What are Black mothers' experiences of postpartum mental health support?" or "What are K-12 school counselors' lived experiences of cultural broaching with students' parents?" Some examples of *how* questions might include: "How do older adult men describe their experiences of navigating unanticipated retirement? or "How do adolescent clients describe their lived experiences of counseling related to a death in their immediate family?"

Ways to Gather Information

Further, phenomenological research methods are a fit with counselors' inherent skill set to seek information through multiple ways (e.g., verbal, observation, drawings, letters) and then synthesize into conceptualizations about human experiences (Hays & Wood, 2011). The first step in gathering data is to consider who may be a fit for participating, sampling method, and number of participants needed. Phenomenological research questions are developed to understand the lived experiences of persons who have been involved with the phenomenon under investigation. Therefore, researchers who conduct phenomenological studies often use criteria-based sampling to ensure participants can speak to the studied phenomenon. Researchers not only need to create the criteria for participation, but they also need to provide rationale for why those are important and fit their study (Merriam & Tisdell, 2015).

Some other sampling methods options that are common include snowball sampling, typical sampling, and convenience sampling (Merriam & Tisdell, 2015). Snowball sampling involves participants providing contact information for others who have experienced the studied phenomenon. Typical sampling involves selecting participants who are the average (i.e., no extreme characteristics) representation of the participant group. Convenience sampling involves selecting participants based on easy access (Merriam & Tisdell, 2015). The number of participants you will need is dependent on several factors such as the specific type of phenomenological study you are conducting. For example, interpretive phenomenological studies can include fewer participants (between 3–10) given that approach is more concerned about depth within a specific context (Smith et al., 2022). Other professional guidance suggests between five and 25 participants (Polkinghorne, 1989). However, other individuals state the number of participants is determined by when you no longer hear any new information (e.g., data saturation) about the phenomenon during data collection (Merriam & Tisdell, 2015). Since there are variations in what is suggested, it is best to refer to guiding scholarly literature and published studies that utilized the phenomenological approach you are considering for your study. For examples of guiding literature and studies, see the resources provided at the end of the chapter.

The methods for gathering information (i.e., data) are somewhat up to you, but it is important to state the rationale and use more than one method to develop thoroughness of findings (Kline, 2008; Vagle, 2018). Additionally, it is helpful to also state the reasons (anchor this in professional literature) for the decisions about how and amount of data-gathering methods you use in your study. According to Creswell and Creswell (2022), methods for investigation under phenomenological approaches include demographic questionnaires, individual interviews, focus groups, pictorial representations, and artifacts (e.g., poems, pictures). According to Denzin and Lincoln (2008), "each practice makes the world visible in different ways. Hence, there is frequently a commitment to using more than one interpretive practice in any study" (p. 5). Although there are many options for gathering information, the most common in phenomenological approaches is conducting individual interviews (Creswell & Creswell, 2022). When reviewing recently published phenomenological studies, you will see some researchers chose to conduct two interviews with each participant for more thoroughness (see Salpietro et al., 2023, for more detail).

Let's consider a phenomenological study in which you decide to conduct interviews. The structure of interviews is important to consider, as it can impact the depth of information provided by participants. Considering phenomenological research aligns with a constructivism viewpoint (i.e., multiple realities), it is important you develop interview protocols in ways that facilitate an open environment for the participant to express their realities. There are three most common interview formats: (1) structured, (2) semi-structured, and (3) unstructured (Creswell & Creswell, 2022). A structured interview involves you asking a predetermined set of questions, exactly as worded, and without asking follow-up questions. A semi-structured interview allows for more flexibility due to you having predetermined questions, but order can be changed, and you can ask follow-up questions during the interview. Last, an unstructured interview is conducted without predetermined questions and allows for follow-up questions. Creswell and Creswell (2022) suggested that semi-structured seems to be the most common, with the use of approximately five open-format questions. Ultimately, the questions in the interview need to be anchored back to the research question(s), and be constructed in an inclusive (e.g., consider the words you use and how those will impact your participants) and informed way by exploring related scholarly literature and having others review the questions and give feedback. Other things to consider during interviews include strategies for bracketing your biases and making notes, ways to record the interview, appropriate length of interview, and mode of interview (e.g., face to face, virtual platform, or over phone; Creswell & Creswell, 2022).

Additional information-gathering strategies can be used to supplement your interviews. For example, you might ask the participants to draw a picture to offer another way to describe their experiences of the phenomenon. Poldma and Stewart (2004) stated visual representations "allow for the creation of new insights using art either as the starting point for creative thought generation or as the means by which new meanings in the research can be expressed" (p. 146). You could also ask your participants to bring in an artifact. For example, Leagjeld et al. (2021) asked counselors who worked with rural women to bring an item (e.g., letters, poem, artwork) to their interviews that represented their work with rural women. Participants brought artifacts such as pictures, poems, stories – all of which enriched the description of their work with rural women clients (see Leagjeld et al., 2021, for more details).

Ways to Conceptualize the Information

Another important step in the phenomenological approach is the information conceptualization (i.e., data analysis) process. The overall goal of the conceptualization process is to develop main themes and subthemes (think of the themes we pull out from client content within and across sessions) that give voice to participants' lived experiences. The research themes need to be linked to the research question(s) (Creswell & Creswell, 2022; Merriam & Tisdell, 2015). We will share about an analysis procedure Moustakas (1994) created, which is a simplified, comprehensive method as modified from Stevick-Colaizzi-Keen (see Creswell, 2012, for more detail):

1. Revisit and expand on the experience you have with the phenomenon under investigation (i.e., researcher statement). This will assist you in setting aside biases and thoughts related to the topic.
2. Find and list important statements made by participants regarding how they experienced the phenomenon. You will need to examine your written notes on transcriptions and other research documents (i.e., margin notes and codes).
3. Group statements into main themes (i.e., research themes) that collapse many of the important statements based on overlap (i.e., meaning units).
4. Describe what happened in relation to the phenomenon (i.e., textural description).
5. Describe how the phenomenon was experienced (i.e., structural description).
6. Narrate the experience by combining the textural and structural descriptions.

It is important to note at the inception of your study idea and during the entire research process that you need to be involved in procedures that hold you accountable to most accurately interpreting the participants' words (i.e., trustworthiness procedures). Trustworthiness procedures are intended to make sure the findings are valid and credible (Giorgi, 1994; Kline, 2008; Moustakas, 1994; Polkinghorne, 1989). Trustworthiness procedures might be compared to the strategies counselors use to acknowledge and bracket their own thoughts about session content and client experiences so they can understand the pure meaning from client stories. Although there are no uniform guidelines on the number of trustworthiness procedures to employ in a phenomenological study, Waalkes et al. (2021) found, on average, researchers used four when conducting qualitative studies.

Some examples of trustworthiness procedures include being transparent about your own experience in relation to the phenomenon being investigated (i.e., researcher statement), prolonged engagement with the data, writing notes about your thoughts during the research process (i.e., research memos, field journal, reflexive journaling), having a peer review the research materials (i.e., peer review), and sending research materials to your participants to have them verify accuracy and give feedback (i.e., member check) (Creswell & Creswell, 2022; Giorgi, 1994). Waalkes et al. (2021) indicated the top four most frequently used trustworthiness procedures included researcher statement, member checking, reflexive journaling, and peer review.

We know this has been a lot of information to consume so let's take a moment to pause. In your moment of pause, consider reflecting on how the information thus far connects with the work you are currently doing or will do with clients or students. Please jot down those thoughts and add to those as we now move into a case example – one which has been informed by our own experiences working in the field as licensed counselors.

Case Example: Where Did the Client Go?

In this section, we present a case example to model the process of designing a phenomenological study that could be directly applied to your work with clients or students. Additionally, this will allow you to see that you already have many of the skills and the researcher mindset to conduct a qualitative study using a phenomenological approach.

Carol (she/her) graduated with a master's degree in clinical mental health counseling two years ago. She is employed as a licensed professional counselor (LPC) and works in a community mental health counseling setting with ten other LPCs, two clinical supervisors, two support staff, and one clinic director. She schedules between 20 and 30 sessions per week. While having weekly case consultations with her LPC colleagues, she notices a trend across counselors that there are clients who end services and never return to counseling after the first session. When talking with her friends in private practice settings, it seems like this might be a more frequent occurrence in community mental health settings. These conversations with counselors make her become curious about understanding what contributes to clients suddenly ending services after their first session. Are there cultural considerations? Issues occurring within agency settings regarding policies and procedures? Carol decides she wants to do research on this topic and asks one of her colleagues, Robyn (she/her), to join as a co-researcher (YAY! The combination of research and social connection!). Robyn says yes! Carol will be the lead researcher and do the majority of the steps, and they will work out the details and roles prior to starting their study (to follow research ethics). Carol feels passionate that if they can learn more through their research, perhaps they can create data-informed interventions counselors can employ during the first session to keep clients coming back to get the services they need ... and the research begins!!

Carol and Robyn Design Their Study

Based on previous information in this chapter, we know that Carol and Robyn will need to consider all of the following: Their beliefs about reality (i.e., philosophical assumptions and phenomenological traditions), what they want to explore (i.e., research questions), with whom and how they will gather information (i.e., participants, sampling, and data collection), research ethics, how they ensure their findings are credible (i.e. trustworthiness procedures), how they will conceptualize the information (i.e., data analysis), and how and with whom they will disseminate the information (i.e., presentation of research findings).

Carol and Robyn's Beliefs About Reality

Carol and Robyn believe there is no absolute answer or truth to the question they have about clients ending counseling after one session, but there might be common shared experiences. Although they both have some existing biases and assumptions (that they will bracket), they believe there has to be multiple and shared reasons. Their beliefs about multiple realities and people being the experts of their own experiences lead them to ask research questions that align with phenomenological methodology.

Carol and Robyn Want to Explore

In the process of talking with their colleagues and conducting a review of scholarly resources (see chapter on literature review for more on this research step), they begin to figure out what they want to explore. The literature review process allows them to develop the need for their study and refine phrasing of what they want to examine (i.e., research questions). The literature review process also helps them confirm they are filling a gap in what currently exists (Creswell & Creswell, 2022). From what they find in the literature, most researchers utilized quantitative methodologies, focused on termination of services across the treatment episode, and examined variables such as gender identity, age, employment status, marital status, family issues, and substance use (Kelly & Moos, 2003; Saxon et al., 2010; Claus & Kindleberger, 2002). That information helps them know the gaps and also think about what setting and contexts they might want to consider when crafting their research question(s). Based on past research and their beliefs about reality, Carol and Robyn decide on the type of phenomenological approach and their research questions.

Carol and Robyn decide they will conduct a transcendental phenomenological study and explore the following research questions: *What are the lived experiences of clients in community mental health agency settings that end counseling after one session?* Other aspects they would like to examine include (i.e., sub-questions): *How do clients come to the decision to end counseling after one session? What role does a client's personal life and experiences play in their decision to end counseling after one session? What role does a client's experiences of their counselor play in their decision to end counseling after one session? What role do elements of the counseling setting play in clients' decisions to end counseling after one session?*

Carol and Robyn Decide About Participants

Carol and Robyn will need to consider previous literature to understand participant contexts and settings that have been previously studied. They will also need to revisit the research question(s) to make sure their participants can inform what they want to explore. Carol and Robyn will sample participants who were being seen in a community mental agency health setting when they decided to end counseling services after one session. In the process of creating other specific participant criteria, Carol and Robyn develop brief criteria for participants that include the following: (1) started a counseling experience in a community mental health agency setting; (2) stopped seeing that same counselor after only one session; (3) that event occurred within the last two years (must have accurate recall of the event); (4) and over the age of 19 (must be able to provide informed consent for self).

Given research is time intensive and finding participants can be difficult, Carol and Robyn decide to use both criteria-based and convenience sampling. Other participant considerations include recruitment and number of participants needed. Since Carol and Robyn are using a convenience sampling approach, they decide they will recruit participants in their agency. They will have study invitation flyers at their agency front desk and posted in the lobby. Carol will take participants who are not her clients through the informed consent and gather data with them as well. Robyn will take any of Carol's clients through the informed consent and gather data with them. These steps will be taken to reduce coercion to participate and avoid dual boundaries between the researchers and their own clients. Lastly, Carol and Robyn will aim for 10–15 participants, but ultimately stop collecting data when they hear no new information from participants (e.g., data saturation).

Carol and Robyn Decide How to Collect Information

Carol and Robyn must also decide how they will go about collecting information (i.e., data) from their participants. Carol and Robyn learn the hallmark of phenomenological research is to conduct interviews, with the most common format being semi-structured. Carol and Robyn decide they will conduct interviews with their participants and request visual representations. Carol and Robyn will also get demographic data (e.g., age, gender identity, racial identity, partnered status, social class identity, sources of relational support, and so on) by having their participants complete a questionnaire. Carol and Robyn will ask the following questions in semistructured interviews (which they have informed by literature and through two rounds of review with counseling colleagues at their agency):

1 Tell me about the counseling experience you ended after one session.
2 What, if anything, did the counselor do that contributed to you wanting to end that counseling experience after one session?
3 What, if anything, happened during that first session that contributed to you wanting to end that counselling experience?
4 What, if anything, did the counseling agency staff do that contributed to you wanting to end that counseling experience after one session?
5 What, if anything, was going on for you that contributed to you wanting to end that counseling experience after one session?
6 What, if anything, happened in the counseling setting that contributed to you wanting to end the experience after one session?
7 Draw a picture of the visual you get when thinking about that counseling experience (explain the picture to me).
8 What, if anything, would you like to share with me about that counseling experience that I have not asked about?

Carol and Robyn decide they will have interviews over a secure virtual platform and record only audio. After interviews are recorded, Carol and Robyn will transcribe each interview they conduct on to a Word document, delete all identifiers and attach participant-selected pseudonyms, number each line, use large text, and put a space between when they speak and when the participants speak. They will attach the picture the participant draws to the associated transcript. All research documents will be stored in a way that follows research ethics.

Carol and Robyn Follow Research Ethics

We have already discussed some research ethics in their study and will share more specifics here regarding other research ethics Carol and Robyn need to follow (See also the chapter in this textbook about research ethics). Just like in our counseling practices, Carol and Robyn need to adhere to research ethics from the inception of their study idea. Carol and Robyn will need to connect with a local Institutional Review Board (IRB) to get specific instructions. They also will need to submit their study information to an IRB to get official approval of the study *prior* to actually collecting data. Staff at that IRB office will walk them through procedures to follow and documents to construct for the study (e.g., informed consent, study invitation, and so on) as well as other research ethics steps. For example, they will need to complete the research ethics training through whatever IRB office they submit their study. Other things Carol and Robyn must think about include how they will recruit in ways that respect the privacy of participants and minimize coercion to participate. They will also need to let participants know interviews will be around 60 to 90 minutes and that participants can drop out of the study at any point. Further, they will need to get documented informed consent from participants, conduct interviews in private locations to promote honest responses and confidentiality, and remove participants' actual names (i.e., use pseudonyms) when reporting the findings.

Carol and Robyn will need to store their hard copy research materials in a locked filing cabinet behind a locked door at their counseling office. They believe Carol's counseling office is a secure location, and having research materials at her office will further accentuate the merging of their professional identities of counselor and researcher. Carol will have separate filing cabinets for her counseling documents and research documents. Any electronic research materials will be stored on a password-protected computer.

Carol and Robyn Ensure Credibility of Their Research

Trustworthiness strategies will help Carol and Robyn stay attuned with their own thoughts, feelings, and biases. This will help them better engage with the data and accurately represent their participants' experiences. They decide to use four trustworthiness procedures. They both will write a researcher statement at the start of their study, keep a researcher journal (i.e., reflexive journaling) during the entire research process, use member checks, and conduct a peer review process. In the process of writing researcher statements, they will write a thorough description about their thoughts and feelings about the reasons clients end counseling after one session, their own professional and personal experiences with the phenomenon, and acknowledge any important cultural identities that may be relevant to the study and their roles as researchers. While both researchers would need to create a researcher statement before they start the study, we will just share a snippet from Carol's here:

> This is my first study, so I am new to research and only have my past experiences in my counseling research methods course to draw on. I have been a counselor in a community mental health agency setting for 2 years. At first, I did not give much thought to clients no-showing sessions. I figured they had other things going on or did not want to commit to counseling. I then noticed a few clients here and there stopped coming after the first session and I never heard from them again. I had actually started counseling before and decided after the first session that it was not a good fit, and I could not travel to see them on a regular basis. I particularly did not like the approach of the counselor because it seemed more like casual dialogue. I also struggled with finances at the time, and ended up realizing I could not pay out of pocket until my deductible kicked in. I had this also occur when I was a child as my parents struggled with money and could not pay for the counseling I needed. Reflecting on my own experience in relation to exiting counseling after one session made me even more curious about this. When it happens with my own clients, I often think it might be because clients do not have time, financial resources, adequate transportation, family support, or a commitment to change. I also wonder if it related to something I did –perhaps my identities were not a best fit for the client, or they did not appreciate my approach to the counseling session.

Member checks will involve Carol and Robyn sending participants their transcribed interviews to make sure there has been an accurate, word-for-word representation of what they said. They will also send themes and associated quotes from each transcript to all participants once they have completed their conceptualization of the information they gather. Additionally, Robyn will serve as the peer reviewer of the research process. This will involve Carol having Robyn read all the transcripts and completing the same process Carol goes through to analyze and conceptualize the information. These steps will be done so Robyn can make an informed review of Carol's conceptualizations and research themes. The peer review process will also include regular meetings for them to talk about and integrate any differences in their conceptualizations. Lastly, both Carol and Robyn will keep a researcher journal throughout the entire research process as a platform for reflecting on biases, observations, and thoughts that come up during their study.

Carol and Robyn Conceptualize Information

In the process of conceptualizing information (i.e., data analysis), Carol and Robyn will individually do these steps and regularly meet to discuss their reflections. Carol will lead the data analysis and Robyn will serve as the peer reviewer to ensure credibility and accuracy of findings. They will start by revisiting and further developing their researcher statements, which will allow them to reflect again on their own beliefs and assumptions about the phenomenon. While reading the transcribed interviews, they will write notes on the transcripts and other research documents (i.e., making margin notes) to put themselves in a reflective state and capture their own thoughts about the process. They will also put a few keywords to the right of sentences to summarize what is being said every few lines to draw out significant statements. They will do this with each transcribed interview. These steps will help Carol and Robyn list important statements made by participants and group those words to create units of meaning. The goal of the information conceptualization process is to create main and subthemes that illuminate common experiences of all participants.

Once Carol and Robyn have the research themes, they will construct text to give meaning to each. This will involve Carol and Robyn describing what happened (i.e., textural description) and how what happened was experienced (i.e., structural description). Let's consider Carol and Robyn discover a main theme of *financial stressors*. Textural descriptions would provide understanding about the types of financial stressors. For example, the furnace went out, a tire blew, a family member got sick and had medical bills, or a vacation is planned. Structural descriptions would provide understanding about how the stressors were experienced by the participants. Financial stressors could cause participants to panic as they realize they do not have enough money to pay for counseling and unexpected costs. On the other hand, financial stressors could also prompt feelings of resolve, as it could help participants better understand their priorities (e.g., traveling being more important than counseling). These examples would highlight that participants share in common that financial stressors contributed to them quitting counseling after one session, but the types of financial stressors may be different and also experienced in different ways.

Carol and Robyn Share the Information

Once Carol and Robyn have conceptualized the information, they will want to write up and disseminate their findings to intended audiences (e.g., clients, colleagues, other counselors, agency staff, clinic directors). They will share the information in ways that connect to their research questions. Carol and Robyn will need to give a synthesis of the textural and structural descriptions to provide a holistic understanding of the lived experiences of clients who ended counseling after one session. They will also feature several quotes from interviewees under each theme to give voice to their participants and accentuate how their words informed the findings. They could also feature a participant's visual representation to describe the main themes (see Figure 12.1).

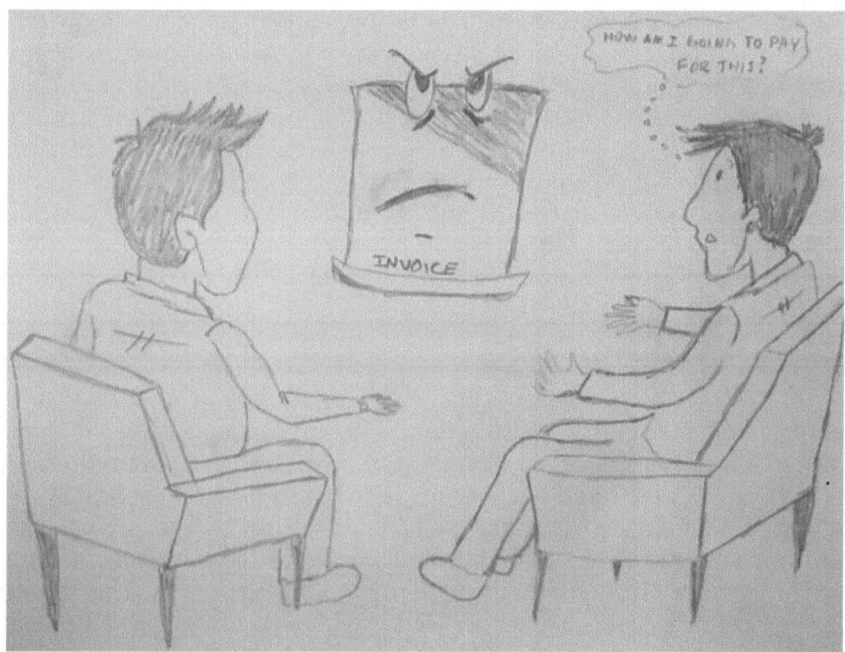

Figure 12.1 Client Drawing.

Note: The participant drew a picture with a focal point of a "mean bill." They said, "I couldn't find a way to pay for counseling, so I had to end counseling after the first session."

Let's continue with finances and say they discover a main theme of *Financial Stressors*. When sharing the findings, they would want to describe how many of their participants indicated financial stressors, contexts from the demographic questionnaire, types of financial stressors, and their experiences of those financial stressors. They would also want to feature quotes to highlight a specific type of financial stressor and how the participant experienced it. Here is an example quote:

> *I found myself feeling very stressed after I attended the first session and got the bill. I was surprised by the cost as that wasn't something discussed during the session. My insurance did not pay for some reason, and I was left with the entire bill of $180.00. I wasn't sure how I was going to afford to pay for counseling. Then, my furnace went out! I was so stressed and now facing the problem of not being able to afford all my bills. I was basically living paycheck to paycheck and I have no have family financial support and my partner could not help. Something had to give, and I didn't know what to do. I ultimately decided that I had to end counseling. I felt really sad about ending because I needed counseling and I really liked the counselor, but I didn't know how else I could solve my money problems. I just wasn't prepared for how expensive counseling was or how to negotiate my health insurance. My counselor never spoke with me about cost. I know I got documents, but I wish they would have talked with me about cost.*

At the onset of their study, Carol and Robyn began thinking about platforms for disseminating their findings. They decided they will share findings in short write-ups and through verbal presentations with their colleagues during case staffing meetings. They will encourage their colleagues to use the information to broach with clients during the first session. For example, should they find social justice issues such as finances are a common reason clients ended counseling, they could give counselors guidance to broach about finances to determine needs and a realistic session frequency. Carol and Robyn also decided they will submit a presentation proposal to their state counseling conference. Additionally, they plan to construct handouts about the findings to share with clients to apply their research directly with their intended audience and with hopes to intercept outcomes of clients ending counseling after first sessions. Carol also has stayed in touch with the professor who taught her counseling research methods course and will reach out to her to ask about research mentorship on pursuing publication (in an open-access, counseling-focused scholarly journal) of their study and interest in joining as a co-author.

Parting Message

Professional counselors in practice have unique insight regarding what will improve client care, and research is a mechanism that can push our profession forward for the betterment of our clients. Further, this methodology is the type of research that is applicable and manageable for you to accomplish in your current practice setting. It also provides an excellent opportunity for you to further develop your clinical expertise by understanding human experience in ways that cannot be captured through the counseling process. The phenomenological approach of exploring and telling the lived experiences of people related to a specific phenomenon (Creswell & Creswell, 2022) is the perfect overlap between counseling and research. In that, what makes you a skilled counselor (e.g., understanding there are multiple realities, asking open questions, bracketing your thoughts and beliefs, desiring to be interactive with people to understand them) makes you already a skilled researcher.

Practice-Based Application

Now, reflect on the prompt in Chapter 1 and the client or student (or something you've seen in your organization, or something that is relevant to your work as a clinician) you've been traveling with throughout this book and consider these application questions:

- What are two examples of phenomenological research questions you could ask about a phenomenon either your client or student (or you, or your organization) is experiencing?
- Let's say you decide to do an interview to gather data. Take one of the research questions you created and develop four interview questions you could include. Describe who you would have review your interview questions and your reasons for selecting that person(s).
- Here's a chance to keep honing your counselor-researcher mindset for getting more and different data. Staying with the same research question, what additional way could you collect data from your clients to integrate with the information you get from interviews? Describe your reasons for selecting that additional data collection method.

Resources for More Information

Conceptual and Empirical Peer-Reviewed Journal Articles

Hays, D., & Wood, C. (2011). Infusing qualitative traditions in counseling research designs. *Journal of Counseling and Development, 89*, 288–295. doi:10.1002/j.1556-6678.2011.tb00091.x
Krennerich, S., Haiyasoso, M., & Flasch, P. S. (2021). Professional counselors' experiences counseling and working in areas repeatedly impacted by hurricanes. *Teaching and Supervision in Counseling, 3*(1), Article 6. https://doi.org/10.7290/tsc030106

Meyer, M., Wiggins, E., & Elliott, G. (2023). Adult adoptees adoption-related experiences of counseling, loss, and grief: A transcendental phenomenological study. *The Professional Counselor*, *13*(2), 129–144. doi: 10.15241/mm.13.2.129

Sackett, C., Mack, H., Sharma, J., Cook, R., & Dogan-Dixon, D. (2023). A phenomenological exploration of counselors-in-training's experiences of microaggressions from clients. *The Professional Counselor*, *13*(2), 145–161. doi: 10.15241/crs.13.2.145

Books

Creswell, J. W., & Creswell, J. D. (2022). *Research design: Qualitative, quantitative, and mixed method approaches* (6th ed.). Sage.

Merriam, S., & Tisdell, E. (2015). *Qualitative research: A guide to design and implementation* (4th ed.). Jossey-Bass.

Moustakas, C. (1994). *Phenomenological research methods*. Sage Publications.

Smith, J., Flowers, P., & Larkin, M. (2022). *Interpretive phenomenological analysis. Theory, method, and research*. Sage.

Vagle, M. (2018). *Crafting phenomenological research* (2nd ed.). Routledge.

Questions for Further Review and Application

1 What is the aim of qualitative phenomenological methodology?
2 What are two reasons a phenomenological approach seems especially fitting for professional counselors to utilize?
3 What are two ethical considerations counseling and phenomenological research have in common?
4 Name and describe the three different formats of interviews that can be used in this research approach.
5. Describe two reasons why it is important to utilize trustworthiness procedures when conducting phenomenological research.

References

American Counseling Association. (2014). *ACA code of ethics*. Author.

Anderson, H., & Goolishian, H. A. (1992). The client is the expert: A not-knowing approach to therapy. In S. McNamee & K. J. Gergen (Eds.), *Therapy as social construction* (pp. 25–39). Sage Publications.

Bedi, R. P., & Duff, C. T. (2014). Client as expert: A Delphi poll of clients' subjective experience of therapeutic alliance formation variables. *Counselling Psychology Quarterly*, *27*(1), 1–18. doi:10.1080/09515070.2013.857295

Claus, R., & Kindleberger, L. (2002). Engaging substance abusers after centralized assessment: Predictors of treatment entry and dropout. *Journal of Psychoactive Drugs*, *34*, 25–31. doi:10.1080/02791072.2002.10399933

Creswell, J. (2012). *Qualitative inquiry and research design: Choosing among five approaches* (3rd ed.). Thousand Oaks, CA: Sage.

Creswell, J. W., & Creswell, J. D. (2022). *Research design: Qualitative, quantitative, and mixed method approaches* (6th ed.). Sage.

Denzin, N., & Lincoln, Y. (2008). *Strategies of qualitative inquiry* (3rd ed.). Sage Publications.

Giorgi, A. (1994). A phenomenological perspective on certain qualitative research methods. *Journal of Phenomenological Psychology*, *25*, 190–220. doi:10.1163/156916294X00034

Haase, T., & Johnston, N. (2012). Making meaning out of loss: A story and study of young widowhood. *Journal of Creativity in Mental Health*, *7*, 204–221. doi:10.1080/15401383.2012.710170

Hays, D., & Wood, C. (2011). Infusing qualitative traditions in counseling research designs. *Journal of Counseling & Development*, *89*, 288–295. doi:10.1002/j.1556-6678.2011.tb00091.x

Husserl, E. (1931). *Ideas pertaining to a pure phenomenology and to a phenomenological philosophy: First book*. K. Kersten (Trans.). Springer.

Jorgensen, M., & Duncan, K. (2015). A grounded theory of master's-level counselor research identity. *Counselor Education and Supervision*, *54*, 17–31. doi:10.1002/j.1556-6978.2015.00067

Kelly, J., & Moos, R. (2003). Dropout from 12-step self-help groups: Prevalence, predictors, and counteracting treatment influences. *Journal of Substance Abuse Treatment, 24*, 241–250. doi:10.1016/S0740-5472(03)00021-7

Kline, B. (2008). Developing and submitting credible qualitative manuscripts. *Counselor Education and Supervision, 47*, 210–217. doi:10.1002/j.1556-6978.2008.tb00052.x

Kocet, M. M., & Herlihy, B. J. (2014). Addressing value-based conflicts within the counseling relationship: A decision-making model. *Journal of Counseling & Development, 92*(2), 180–186. doi:10.1002/j.1556-6676.2014.00146.x

Miller, R., Chan, C., & Farmer, L. (2018). Interpretive phenomenological analysis: A contemporary qualitative approach. *Counselor Education and Supervision, 57*, 240–254. DOI: 10.1002/ceas.12114

Leagjeld, L., Waalkes, P., & Jorgensen, M. (2021). Mental health counselors' perceptions of rural women clients. *The Professional Counselor, 11*(1), 86–101. doi: 10.15241/lal.11.1.86

Merriam, S., & Tisdell, E. (2015). *Qualitative research: A guide to design and implementation* (4th ed.). Jossey-Bass.

Moustakas, C. (1994). *Phenomenological research methods*. Sage Publications.

Patton, M. (2014). *Qualitative research and evaluation methods* (4th ed.). Sage Publications.

Poldma, T., & Stewart, M. (2004). Understanding the value of artistic tools such as visual concept maps in design and education research. *Art Design & Communication in Higher Education, 3*, 141–148. doi:10.1386/adch.3.3.141/1

Polkinghorne, D. (1989). Phenomenological research methods. In R. S. Valle & S. Halling (Eds.), *Existential-phenomenological perspectives in psychology: Exploring the breadth of human experience* (pp. 41–60). Plenum Press.

Rogers, C. (1980). *A way of being*. Houghton Mifflin Company.

Salpietro, L., Ausloos, C. D., Clark, M., Zacarias, R., & Perez, J. (2023). Confidential grief: How counselors cope with client suicide. *Journal of Counseling & Development, 101*, 461–474. https://doi.org/10.1002/jcad.12484

Saxon, D., Ricketts, T., & Heywood, J. (2010). Who drops-out? Do measures of risk to self and to others predict unplanned endings in primary care counselling? *Counselling and Psychotherapy Research, 10*, 13–21. doi:10.1080/14733140902914604

Smith, J., Flowers, P., & Larkin, M. (2022). *Interpretive phenomenological analysis. Theory, method, and research*. SAGE Publications.

Vagle, M. (2018). *Crafting phenomenological research* (2nd ed.). Routledge.

Waalkes, P., DeCino, D., & Flynn, S. V. (2021). A content analysis of qualitative dissertations in counselor education. *Counselor Education and Supervision, 60*(3), 209–223. https://doi.org/10.1002/ceas.12212

13 Photovoice

Heather Trepal and Yuliya Cannon

Introduced originally by Wang and Burris (1994) as *photo novella* (meaning photo story), photovoice has emerged as an innovative and participatory qualitative research method. In this method, individuals take pictures of their experiences and use written reflections to express themselves with the goal of promoting insight, action, and change. In creating the term *photovoice*, Wang and Burris (1997) used the word "VOICE" intentionally to represent "Voicing Our Individual and Collective Experience" (p. 381). The goals of inspiring personal and community change and taking grassroots actions lie at the heart of photovoice research. Photovoice aims to achieve the following three goals: (a) capture concerns and strengths using pictures/photographs; (b) facilitate critical reflection and dialogue about individual and community concerns; and (c) reach and engage policy makers with a goal of making social change (Wang, 1999). Along with using photovoice as a research methodology, it can also be used as a clinical intervention with individual clients who are facing barriers to their growth (Sackett & Jenkins, 2015).

Remember, photovoice is not research "on" or "about" something but rather research "with" your participants. They are involved as co-researchers in all steps of the process including designing what you will research, approaching the research, analyzing the data, and communicating the findings.

When you use photovoice with individuals or even with your clients as an intervention, the combination of narrative and visual data in photovoice research allows you to capture individuals' realities from their own perspectives (McIntire, 2003). We will talk a little about how you get both forms of data in photovoice and how you would combine them. Before we begin giving more depth about the methodology itself, there are some other important points to know. First, in photovoice, people are viewed as the experts on their own lives, and they need to have a say in the creation of policies that impact their communities (Wang & Burris, 1997). Thus, an essential step in photovoice is connecting participants and policy makers, with the goal of raising policy makers' awareness about critical community issues. This awareness raising, in turn, could potentially lead to changes in policy that could positively impact the community. In this chapter, we provide some information about the theoretical underpinnings of photovoice methodology, walk the reader through the steps of conducting a photovoice study, illustrate the process through a case study, and discuss the limitations of this research design.

DOI: 10.4324/9781032706139-13

Theories That Influenced Photovoice

Three theoretical sources that influenced the development of photovoice include (a) key theoretical concepts of critical consciousness, (b) feminist theory, and (c) contemporary and documentary photography. All three sources aim to inspire community participation and action.

The Brazilian theorist Paulo Freire's approach to education for critical consciousness was an important lens in the creation of photovoice. The central idea of Freire's praxis lies in the premise that education cannot be viewed outside of the context within which it occurs. The theorist believed that education could liberate individuals and empower them to have a voice in their own lives. In his work, Freire engaged participatory strategies in designing and conducting adult literacy programs (Carlson et al., 2006). Embracing social knowledge is an important part of education that inspires people to gain control over their lives. In participatory strategies, a dialogue approach is used to empower individuals to critically evaluate the root causes of their concerns. Freire's ideas have been instrumental in informing the development of education, literacy, community development, and health education programs worldwide. Although Freire utilized drawings or photographs that captured individuals' realities, photovoice methodology extends his approach of using photographs and drawings by allowing people to create images themselves (Wang & Burris, 1997).

Photovoice is also rooted in feminist inquiry (Wang, 1999). Feminist scholars focus on giving voice to underserved and vulnerable populations by illuminating how the dominant forms of power act in tandem to silence and oppress these voices. Another important aspect in feminist methodology is the honoring of women's experiences. Wang (1999) maintained that photovoice challenges the traditional notions of positivistic research by honoring women's knowledge and experience and including them as co-researchers, advocates, and participants in the process of scientific inquiry. Through photographs, women are empowered to express their unique experiences and challenges and engage in critical discussions about the nature of these issues.

The third theoretical root of photovoice is contemporary and documentary photography. Photography captures the lives and struggles of vulnerable populations, giving voice to those who otherwise may feel unheard (Rose, 1997). In photovoice, individuals "who may otherwise not have access to such a tool" use cameras to capture a range of experiences that may be difficult to express using words (Wang & Burris, 1997, p. 370). The creators of photovoice believed that pictures allow people to take a deeper look at experiences from a perspective of a person other than a professional photographer. The main distinction between photovoice and traditional documentary photography is in its prominent focus on empowering individuals to become active participants in discussing the issues they face rather than the passive subjects of photographs captured by others. For a more in-depth history on the development of photovoice, readers can refer to the original article by Wang and Burris (1997) referenced at the end of this chapter.

When to Use Photovoice

When you consider your clinical practice, you may be wondering when photovoice is most appropriate to use and what types of questions you might ask that photovoice would be particularly useful to answer. Photovoice is a flexible research method that has been used by researchers from various disciplines with a common goal of addressing the health and social needs of diverse populations and cultures (Box 13.1).

Box 13.1   Goals and Uses of Photovoice

Photovoice can be used to:

- Teach, influence, highlight/provide voice, create action
- Identify, represent, and enhance a community through a specific photographic technique/process
- Understand (deeper participant awareness), transform (participants' social action), or both

There are three main goals:

- Enable people to record or reflect something (e.g., community strengths, barriers, concerns, experiences)
- Promote critical dialogue and knowledge about an issue
- Reach policy makers and/or others

Essentially, photovoice can be used when you or your clients see a potential problem. That problem may be one for which the client may or may not have words to express or a problem they experience that others may not understand fully. As a mental health practitioner, you can't follow the client's day-to-day life and see all the things that your client is expressing or experiencing. This is true for others in the community who may not understand the client's experience, either. Thus, photovoice can become a way to show others what the experience is, what barriers they may face, and what strengths and assets they possess. So, there are many considerations about when to use photovoice as a methodology in your practice. Photovoice is something to consider using when you need more depth, a different perspective, or a framework that can allow your clients or other individuals with whom you are working to engage in social action.

A Discussion About Social Action

Due to the focus on social action, some assert that photovoice is a research method that has implications for social justice and advocacy (Sackett & Jenkins, 2015; Smith, et al., 2012). Thus, this is a methodology that can fall within advocacy-based research (which you will read more about in Chapter 14). Sanon et al. (2014) examined photovoice studies and found that there were three categories of social justice: Awareness, amelioration, and transformation. Some researchers are interested in raising social justice awareness at the individual or community level – or, more specifically, highlighting personal insights which can result in making people aware of an issue. Others are more interested in ameliorating a social condition, pointing out the factors or barriers leading to injustice, or actually promoting change with social transformation.

Of course, you could gain this same information about participants' perceptions of their concerns through needs assessments, surveys, or even interviews. Photovoice, however, offers the possibility of *perceiving* the world through the lens of the participant. In some ways, photovoice is the methodological representation of the saying "a picture is worth 1,000 words."

The photovoice method values the knowledge put forth by individuals as the experts around an issue, but it does so in a way through which you can not only hear what individuals are saying but see how they perceive their world through pictures. Through this lens, participants' pictures can affirm the world of individuals who may be vulnerable, oppressed, or marginalized. In addition, photovoice goes beyond the typical needs assessment by inviting participants to become their own advocates, allowing them to engage with you and with others around them to create social action. Remember that social action is an important goal of this method, and that action may take the form of awareness, amelioration, or transformation (Sanon et al., 2014).

Photovoice has been utilized to examine social and health issues (McIntyre, 2003), issues related to youth (Wang, 1999), poverty (Willson et al., 2006), experiences of living with mental illness (Thompson et al., 2008), employment-seeking behaviors of individuals with various diseases (Rhodes, 2006), experiences of people with intellectual disabilities (Jurkowski & Paul-Ward, 2007), exploring barriers and supportive resources when considering revealing affectional orientation (Sackett & Jenkins, 2015), in after-school youth programs (Smith et al., 2012), and immigration (Schwartz et al., 2007). There have been reviews of photovoice studies specifically in mental health (Han & Oliffe, 2016), which can provide you examples of how photovoice has been adapted to meet the needs of different topics or contexts.

Wester et al. (2021) contend that photovoice can be used for helping counselors understand client experiences. There have been recent studies examining how queer womxn of color experience microaggressions in counseling (Reyes et al., 2022), and what one family experienced as barriers to implementing mindfulness skills used in counselling (Sackett et al., 2023). Photovoice has also been used in counselor training to examine students' internship experiences (Wells & Hunt, 2021) and to process race-based topics in a multicultural course (Paone et al., 2018).

Other benefits of this research method in clinical practice include that photovoice can be used with clients of all ages and who speak different languages. It can also be used with clients who feel like others don't understand them or by those who are having difficulty expressing their experience verbally. These examples suggest that photovoice is especially valuable in examining and affirming the experiences of individuals who are marginalized. While we have been focusing primarily on the photographs of photovoice, it should be noted that the photovoice methodology is much more than that. It contains aspects of critical dialogue, which we will talk more about later in this chapter. But know that by using photovoice, you have a unique opportunity to encourage people to come together to share their concerns and discuss ways to generate change. In some situations, when clients come together with a similar concern and talk through their photographs, it can provide a normalizing experience. Ultimately, photovoice aims to empower individuals to advocate for their rights. Thus, an important part of a photovoice study is capturing individuals' strengths and assets (Wang & Burris, 1997). Knowing these qualities allows you to capitalize on the existing strengths of the community in reaching policy makers and generating change.

Outside of the impact that photovoice can have as a powerful research tool, there are many unique benefits for participants who become active collaborators in the research process. In photovoice, you intentionally offer individuals a safe place to reflect on their unique experiences and challenges. Through this process, participants may develop a greater sense of awareness and in-depth knowledge of sociopolitical issues that impact their communities. Participants may gain skills and confidence in self-advocacy, lobbying, and empowerment (Blackman & Fairey, 2007). In addition, by engaging in photovoice research, participants can gain immediate benefits by cultivating relationships with each other (Wang & Burris, 1997).

Photovoice Methodology

While photovoice investigations may differ from one another depending on the focus of a particular study, the overall design of photovoice research can be implemented in a sequential fashion. Although in some instances these process steps may overlap, the guide in Table 13.1 can help you design and implement a photovoice study.

Preparation Stage

Planning the Project

The planning of the project is a critical part in the execution of a successful photovoice study. It requires you to create a timeline for the study, organize necessary resources, and define ways to address potential challenges that may arise. This process will depend on who your participants are but also on what the topic of the photovoice project is. During the planning phase, you need to consider ways of accessing communities to recruit participants for the study. In this effort, it is advisable to target a group or community that can directly speak to the phenomenon under investigation or one with which you directly work. For example, if you work in a school or run counseling groups, there may already be students/clients who work together as part of a community. Other populations or groups of individuals may be more difficult to access, and finding ways to build relationships with these groups is an important step in planning when considering your timeline, resources, and challenges.

Developing trust is an essential aspect of photovoice research because many communities may be hesitant to speak with researchers, viewing them as outsiders unable to understand their unique needs and challenges. Establishing relationships requires researchers to connect with communities and gain their trust. Building relationships with stakeholders in the community establishes the foundation for a lasting collaborative coinvestigation and community involvement during the research process (Palibroda et al., 2009). Building genuine relationships often takes time, commitment, and effort on behalf of the investigator. Therefore, you may be required to spend time observing communities, possibly attending their meetings, and, in general, learning about the community culture. Getting involved with the community is a good way to develop relationships, not only with individual members but also with the community as a whole (Palibroda et al., 2009). Furthermore, you should begin involving community members when clarifying the goals for their photovoice projects. Most photovoice

Table 13.1 Photovoice Step Process Guide

Preparation Stage	
	Planning the project
Implementation Stage	
	Recruiting participants
	Data collection
Data Analysis	
	Selection of photographs
	Contextualization of photographs
Action Stage	
	Preparing and sharing photovoice project
	Reaching policy makers or others to create social change

projects begin with conversation about the issue in the community that will be the focus of the team's collaborative work.

A photovoice investigation may require additional resources to cover the cost associated with the execution of the study. You should anticipate allocating resources to purchasing cameras (or making sure those without access to cameras on cellular phones have them), covering participant traveling expenses associated with the study, and securing a place for group discussions. Depending on the focus of a study, additional expenses may be necessary; therefore, you should address any financial or resource matters during the planning phase of a photovoice project.

Another important part of the planning phase is to begin identifying the target audience for this research. Who do you want to reach as a result of the project? People who have the power to make decisions and implement change should ideally represent a target audience. You should consider ways to approach and to engage the target audience (Wang, 1999). Who represents the target audience? How will you and the participants be able to meet the decision makers? Taking concrete steps to reach the target audience should be a collaborative process that involves community members and leaders. Palibroda and colleagues (2009) suggest seeking the target audience within city or town councils, human service agencies, schools, and/or various government and community agencies and departments.

Last, an ethical researcher tries to anticipate how any barriers and issues may be addressed if they should arise during a photovoice investigation. Although various challenges may come up in the process of a photovoice study, some may be associated with (a) the cost of materials, (b) securing of the space for group meetings, (c) facilitation of the group process, (d) potential conflicts that may emerge within group members, and (e) participants losing interest in the group process and the study (Palibroda et al., 2009).

Implementation Stage

Participant Recruitment

As stated earlier, an important consideration in the recruitment phase of the project is to ensure that the potential participants have a first-hand experience with the phenomenon under investigation. Depending on the focus of their study, participants can be recruited using formal or informal ways. Sending emails, brochures, or posting flyers may be a more formal way of recruiting participants, while personally inviting participants to take part in the study can be viewed as informal recruitment (Palibroda et al., 2009). Participants can be recruited in the community or even from your clinical practice or school setting. Make sure to abide by all ethical principles when you recruit participants (see Chapter 3 for more on ethics in research).

Wang (1999) believes that an ideal size of a photovoice study is seven to ten people. In a group of that size, you can facilitate a more personal and in-depth discussion among participants. In addition, participants may feel more comfortable and safer discussing their concerns and issues in a group of a smaller size. Since photovoice empowers community members to advocate for themselves, participants may play multiple roles in the research process (Wang, 1999). Specifically, participants in the photovoice investigation assume the responsibility of becoming co-researchers who discuss research goals and engage in the data collection and data analysis processes (Wang, 1999). You should keep that information in mind during the recruitment process and be able to discuss the importance of their coinvestigation roles with potential participants. In addition, you need to discuss any ethical issues that may be associated with this type of research and obtain a written consent from participants that clearly explains the significance of the study and all potential risks and benefits associated with it, as well as the voluntary nature of research (Wang, 1999).

Data Collection

The data collection process starts with organizing a meeting with research participants. During the initial meeting, you can introduce the contributors to the study and present the topic under investigation with the goal of initiating a group dialogue. Carlson and colleagues (2006) suggested that the expected participation may not occur without active facilitation from the researcher. Therefore, you should be intentional in creating a safe environment for participants to engage in a reflective discourse. To facilitate a thoughtful dialogue with participants, a variety of communication methods can be utilized. For instance, you may show a movie or video clip or PowerPoint or read an article on the issue to explore with participants. The material used in the presentation should be relevant for participants and their community. Following the presentation, you can invite participants to share their reflections about the presented issue. Participants are also encouraged to explore ways to use the research findings to advocate for their communities through reaching various policy makers (Wang & Burris, 1997). Once the goal of the investigation is clarified and the participants' commitment is gained, you introduce participants to the concept of photovoice (Wang, 1999). You also discuss with participants the importance of recording their meetings, noting that the information from these meetings will serve as additional forms of data in the following analysis process.

Depending on the technology that is used to capture images, participants may need to be trained in the use of a particular tool. Some photovoice experts recommend inviting a professional photographer to teach participants about the principal techniques in photography. Using photographic techniques may allow participants to capture images that more vividly and creatively represent what they want to express. However, given the common nature of smartphones, tablets, and social media, many participants may already be very comfortable with taking pictures. It is also important to discuss the type of images participants can take. Photographs have the unique power to leave an indelible impression on people. Considering that, you should discuss the importance of an ethical photo practice and explain ethical concerns associated with taking and using certain images (e.g., confidentiality, safety of participants and people around them, emotional reactions evoked by certain images). You should instruct participants not to take images that may potentially embarrass or stigmatize subjects. Last, you need to establish a timeframe for participants to turn in their photographs for the analysis (e.g., a few days; within 2 or 3 weeks). Keep in mind that during this time frame, when you ask participants to go back into the community and take photographs about the problem or experience they are representing, you can often ask participants to take as many pictures as they would like. You will find in the data analysis phase that not all pictures will be used, but opening the possibility of taking an infinite number of pictures can provide participants with freedom and not make them feel constrained to represent their experience within just one or two monumental photographs.

Data Analysis

The data analysis stage involves selecting images that can be contextualized to represent a story and then codifying these images (Wang, 1999). This process requires a great deal of the participants' collaboration with you and can be done either individually or during the group discussion. The group context may be particularly beneficial for establishing relationships between group members (Palibroda et al., 2009). There are multiple steps within data analysis in terms of receiving, contextualizing, and discussing photographs, which results in selecting and coding themes.

Selection of Photographs

Once the images are returned from participants to you, a follow-up meeting with participants is scheduled. The goal of that meeting is to invite participants to discuss the images they produced. You can ask participants to select one or two images they believe best represent the issues under investigation (Wang, 1999). As mentioned earlier, this can be done between you and the participant or between participants as more of a critical dialogue within a group setting. The ultimate goal of photovoice is to embolden participants to have a voice and feel empowered to advocate for their needs. A critical dialogue that inspires action is at the heart of photovoice research. In this critical dialogue, participants are invited to actively participate in the discussion about the way their images/stories should be presented to policy makers (Wang, 1999). This can be done through a slideshow or exhibit but has also been done in the way of books, websites, or pamphlets. Keep in mind that while social action is one of the goals for photovoice, this action of presenting the photographs and findings to others may also be viewed as political activism and evoke reactions that may lead participants to face various consequences, whereas you (the researcher) may not be directly impacted by the study. For this reason, Wang and Burris (1997) suggested allowing participants to choose the images they are willing to share. This means that while participants may have consented at the start of the photovoice study, another consent process occurs at the close of the photovoice process by allowing them to select which pictures they are comfortable with you sharing with others.

Contextualization of Photographs

During the critical dialogue process noted already, defining the image is a critical step in contextualizing the data (Wang, 1999). Rather than interpreting participants' images in isolation, your job is to encourage a critical dialogue on the meaning participants attribute to their images. How do these photos represent their world? Participants may be encouraged to reflect on and express their feelings associated with photographs. You must be sensitive to participants' feelings and create a safe environment for them to process various emotions that may arise (Palibroda et al., 2009). This requires you to utilize group facilitation skills.

To contextualize photographs, first – as noted – have participants select the photographs they are going to show to you or the larger group. These selected image(s) should be pictures that most descriptively capture their concerns. Once they have a few photographs, invite participants to reflect on them. The SHOWeD method can be used to engage participants in critical reflection on their realities. The questions in this method include (a) What do you *S*ee here? (b) What is really *H*appening here? (c) How does this relate to *O*ur lives? (d) *W*hy does this situation, concern, or strength exist? (e) How can we become *E*mpowered by new social understanding? and (f) What can we *D*o about it? Using the SHOWeD method allows participants to discuss concerns depicted in their photos and to seek action strategies to create change (Wang, 1999). While most photovoice studies use some version of the SHOWeD method, you can also be creative and use other means to promote reflection, such as having participants caption their pictures.

Coding Themes

The codification of themes involves identifying the topics or issues that emerge from the participants' photo stories and sorting them into categories of issues (Palibroda et al., 2009). Wang and Burris (1997) maintained that in photovoice research, participants play an active role in selecting and contextualizing images with stories they tell as well as identifying themes or key issues in these images that serve as a medium for their voices to be heard. Depending on the goal of the study, you and the participants may choose a specific way to organize the images that represent specific themes or issues. The investigation ensures that the team (which, remember, includes both you and the participants) focuses on selecting the issue or theme that can be realistically targeted and addressed (Wang & Burris, 1997).

During this phase of coding, the group can discuss their hopes and desires for the outcome of the project. We mentioned this earlier in selection of photographs, but this is a good time for participants to determine which pictures they would like to be used to represent the themes and potentially which pictures they would like to remain private – thus not displayed for others to see. Last, you and the participants discuss ways to organize the selected images that tell stories about their communities and their unique concerns. This can be done, as noted, in a slideshow or exhibit or any other format that best matches the data that you would like to show, respects your participants, and reaches the target audience. Another consideration other than just exhibiting the photographs is to provide contextual data, which can include both themes and captions. One way to organize and tell these stories is through the SHOWeD method that was described earlier. However, you may select a less structured way to organize your data.

Action Stage

Taking action is the last step in a photovoice study, but it is a critical step. During the action stage, participants have a unique opportunity to provide input and bring forward their concerns about a policy they would like to address and change (Palibroda et al., 2009). As Wang (1999) stated, "using photovoice as a tool for action reflects the [participatory action research] PAR's commitment to meaningful social change" (p. 190). The data analysis process in photovoice produces rich knowledge. But how can this knowledge and the pictures that capture it influence policy and generate change? Without a concrete plan of how to reach the target audience and a way of accessing the decision makers, the photovoice research may not realize its goal of stimulating action. Thus, creating an individual and communal action plan is an important part of photovoice research. As noted earlier, starting this part of the process begins in the planning stage, but it can also be brought into conversations with participants in the critical dialogue phase once experiences have been discussed and themes have been generated.

Finding a way to present the findings of a photovoice study with people in power may be a challenging process. One way that participants can share their experiences with policy makers is through the organization of community forums. To prepare for the forum, participants need to prepare their photovoice exhibit in a way that will help them to discuss issues with the target audience. Palibroda et al. (2009) make some useful recommendations that you may want to keep in mind when preparing for a photovoice exhibit. For instance, they suggest that you ensure the images that are selected for the exhibit are vividly speaking to the issue that will be raised during the exhibit. Once selected, the organization of images should not be done haphazardly. Hanging pictures separately and making sure that captions are attached to the right photograph can ensure the target audience is engaged and not overwhelmed by the presented exhibit. Additional consideration should be given to the size of the photovoice exhibit, because it needs to be transportable to a location where the meeting with the target audience will take place (Palibroda et al., 2009). Last, you should have a discussion with the participants (who are your coresearchers) about their participation in the exhibit and their ability/desire to speak about the images they captured. You may find that some participants want to attend and be present in the exhibit, while others may not. After the presentation, a debriefing with all participants about their experiences during the presentation should be held.

The photovoice process we just described is further detailed in what follows using a case study from a project that we completed. In each section, we describe how the method was used in our project. We hope that having these concrete examples will help to clarify the steps.

Case Study: Body Image Resilience in College Women

Preparation Stage

Planning the Project

Planning for the Body Image Resilience Project began during a class discussion about women's struggles with body image in the face of media pressure. The students shared an idea that women were the best voices on their own experiences of body image resilience. We decided that we wanted to create a project in which women could express their ideas about body image resilience. The goal of the project was to raise awareness about this important issue. We (a group of four researchers) met and planned the project. We developed a media presentation to get participants talking about the issue. We also prepared instructions for completing the photovoice projects.

Implementation Stage

Recruitment of Participants

Our team developed a flyer advertising the photovoice project and spread copies all over campus. The flyer instructed women over the age of 18 to call or email one of us if they were interested in learning more about the project. When someone contacted us, we gave them the information about the project including the time involved. The project involved two groups of women (8–10 in each group). During a two hours meeting on campus, the women listened to a PowerPoint presentation about media and body image and were engaged in a lively discussion about the topic.

Data Collection

Afterward, photovoice was introduced and the women were given oral and written instructions on how to complete their projects. We asked them to take a series of three pictures and develop the accompanying written reflections in a modified version of the SHOWeD method mentioned earlier. See Figure 13.1 for a sample photovoice picture and reflection.

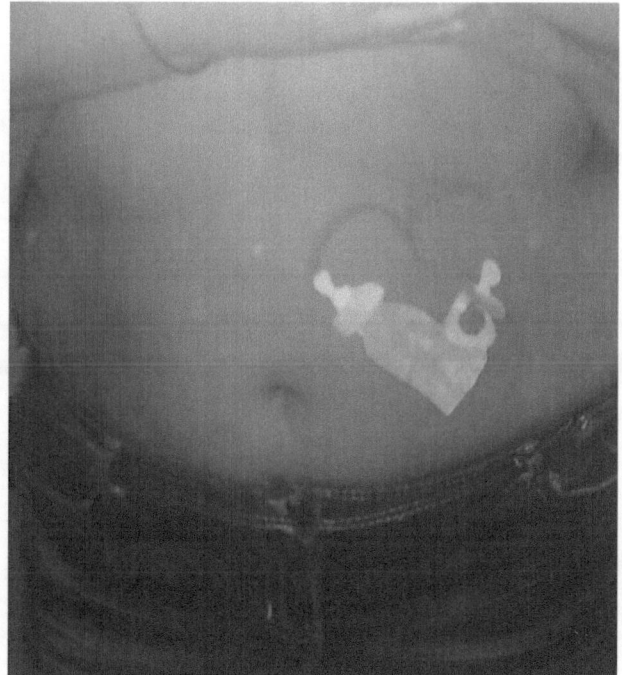

Figure 13.1 Example Photovoice Picture and Reflection.

Participant Caption

My stomach does not have "abs of steel," it is more like a flabby pit. However, I am not ashamed of this. In fact, I love my stomach because one day it will hold inside it another life. It will be the home and shelter of another human being. It will guard and protect and grow another person. One day, I will have a precious baby growing inside my stomach, and the extra flab will help to protect the innocence of my baby. I love my stomach because it will be the place I rest my baby when he/she is born. I love my stomach because when he/she grows up and needs some comfort they will wrap their arms around me and feel a sense of peace. I love my stomach because it gives me the ability to love unconditionally a child who has not yet been conceived, but that will one day need me. I love my stomach because it is a part of my past and will be a part of my future.

Data Analysis Stage

Selection of Photographs

Both groups of women met a second time, separately, to discuss their photovoice projects. Each woman in the group was asked to select her favorite picture, which was then projected to the group on a large screen. When their picture was displayed, each participant was able to read their reflection (from the modified SHOWeD reflection that they were instructed to complete in the data collection phase) out loud and add anything else that they wanted to share. Other women in the group were able to ask questions and comment on each person's photo and reflections.

Contextualization of Photographs

During this meeting of selecting and displaying photographs, the women were also asked to talk about commonalities (themes) that they saw between and among their photovoice projects. The research team was present at the group discussions, so they participated in the discussions and guided the participants to facilitate sharing. The group decided that the photovoice projects and our group discussion resulted in two distinct themes: (1) Beauty Ideals (created and reinforced by the media) and (2) Self (self-awareness and self-criticism). Note Figure 13.1 to see if you can observe how the themes were represented in this photovoice picture and reflection.

Once the groups were over, the team met separately and reviewed the themes the participants created. We (the four members of the research team) created a visual model of the themes and emailed all the participants to get their feedback and input, ensuring that they continued to be active with the research team as well.

Action Stage

Preparing and Sharing the Photovoice Project

We decided to partner with a student organization that was holding events for Eating Disorders Awareness Week on campus. Our overarching social justice goal and the focus of the exhibit was to raise awareness about body image resilience in the face of pressure and messages from the mainstream media. The intended target audience was other students on campus. The participants' photovoice projects and their reflections were printed out and displayed on poster board in the main lobby of our classroom building. The participants purposely chose pictures that represented the themes (Beauty Ideals and Self). The student organization had several speakers about the media, eating disorders, and body image.

Ethical Considerations in Photovoice Research

Like any research method, a photovoice study must be conducted within ethical guidelines that govern the process of designing and executing a study. Thus, a solid understanding about how to adhere to ethical research guidelines is critical. As stated previously, it is important for you to have clear steps to address any potential barriers that may emerge in a photovoice study. These steps must be created during the planning phase of the project and be clearly outlined in the project proposal, which will then be evaluated by the institutional review board or another ethical entity.

Informed Consent

You should provide complete information about the study to participants and discuss potential risks and benefits of engaging in this type of research. Keep in mind that providing photographs of one's experience and life can be identifying in ways that responding to a needs assessment may not be. Thus, participants should be able to consent to the study understanding what to expect and how to voluntarily withdraw from the study (Palibroda et al., 2009). Participants should also be aware of potential emotional distress that may occur during the photovoice study, as powerful pictures and images can sometimes cause difficult emotions to arise. Thus, it is important to prepare your participants for this potential result, as well as to have a plan in place for when or if this does occur (e.g., having more than one research team member in the group discussion or offering information about counseling resources in the community). Additionally, a negative outcome of the study may be associated with an inability to reach the target audience. Thus, participants should be made aware about this important limitation (Wang, 1999). Finally, if your participants are minors, the parents/guardians need to be involved in the informed consent process.

Privacy and Safety Issues

Anonymity, safety, and confidentiality are the critical aspects of photovoice. You need to educate participants about the importance of respecting individual privacy when taking images during the data collection phase (Wang & Redwood-Jones, 2001). During that process, it is important to educate participants on the risks of taking pictures that may identify individuals. Depending on a particular project, you may instruct participants to avoid taking photos that may link an individual to the image. Yet in some studies, pictures of human subjects will be permitted. Gaining informed consent from these subjects is critical; therefore, participants need to be trained on the proper way to facilitate this process. The use of personal devices (e.g., cell phones, personal cameras) also needs to be addressed as a special ethical issue.

The safety of participants and their subjects is an important part of an ethical photovoice research study. You need to instruct participants about the importance of maintaining safety throughout the research process and teach them skills to safely take pictures (Palibroda et al., 2009). Wang and Redwood-Jones (2001) maintain that the use of cameras allows participants to hold a certain level of power. Participants need to be always aware of their environment and any potential risks. Thus, the discussion about the responsibility, as well as the ethics and power of using cameras, should precede the training on the use of cameras (Wang & Redwood-Jones, 2001).

Photo Selection

During the training phase, participants are encouraged to take images that represent their communities authentically and respectfully. Depending on the number of participants, a photovoice study may produce a large volume of visual images. Selecting the most representative images that can expressively communicate with the target audience is an essential step in the photo selection phase (Wang & Redwood-Jones, 2001). You need to determine the number of images that will be selected for the exhibition. However, this should be a consent process with each participant. Specifically, each participant needs to consent to each image they would like to bring into the group discussion and photo selection phase. While this may seem like it is under their control, as participants may bring their images to the group, some researchers have participants email or send photographs prior to the group so that they are ready to be viewed or projected on a larger screen. Thus, it is important to ensure the specific photo(s) that are presented in the larger group are the ones that the participant consented to be used and displayed.

Photo Storage

You also need to have a clear plan for how you will safely and securely store the data collected during the study. Maintaining a clear organizational framework for tagging, organizing, and storing participants' images and meeting notes are an essential step in conducting an ethical photovoice research project.

Limitations of Photovoice

Every research methodology presents limitations that need to be taken into consideration when constructing a study. In what follows, we list some of the challenges that you need to take into consideration when designing a photovoice study.

Challenges for Participants

Time Commitment

Engaging in photovoice may require participants to dedicate a significant amount of their time to the project. Therefore, you need to discuss time commitment during the recruitment phase of the process.

Taking Photos

Participants may not be able to find images that represent their unique experiences. For this reason, educating participants on the symbolism of photography may be helpful in addressing this particular challenge.

Contextualizing Images

Reflecting on the content of the photos can evoke strong emotions from participants, who may also struggle to contextualize the images they select. You should rely on your group facilitation skills to allow participants to safely process their emotions.

Potential Challenges for You as a Photovoice Researcher

Time Commitment

Constructing and executing a photovoice study can take a significant amount of time. Therefore, you need to factor this in when thinking about a potential photovoice project.

Finding Participants

You may find yourself needing to take a significant amount of time to establish relationships with individuals prior to conducting a study.

Resources

Another challenge may be associated with the cost of organizing a photovoice study. The cost may be associated with buying cameras, printing out photovoice projects, or securing space to invite participants into group discussions. However, the use of smartphone cameras, tablets, and digital sharing may mitigate some of the costs.

Putting It All Together

Photovoice can be a powerful tool for researchers who want to bring their participants' voices to life. This method involves participants documenting their reflections on their own perspectives with photographs and then contextualizing them with written reflections. The participants work together as co-researchers to interpret the photographs and decide what perspectives and information to present. Further, photovoice can be an effective tool for reaching stakeholders in the community with participants' ideas about change. Now that you have learned about the photovoice method, what communities or clients do you think this method may work best with? The resources that follow can help you design your photovoice project.

Practice-Based Application

Think about the client-presenting concern, symptom, or situation that you identified in Chapter 1, and use that to answer the following questions:

- Describe how you might incorporate photovoice as a form of homework to both empower your client and better understand their experiences in counseling.
- What would be some of the guidelines or parameters that you would use with your client when talking with them about taking photos? How would you plan to work with your client when showing, sharing, and contextualizing photos in session?
- Thinking about the action-oriented goals of photovoice, how would you make sure to incorporate this into their sessions to effect change?

Resources for More Information

Books and Manuals

Blackman, A., & Fairey, T. (2007). *The photovoice manual: A guide to designing and running participatory photography projects*. London: PhotoVoice.

Palibroda, B., Krieg, B., Murdock, L., & Havelock, J. (2009). *A practical guide to photovoice: Sharing pictures, telling stories and changing communities*. Winnipeg, MB: Prairie Women's Health Network.

Peer-Reviewed Journal Articles

Becker, K., Reiser, M., Lambert, S., & Covello, C. (2014) Photovoice: Conducting community-based participatory research and advocacy in mental health. *Journal of Creativity in Mental Health, 9*(2), 188–209. doi:10.1080/15401383.2014.890088

Smith, L., Bratini, L., & Appio, L. M. (2012). "Everybody's teaching and everybody's learning": Photovoice and youth counseling. *Journal of Counseling and Development, 90*, 3–12. doi:10.1111/j.1556-6676.2012.00001.x

Wang, C. C. (1999). Photovoice: A participatory action research strategy applied to women's health. *Journal of Women's Health, 8*(2), 185–192. doi:10.1089/jwh.1999.8.185

Wang, C. C., & Burris, M. (1997). Photovoice: Concept, methodology, and use for participatory needs assessment. *Health Education & Behavior, 24*, 369–387. doi:10.1177/109019819702400309

Questions for Further Review and Application

1 What types of research questions or concerns are best addressed by photovoice? How can you see this methodology being used in your work setting?
2 Note the photovoice picture in Figure 13.1. Can you see how important the reflections and group discussion/identification of themes are in a photovoice study? What do you think might happen if you just collected the participants' photos without the contextualization or group sharing aspects of this method? What opportunities might be lost for group/community participation, connection, and action?

3   What are some potential ethical concerns related to the use of photographs? How would you plan early to cover these potential pitfalls with participants?
4   What strategies would you use to engage stakeholders?

References

Blackman, A., & Fairey, T. (2007). *The photovoice manual: A guide to designing and running participatory photography projects.* London: PhotoVoice.

Carlson, E. D., Engebretson, J., & Chamberlain, R. M. (2006). Photovoice as a social process of critical consciousness. *Qualitative Health Research, 16*(6), 836–852. doi:10.1177/1049732306287525

Han, C. S., & Oliffe, J. L. (2016). Photovoice in mental illness research: A review and recommendations. *Health, 20*(2), 110–126. doi:10.1177/1363459314567790

Jurkowski, J. M., & Paul-Ward, A. (2007). Photovoice with vulnerable populations: Addressing disparities in health promotion among people with intellectual disabilities. *Health Promotion Practice, 8*(4), 358–365. doi:10.1177/1524839906292181

McIntyre, A. (2003). Through the eyes of women: Photovoice and participatory research as tools for re-imagining place. *Gender, Place & Culture, 10*, 47–66. doi:10.1080/0966369032000052658

Palibroda, B., Krieg, B., Murdock, L., & Havelock, J. (2009). *A practical guide to photovoice: Sharing pictures, telling stories and changing communities.* Winnipeg, MB: Prairie Women's Health Network.

Paone, T.R., Malott, K.M., Pulliam, N., & Gao, J. (2018). Use of photovoice in processing race-based topics in a multicultural counseling course. *Journal of Creativity in Mental Health, 13*, (1), 92–105, https://doi.org/10.1080/15401383.2017.1294517

Reyes, A. G., Lindo, N. A., Allen, N., & Rodríguez, M. (2022). Centralizing the voices of queer womxn of color in counseling. *Journal of Counseling & Development, 100*, 171–182. https://doi.org/10.1002/jcad.12417

Rose, G. (1997). Engendering the slum: Photography in East London in the 1930s. *Gender, Place & Culture, 4*(3), 277–301. doi:10.1080/09663699725350

Rhodes, S. D. (2006). Visions and voices: HIV in the 21st century. Indigent persons living with HIV/AIDS in the southern USA use photovoice to communicate meaning. *Journal of Epidemiology and Community Health, 60*(10), 886.

Sackett, C., & Jenkins, A. (2015). Photovoice: Fulfilling the call for advocacy in the counseling field. *Journal of Creativity in Mental Health, 10*, 376–385. doi:10.1080/15401383.2015.1025173

Sackett, C.R., Jenkins, A. M., & Gambrel, L.E. (2023). Photovoice as counselling intervention and research method: One family's experience of barriers to implementing mindfulness skills. *Counseling Outcome Research and Evaluation, 14*, 2, 89–107. https://doi.org/10.1080/21501378.2023.2206952

Sanon, M. A., Evans-Agnew, R. A., & Boutain, D. M. (2014). An exploration of social justice intent in photovoice research studies from 2008 to 2013. *Nursing Inquiry, 21*(3), 212–226. doi:10.1111/nin.12064

Schwartz, L. R., Sable, M. R., Dannerbeck, A., & Campbell, J. D. (2007). Using photovoice to improve family planning services for immigrant Hispanics. *Journal of Health Care for the Poor and Underserved, 18*(5), 757–766. doi:10.1353/hpu.2007.0107

Smith, L., Bratini, L., & Appio, L. M. (2012). "Everybody's teaching and everybody's learning": Photovoice and youth counseling. *Journal of Counseling and Development, 90*, 3–12. doi:10.1111/j.1556-6676.2012.00001.x

Thompson, N. C., Hunter, E. E., Murray, L., Ninci, L., Rolfs, E. M., & Pallikkathayil, L. (2008). The experience of living with chronic mental illness: A photovoice study. *Perspectives in Psychiatric Care, 44*(1), 14–24. doi:10.1111/j.1744-6163.2008.00143.x

Wang, C. C. (1999). Photovoice: A participatory action research strategy applied to women's health. *Journal of Women's Health, 8*(2), 185–192. doi:10.1089/jwh.1999.8.185

Wang, C. C., & Burris, M. A. (1994). Empowerment through photo novella: Portraits of participation. *Health Education Quarterly, 21*(2), 170–186. doi:10.1177/109019819402100204

Wang, C. C., & Burris, M. A. (1997). Photovoice: Concept, methodology, and use for participatory needs assessment. *Health Education & Behavior, 24*(3), 369–387. doi:10.1177/109019819702400309

Wang, C. C., & Redwood-Jones, Y. A. (2001). Photovoice ethics: Perspectives from Flint photovoice. *Health Education & Behavior, 28*(5), 560–572. doi:10.1177/109019810102800504

Wester, K. L., Wachter Morris, C. A., Trustey, C. E., Cory, J. S., & Grossman, L. M. (2021). Promoting rigorous research using innovative qualitative approaches. *Journal of Counseling & Development*, *99*(2), 189–199. doi:10.1002/jcad.12366

Wells, P.C., & Hunt, B. (2021). A qualitative research study of counseling students' Journeys through internship using photovoice, *Journal of Creativity in Mental Health*, *16* (4), 444–455. doi:10.108 0/15401383.2020.1790455

Willson, K., Green, K., Haworth-Brockman, M., & Rachel, R. B. (2006). Looking out: Prairie women use photovoice methods to fight poverty. *Canadian Woman Studies*, *25*(*3*), 160–166. ISSN: 07133235

14 Mixed-Methods Research

Ye He

Up to this point, you have learned about various quantitative and qualitative methodologies that, for the most part, are used in isolation. This means that you would be conducting solely a quantitative study or solely qualitative study. In this chapter, you will learn about the design of mixed-methods (MM) research, through which quantitative and qualitative data collection and analysis methods can be combined. This chapter introduces commonly used MM terms and approaches and illustrates how to apply MM research design. The use of the three core MM design typologies is elaborated through a case example. Additional resources are provided for further exploration of specific application of MM in your research.

Overview of Mixed-Methods Research

MM emerged from the movement against the dominant use of quantitative research in the 1980s (Gage, 1989; Hammersley, 1992). Researchers such as Guba (1990) promoted the use of qualitative research methods. However, qualitative researchers also argued that there was a systematic set of beliefs guiding the use of research methods (Lincoln & Guba, 1985) and suggested that the use of both quantitative and qualitative methods in one research study is not appropriate (Guba, 1990; Howe, 1988). MM researchers challenged this perspective and proposed the compatible use of both quantitative and qualitative methods and established MM as "a distinct third methodological movement" (Teddlie & Tashakkori, 2003, p. 24).

A variety of MM definitions have been crafted and used by researchers and methodologists in the field. Two most commonly used definitions were proposed by Johnson, Onwuegbuzie, and Turner (2007) and through the *Journal of Mixed Methods Research* (*JMMR*), the official journal including studies using MM and discussions regarding the use of MM at the methodological level.

Johnson et al. (2007) proposed a general MM definition based on the review of MM definitions used by 21 highly published MM researchers:

> Mixed methods research is the type of research in which a researcher or team of researchers combines elements of qualitative and quantitative research approaches (e.g., use of qualitative and quantitative viewpoints, data collection, analysis, inference techniques) for the broad purposes of breadth and depth of understanding and corroboration.
>
> (p. 123)

DOI: 10.4324/9781032706139-14

JMMR shared an even more general MM definition with its authors and readers:

> mixed methods research is defined as research in which the investigator collects and analyzes data, integrates the findings, and draws inferences using both qualitative and quantitative approaches or methods in a single study or a program of inquiry.
>
> (Tashakkori & Creswell, 2007, p. 4)

While these general definitions are commonly used by MM practitioners, it is important to note that the tradition of MM varies across different disciplines and geographic regions. Instead of adopting a single definition, some MM methodologists suggested detailing the characteristics of MM research instead (Tashakkori & Teddlie, 2010).

In their third edition of *Designing and Conducting Mixed Methods Research*, Creswell and Plano Clark (2017) included core characteristics of MM such as:

- collects and analyzes both qualitative and quantitative data rigorously in response to research questions and hypotheses,
- integrates (or mixes or combines) the two forms of data and their results,
- organizes these procedures into specific research designs that provide the logic and procedures for conducting the study, and
- frames these procedures within theory and philosophy.

(p. 5)

Similarly, in a report presented by the Mixed Methods International Research Association (MMIRA), Mertens et al. (2016) highlighted two core criteria for MM including (1) "the use of more than one method, methodology, approach, theoretical or paradigmatic framework"; and (2) "integration of results from those different components" (p. 4).

Appropriate Use of Mixed-Methods Research Design

Combining the strengths of quantitative and qualitative methods you have learned, MM research presents many benefits. The major purposes of MM research include corroboration, elaboration, and development (Arnault & Fetters, 2011; Creswell & Plano Clark, 2017; Tashakkori & Teddlie, 2010). *Corroboration* refers to the use of multiple methods (e.g., quantitative survey and focus group discussion) to triangulate and test the consistency of findings. *Elaboration* refers to the use of one method (e.g., follow-up interview) to substantiate the interpretation of data collected using another method (e.g., test scores). *Development* refers to the use of results from one method to inform the data collection and/or analysis of the other method (e.g., quantitative instrument development based on qualitative data; Arnault & Fetters, 2011).

Utilizing both quantitative and qualitative theoretical orientations, methodological designs, data collection, and data analysis tools, MM design offsets the weaknesses of studies using only quantitative or qualitative methods and can address research questions that may not be answered by one method alone. In addition, the mixing of quantitative and qualitative data, analysis procedures, display, and interpretation also offers new insights that may not be attainable using quantitative or qualitative research alone. As Creswell and Plano Clark (2017) summarized, you may think about using MM design if you think one type of data source (either quantitative or qualitative) may not be sufficient to address your research questions; the results you report based on quantitative data may need to be further explained and substantiated; you may want to further generalize findings from your qualitative data; or you may need to consider conducting your research in multiple phases to address your overall research objective.

Writing MM Research Questions

If you were to use a MM approach, you would typically take one of two general positions in terms of the role of research questions: (1) the dictatorship model; and (2) the reciprocal approach (Mertens et al., 2016). The dictatorship model states that the research questions drive the selection of MM design, sample procedures, data collection, and analysis processes. This position would also designate MM as only appropriate when the research questions call for the use of both quantitative and qualitative methods. The reciprocal approach, on the other hand, positions research questions in the center as the "hub of the research process" (Plano Clark & Badiee, 2010, p. 280). This position assumes an interactive and reciprocal relationship between research questions and other components of the research study including its purposes, theories, methods, and validity considerations. Based on this position, the research questions may shift and evolve as you carry out the literature review, data collection, analysis, and interpretation throughout the study. In other words, if you adopt the dictatorship model, you will typically specify a MM design once you identify the research questions. If you choose to apply the reciprocal approach, you may be more open to the modifications of the research questions and allow MM design to emerge during the research process.

MM research questions may take on different formats and rhetorical styles depending on the field of the study, the theoretical orientation used, and the specific MM design selected. In general, it is important to ensure that (1) your MM questions, design, and results are clearly aligned; and (2) the need for integration of quantitative and qualitative approaches is conveyed (Plano Clark & Badiee, 2010).

You may include separate quantitative, qualitative, and MM questions; or you can write all MM research questions for your study. For example, if you are interested in exploring the impact of a research methods course on graduate students' research self-efficacy based on a quantitative survey such as the Research Self-Efficacy Inventory (RSEI) (Chesnut, Siwatu, Young, & Tong, 2015) and focus group data, you may ask different sets of research questions that indicate the various levels of MM integration. Table 14.1 includes some sample MM research questions.

Table 14.1 Sample Mixed-Methods Research Questions With Various Levels of Integration

Separate Questions – quantitative, qualitative, and MM questions are separate	• Is there a statistically significant difference between the pre/post RSEI scores? (quantitative) • How do participants describe the impact of the research methods course? (qualitative) • What is the relationship between participants' RSEI scores and their description of the impact of the research methods course? (MM)
Integrated Questions – MM questions imply the use of both quantitative and qualitative approaches	• How do participants with significant increase of RSEI scores describe the impact of the research methods course?

The sample integrated MM question in Table 14.1 also predetermines a specific sequential MM design of the study, in which the researchers would implement the RSEI instrument during the first phase of the research and select participants who illustrated a significant increase of pre/post scores for focus group discussions in the second phase in order to address the overarching MM research question. We will elaborate on the research design typologies in the next section through a case study.

Case Study

MM research may be designed in a variety of ways. In this chapter, we will focus our discussion on three core MM designs, including (1) convergent design, (2) explanatory sequential design, and (3) exploratory sequential design (Creswell & Plano Clark, 2017). In addition, we explore the complex applications of these core designs. To further illustrate the design considerations, we use a research example examining the acculturative stress of international students in the United States. For each design type, we introduce the design prototype, sampling considerations, data collection, analysis, display options, and validity concerns that may need to be addressed.

Mixed-Methods Research Design

Convergent Design

Design Prototype

The convergent design is set up so that you can implement quantitative and qualitative methods during the same phase of the research study in a concurrent manner. You can collect and analyze the quantitative and qualitative data separately and then mix your interpretation of the results. The purpose of this type of design typically is to elaborate or corroborate results using one method with another to reach a more comprehensive understanding of the topic.

For the case study, you may use one quantitative measure, the Acculturative Stress Scale for International Students (ASSIS) (Sandhu & Asrabadi, 1994, 1998), to collect quantitative data, and you may also conduct individual interviews to collect more information regarding students' acculturation experiences. Figure 14.1 illustrates the overall design.

Sampling Considerations

You may include either one or two sample frames in a convergent design. If you use one sample frame, you will collect both quantitative and qualitative data from the same sample. For example, you may want to draw a stratified sample of international students at five local

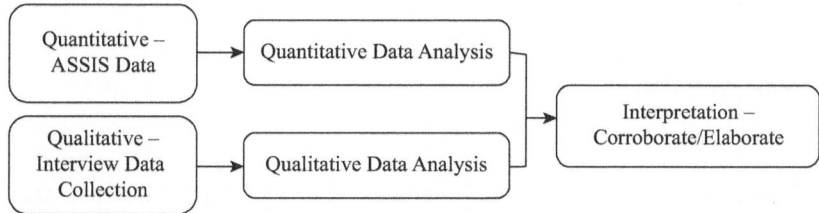

Figure 14.1 Convergent Design.

universities and colleges that represent various higher education institution types for the purpose of this study. You need to take the feasibility of both quantitative and qualitative data collection and analysis into consideration when determining your sample size. While 500 students may be a reasonable number for quantitative data collection, it may not be practical to conduct 500 interviews within the time frame of the study. Similarly, while 15 students can be a manageable sample of interview participants, the small number will likely limit the type of analysis you can use when analyzing your quantitative data.

To optimize the sample size for quantitative and qualitative data collection and analysis methods, you can identify two different sample sizes. You will then need to decide whether the two samples include the same set of participants (i.e., the qualitative sample is a subset of the quantitative sample) or include two independent samples of participants. If your goal is to corroborate the findings across quantitative and qualitative methods and your quantitative and qualitative share the same purpose, identifying a subset of the sample for qualitative data collection may be more appropriate.

Data Collection, Analysis, and Display

The convergent design assumes separate data collection and analysis processes for quantitative and qualitative data, so you can use various quantitative and qualitative methods appropriate for the purpose of the study. The MM interpretation of the data occurs after the completion of independent quantitative and qualitative analysis. Depending on your research questions and initial findings, you need to specify what aspects you want to compare and represent the findings and interpretation of the comparison.

In our case example, you may find that *Homesickness* is the major source of international students' acculturative stress based on ASSIS results. Based on your interview data, you noted that students from a home country where the time difference presents challenges for them to connect with families and friends in real time expressed their experience of homesickness differently than others. The comparison of the quantitative and qualitative data in this case may allow you to elaborate on quantitative findings and draw further interpretation of your data.

Validity Concerns

The data collection and analysis procedure in the convergent design may introduce some validity concerns that need to be addressed. During data collection, the potential use of unequal sample size may introduce validity threat. Strategic subset sampling for the qualitative data collection can be a strategy to address this concern. During data analysis, it is important to make logical comparisons of the results of quantitative and qualitative data analysis and focus on the research purposes and research questions. When interpreting the results, it is critical that you address any divergent findings and be mindful of the weight you give to quantitative and qualitative results.

Explanatory Sequential Design

Design Prototype

The MM sequential design assumes at least two phases of data collection and analysis in one study. The purpose of the explanatory sequential design is to use the qualitative method to explain the initial quantitative results from the first phase of the study (Creswell &

Plano Clark, 2017). Quantitative results can also be used to guide the sampling, data collection, and analysis procedures for the second qualitative phase.

For the case example, ASSIS measure may be used during the first phase, and the sampling procedure and interview protocol during the second phase of the research may be determined based on the first-phase results. Figure 14.2 illustrates the explanatory sequential design.

Sampling Considerations

One of the key features of the sequential design is that the results of the first-phase analysis impact the research questions, sampling, data collection and analysis in the second phase. In the explanatory sequential design, the quantitative findings may identify specific subsets of participants for the follow-up qualitative data collection; may result in statistically significant findings that may become the focus for qualitative data collection, and may inform the data analysis procedures and framework in the qualitative phase.

In the case example, the ASSIS data analysis may result in the identification of the group of international students who expressed the highest level of acculturative stress and be identified as the subset of the participants for the second qualitative interview data collection. The use of extreme case sampling in this case helps explain the responses from this specific subgroup of participants. Major factors that lead to acculturative stress reported by the participants based on ASSIS can also inform the design of the interview protocol in the qualitative phase.

Just as in the convergent design, you can use different samples for each phase of the study. The quantitative results in the first phase may not impact the sampling decision for data collection in the second phase.

Data Collection, Analysis, and Display

The quantitative and qualitative data collection and analysis are conducted in phases. Appropriate quantitative data collection and analysis methods can be used in the first phase, and relevant qualitative design can be used in the second phase. It is important to articulate the connection between the quantitative results and the second qualitative phase. The qualitative results are interpreted to explain and offer additional insights to the quantitative results.

Because the design of the second qualitative phase is dependent on the results of the first quantitative phase, you may not have a finalized qualitative research question, sampling procedure, qualitative instrument, or analysis method identified as you start the research study. The qualitative design emerges as you have a better understanding of the quantitative results.

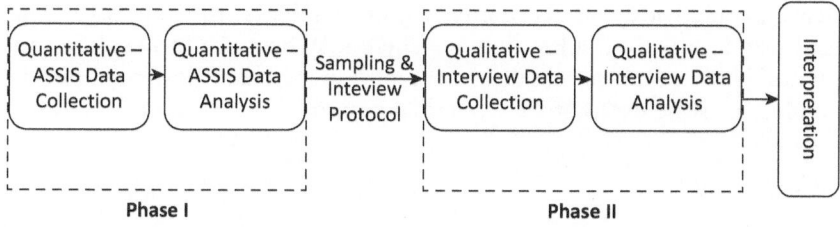

Figure 14.2 Explanatory Sequential Design.

You may need to modify your overall research proposal and documentation for the institutional review board (IRB) as the study progresses.

In the case example, you may draft an interview protocol and determine a cut score that identifies a high level of acculturative stress based on the literature review. The quantitative results may alter your predetermined design. For example, according to the literature, a mean score above 109 on ASSIS indicates evidence of acculturative stress (Sandhu & Asrabadi, 1998). You may adjust the mean and standard deviation used as the cut score for your study depending on the overall group mean and standard deviation. In addition, your interview protocol may also be altered to highlight areas of significant findings based on your quantitative analysis.

Validity Concerns

The sequential design introduces unequal sample size that may be a validity concern. You need to be cautious when interpreting the qualitative results in explaining any significant quantitative findings, especially if sampling during the second qualitative phase is restricted by study context. It is important to keep in mind that even though qualitative results help explain the quantitative findings, causations may not be established through this type of design.

Potential bias may be introduced by overemphasizing the results of the quantitative data. In other words, it is possible that you may focus on the existing quantitative results when conducting the qualitative phase and find it hard to keep an open mind for potential divergent findings. On the other hand, there might be a tendency to keep the second qualitative phase too exploratory in nature and overlook the necessary connection to the quantitative results from the first phase.

Exploratory Sequential Design

Design Prototype

The exploratory sequential design is similar to the explanatory sequential design in terms of the assumption of two sequential phases in the research design. Different from explanatory design, the exploratory design starts with the qualitative exploratory phase. The purpose of the design is to generalize qualitative findings from the first phase to a larger sample with data collected and analyzed in the second quantitative phase. The initial qualitative phase is typically needed for three reasons: (1) lack of measures or instruments on the topic; (2) unknown variables for the purpose of study; and (3) lack of a comprehensive theoretical framework to guide data collection and analysis (Creswell, Plano Clark, Gutmann, & Hanson, 2003).

In the case example, you may observe that even though there is a literature base for the study of international students' acculturative stress, the ASSIS instrument is dated. In addition, the demographic backgrounds of international students studying in the United States have changed significantly in the last decade. There may be a need to explore various social, cultural, and academic variables revealed in recent literature and develop a new instrument. Figure 14.3 illustrates the exploratory sequential design.

Sampling Considerations

The exploratory sequential design typically involves two different sample sizes at the two phases. The qualitative phase typically involves a purposeful sampling procedure with a

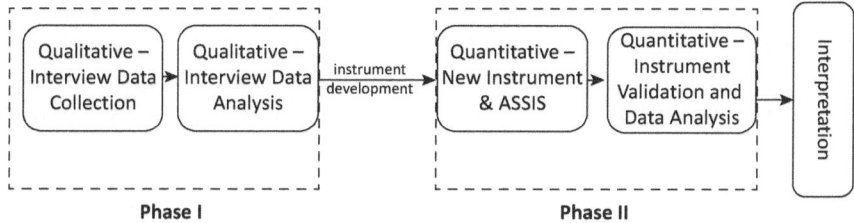

Figure 14.3 Exploratory Sequential Design.

relatively small sample size, while the quantitative phase typically requires a much larger representative sample to achieve the generalizability of the study. Depending on the purpose of the study, the two samples may or may not involve the same subset of participants.

In the case example, you may purposefully select international students from different regions of the world, with different educational backgrounds and working experiences and seeking different degrees and majors in the United States as samples for your qualitative interview data collection during the first phase. During the second phase, you may draw a convenient sample from all international students in the United States who may respond to an online survey distributed through a listserv. The sample size in the first phase of the study is much smaller than the second phase.

Data Collection, Analysis, and Display

Appropriate qualitative data collection and analysis are conducted during the first phase. The qualitative analysis results inform the research questions, sampling, instrument, and data analysis framework in the second quantitative phase. During the second phase, appropriate quantitative data collection and analysis are conducted and the results are interpreted, considering both quantitative and qualitative results. Similar to explanatory sequential design, the exploratory sequential design also involves emergent research design. Sampling procedures, instruments, and data analysis procedure may not be predetermined at the beginning of the study.

In the case example, you may uncover through your interviews that the major themes of acculturative stress include *Homesickness*, *Cultural Shock*, *Perceived Discrimination*, and *Academic Shock*. *Fear* and *Guilt* as defined in the original ASSIS may not emerge as major themes among the selected international students. *Academic Shock*, on the other hand, emerged as a major theme where participants commented on the specific challenges that resulted from the different academic expectations and career readiness preparations (e.g., internships). The interview results can lead to the development of new items for the instrument, and modifications for the IRB may need to be submitted to reflect the change of study protocol.

Validity Concerns

Unequal sample size is typically introduced with the exploratory sequential design. The goal of the first qualitative phase is to explore theories and variables. However, due to the relatively small sample size typically involved in qualitative studies, themes drawn from the qualitative analysis may not be representative for the larger sample you intend to address during the second phase. Overall findings of the study may be restricted by the nature and size of the sample in the qualitative phase.

In the case example, it is also important to note that instrument development is a comprehensive and iterative process. Studies involving instrument development may be designed as multiphase MM studies involving iterative process of quantitative and qualitative data collection, analysis, and validation beyond a simple two-phase exploratory sequential design.

Complex Applications of Core Designs

Design Prototype

Building upon the three MM core designs, you may consider various complex applications. Plano Clark and Ivankova (2016) presented various ways MM design can intersect with another methodology or with a theoretical framework. For example, scholars have proposed mixed-methods–grounded theory (MM-GT) design to emphasize the integration of both quantitative and qualitative philosophy and approaches through the grounded theory inquiry (Johnson et al., 2010; Shim et al., 2021).

Embedding a secondary quantitative or qualitative method within a primary qualitative or quantitative design is another complex application of the core designs (Creswell & Plano Clark, 2017). The embedded element may be introduced before, during, or after the primary quantitative or qualitative design (Sandelowski, 1996). The purpose of the embedded design is to offer supplementary data to enrich findings from the primary design. Embedded design is most often applied with qualitative methods embedded in primary quantitative designs.

In the case example, you may be curious whether and how living on campus may impact international students' acculturative stress over time during their first year in the United States. To set up such a study, you can employ a quasi-experimental design to collect ASSIS data in a pre and post manner over one year from two groups of participants, one group residing on campus and the other off campus. In addition, you may want to collect supplementary qualitative data during the year of this study to explore experiences that may reflect or impact their acculturative stress through participant interviews and written journals. Figure 14.4 illustrates the embedded design.

In embedded design, the qualitative sample is either the same as the quantitative sample or a purposefully selected subset. In the case example, where the qualitative method is embedded in the overarching quantitative design, the qualitative sample may be identified based on initial analysis of the pre ASSIS data. While all participants may be instructed to maintain a journal, interviews may only be conducted with a selected group of participants for the purpose of the study.

In embedded designs where qualitative design is the overall design and quantitative methods are used to collect supplementary data, using the same sample may assist you in building

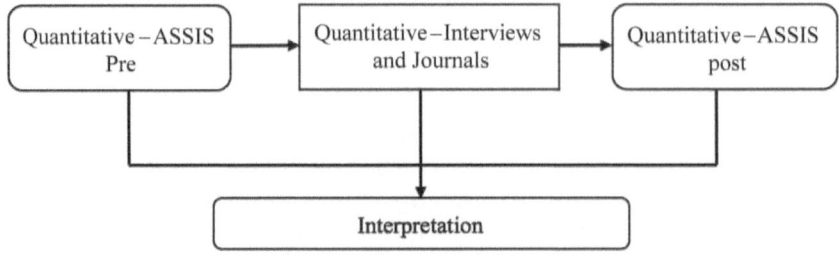

Figure 14.4 Embedded Design Sampling Considerations.

a more comprehensive participant profile to support data analysis and interpretation in general.

Data Collection, Analysis, and Display

Depending on the specific setup of the study, in embedded design, quantitative and qualitative data may be collected in a concurrent manner or a sequential manner. In the case example, the design specifies a sequence of data collection. The pre ASSIS survey data is collected at the beginning of the academic year. During the year, qualitative data including interviews and participant journals are collected. Finally, at the end of the academic year, the post ASSIS data is collected.

Quantitative and qualitative data may be analyzed separately in embedded design and combined for interpretation as in convergent design. In the case example, quantitative pre and post ASSIS data can be analyzed independently from the qualitative data. To further integrate both quantitative and qualitative data to address the research questions, you may consider data conversion. Data conversion occurs when you turn quantitative data into qualitative data or qualitative into quantitative data. In the case example, we may design a rubric based on the ASSIS instrument to record the occurrence of acculturative stress experiences. For example, any description in the journal or interview responses that is related to *Homesickness* receives a "1" on the rubric to tally for frequency by individual and then by group. You can then use this quantified qualitative data in quantitative analysis together with data collected using ASSIS to address MM research questions.

Validity Concerns

The selection of participants is a validity consideration in embedded design, especially if unequal sample size is used. When quantitative and qualitative data are collected and analyzed in a concurrent manner in an embedded design, it is especially challenging to identify specific rationale for sampling decisions.

In addition, you need to consider the meaningful use of supplementary data in an embedded design. In the case example, without a clear focus of the interview and instructions for the participant journal, you may not be able to successfully integrate your qualitative data in the integrated analysis to address the MM research questions.

Data conversion can be used in many MM designs beyond embedded design. However, the data conversion process may introduce validity concerns. When transforming quantitative data to qualitative data or qualitative data to quantitative data, it is critical that you specify the rationale and procedures for such transformation. You also need to be aware of the use of appropriate statistical analysis procedures (e.g., nonparametric statistics) when working with the quantitative data converted from qualitative findings.

Summary

You may consider MM research designs when using either quantitative or qualitative methods alone cannot sufficiently address your research questions. Before starting the MM research design, it is a good idea to review MM studies in your field. You can begin your search of these studies either using "mixed methods" as the key word in journals related to your field or using your disciplinary key word (e.g., counseling) to search in *JMMR*. As you read these MM studies, you want to pay attention to why the authors used MM and what MM definition they used. Whether you adopt the dictatorship model or reciprocal approach for your MM research questions, keep in mind that the congruence between your research questions and the MM design is critical. Throughout your research design and implementation, you also need to be aware of the validity considerations in the sampling, data collection, data analysis, display, and reporting decisions you make.

Effective design and implementation of the MM design rely on researchers' skills and having sufficient time and resources (Creswell & Plano Clark, 2017). If you are considering using MM design for your next project, make sure you take the time to assess your research strengths and readiness and establish a manageable research project plan to ensure the allocation of time and resources for your MM project. While more experienced researchers may use more complex MM designs, it is recommended that beginning researchers start with the basic MM designs such as those introduced in this chapter. You may also consider replicating the design from an MM study in your field. The growing MM literature research projects serve as great resources as you start to design MM studies in your area of study.

Practice-Based Application

Think about the clinical practice topic you identified in Chapter 1, and use that to answer the following questions:

- How would you use each of the three core MMR designs to study the topic you identified in Chapter 1?
- Which core design type is the most appropriate for your research topic? Why?
- Draw a diagram to illustrate your design choice.

Resources for More Information

Online

Mertens, D. M., Bazeley, P., Bowleg, L., Fielding, N., Maxwell, J., Molina-Azorin, J. F., & Niglas, K. (2016a). The future of mixed methods: A five year projection to 2020. *Mixed Methods International Research Association (MMIRA) Task Force Report*. Retrieved from www.mmira.wildapricot.org/resources/Documents/MMIRA%20task%20force%20report%20Jan2016%20final.pdf

Sage Research Methods Video Resource (n.d.) https://methods.sagepub.com/Search/Results?content Types=Videos&methods=Mixed%20methods

Books

Creswell, J. W., & Plano Clark, V. L. (2017). *Designing and conducting mixed methods research* (3rd ed.). Thousand Oaks, CA: Sage Publications.

Tashakkori, A., & Teddlie, C. (2010). *Handbook on mixed methods in the behavioral and social sciences* (2nd ed.). Thousand Oaks, CA: Sage Publications.

Peer-Reviewed Journal Articles

Cooper, A. L., Brennan, M. C., Leslie, G. D., & Brown, J. A. (2023). Integrating literature as a data source in mixed methods research. *Journal of Mixed Methods Research*. doi:10.1177/15586898231188500

Creswell, J. W. (2016). Reflections on the MMIRA the future of mixed methods task force report. *Journal of Mixed Methods Research, 10*(3), 215–219. doi:10.1177/1558689816650298

Dellinger, A. B., & Leech, N. L. (2007). Toward a unified validation framework in mixed methods research. *Journal of Mixed Methods Research, 1*(4), 309–332. doi:10.1177/1558689807306147

Fetters, M. D. (2022). A comprehensive taxonomy of research designs, a scaffolded design figure for depicting essential dimensions, and recommendations for achieving design Naming conventions in the field of mixed methods research. *Journal of Mixed Methods Research, 16*(4), 394–411. doi:10.1177/15586898221131238

Guetterman, T. C., Molina-Azorin, J. F., & Fàbregues, S. (2023). The need to rigorously develop common quality guidelines for reporting mixed methods research. *Journal of Mixed Methods Research, 17*(1), 6–11. doi:10.1177/15586898221143561

Heyvaert, M., Hannes, K., Meas, B., & Onghena, P. (2013). Critical appraisal of mixed methods studies. *Journal of Mixed Methods Research, 7*(4), 302–327. doi:10.1177/1558689813479449

Mertens, D. M., Bazeley, P., Bowleg, L., Fielding, N., Maxwell, J., Molina-Azorin, J. F., & Niglas, K. (2016b). Expanding thinking through a kaleidoscopic look into the future: Implications of the mixed methods international research association's task force report on the future of mixed methods. *Journal of Mixed Methods Research, 10*(3), 221–227. doi:10.1177/1558689816649719

Onwuegbuzie, A. J., Johnston, R. B., & Collins, K. M. (2011). Assessing legitimation in mixed research: A new framework. *Quality and Quantity, 45*, 1253–1271. doi:10.1007/s11135-009-9289-9

Plano Clark, V. L., Anderson, N., Wertz, J. A., Zhou, Y., Schumacher, K., & Miaskowski, C. (2014). Conceptualizing longitudinal mixed methods design: Methodological review of health science research. *Journal of Mixed Methods Research*, 1–23. doi:10.1177/1558689814543563

Poth, C. N., Molina-Azorin, J. F., & Fetters, M. D. (2022). Virtual special issue on "Design of mixed methods research: Past advancements, present conversations, and future possibilities". *Journal of Mixed Methods Research, 16*(3), 274–280. doi:10.1177/15586898221110375

Wisdom, J. P., Cavaleri, M. A., Onwuegbuzie, A. J., & Green, C. A. (2012). Methodological reporting in qualitative, quantitative, and mixed methods health services research articles. *Health Research and Educational Trust, 47*(2), 721–745. doi:10.1111/j.1475-6773.2011.01344.x

Review Questions

1   In your area of study, how do researchers define MM research? What are the key characteristics of MM research recognized in your field?
2   For your future work, what are some advantages of using MM? What are some challenges?
3   If you were to develop a study in your field using MM, would you adopt the dictatorship model or reciprocal approach to writing your research questions? Why?
4   What would be the specific validity considerations you need to be aware of when applying the four commonly used MM designs to your research?

References

Arnault, D. S., & Fetters, M. D. (2011). ROI funding for mixed methods research: Lesson learned from the "mixed method analysis of Japanese depression" project. *Journal of Mixed Methods Research, 5*(4), 309–329. doi:10.1177/1558689811416481

Chesnut, S. R., Siwatu, K. O., Young, H. A., & Tong, Y. (2015). Examining the relationship between the research training environment, course experiences, and graduate students' research self-efficacy beliefs. *International Journal of Doctoral Studies, 10*, 399–418. Retrieved from http://ijds.org/Volume10/IJDSv10p399-418Chesnut0914.pdf

Creswell, J. W., & Plano Clark, V. L. (2017). *Designing and conducting mixed methods research* (3rd ed.). Thousand Oaks, CA: Sage Publications.

Creswell, J. W., Plano Clark, V. L., Gutmann, M., & Hanson, W. (2003). Advanced mixed methods research designs. In A. Tashakkori & C. Teddlie (Eds.), *Handbook of mixed methods in social and behavioral research* (pp. 209–240). Thousand Oaks, CA: Sage Publications.

Gage, N. L. (1989). The paradigm wars and their aftermath: A "historical" sketch of research on teaching since 1989. *Educational Researcher, 18*(7), 4–10.

Guba, E. G. (1990). *The paradigm dialog.* Newbury Park, CA: Sage Publications.

Hammersley, M. (1992). The paradigm wars: Reports from the front. *British Journal of Sociology of Education, 13*(1), 131–143.

Howe, K. R. (1988). Against the quantitative-qualitative incompatibility thesis or dogmas die hard. *Educational Researcher, 17*(8), 10–16.

Johnson, R., McGowan, M., Turner, L. (2010). Grounded theory in practice: Is it inherently a mixed method? *Research in the Schools, 17*, 65–78.

Johnson, R. B., Onwuegbuzie, A. J., & Turner, L. A. (2007). Toward a definition mixed methods research. *Journal of Mixed Methods Research, 1*(2), 112–133.

Lincoln, Y. S., & Guba, E. G. (1985). *Naturalistic Inquiry.* Beverly Hills, CA: Sage Publications.

Mertens, D. M., Bazeley, P., Bowleg, L., Fielding, N., Maxwell, J., Molina-Azorin, J. F., & Niglas, K. (2016). *The future of mixed methods: A five year projection to 2020.* Mixed Methods International Research Association (MMIRA) Task Force Report. Retrieved from www.mmira.wildapricot.org/resources/Documents/MMIRA%20task%20force%20report%20Jan2016%20final.pdf

Plano Clark, V. L., & Badiee, M. (2010). Research questions in mixed methods research. In A. Tashakkori & C. Teddlie (Eds.), *Handbook of mixed methods in social & behavioral science* (2nd ed., pp. 275–304). Thousand Oaks, CA: Sage Publications.

Plano Clark, V. L., & Ivankova, N. V. (2016). *Mixed methods research: A guide to the field.* Thousand Oaks, CA: Sage Publications.

Sandelowski, M. (1996). Using qualitative methods in intervention studies. *Research in Nursing & Health, 19*(4), 359–364.

Sandhu, S., & Asrabadi, R. (1994). Development of an acculturative stress scale for international students: Preliminary findings. *Psychological Report, 75*, 135–448.

Sandhu, S., & Asrabadi, R. (1998). An acculturative stress scale for international students: A practical approach to stress management. In C. P. Zalaquett & R. J. Wood (Eds.), *Evaluating stress: A book of resources* (pp. 1–33). Lanham, MD: Scarecrow Press.

Shim, M., Johnson, B., Bradt, J., & Gasson, S. (2021). A mixed methods–grounded theory design for producing more refined theoretical models. *Journal of Mixed Methods Research, 15*(1), 61–86. doi:10.1177/1558689820932311

Tashakkori, A., & Creswell, J. W. (2007). The new era of mixed methods [Editorial]. *Journal of Mixed Methods Research, 1*(1), 3–7.

Tashakkori, A., & Teddlie, C. (2010). *Handbook on mixed methods in the behavioral and social sciences* (2nd ed.). Thousand Oaks, CA: Sage Publications.

Teddlie, C., & Tashakkori, A. (2003). Major issues and controversies in the use of mixed methods in the social and behavioral sciences. In A. Tashakkori & C. Teddlie (Eds.), *Handbook of mixed methods in social & behavioral research.* Thousand Oaks: Sage Publications.

15 Bringing It All Together
Effective Program Evaluation

Michael Walsh and Amy Allison

Introduction of Methodology

Program evaluation. The very words can strike fear and dread into the hearts of program staff and administrators alike. Visions of audits and reviewers, forms to fill out, onerous processes to follow ... dogs and cats living together ... ahhh!!! Stop the madness!!!

Relax! We have some good news for you: program evaluation doesn't have to be scary or a big hassle. Program evaluation can actually become one of a clinician's best tools. The secret is to design a program evaluation process that is both efficient and effective.

But ... I trained as a professional counselor, not a program evaluator. In recent years, there has been suggestion in the professional literature that professional counselors have a unique set of skills that lend themselves to effective program evaluation (Coleman, 2022). The ability to effectively join with and engage the needs, cultural values, and desires of clients is central counseling training. Here's the good news: According to the president of the American Evaluation Association, John Gargani (2016), these are the very same skills that can be effective in program evaluation! So, take heart. You can do this!

While there are a number of different definitions of program evaluation floating around in the professional literature, the streamlined definition is often the most useful. For our purposes, program evaluation can be defined as *a systematic collection of information about a program, or aspects of a program, in order to make decisions about that program* (Walsh & Balkin, 2017, Walsh & Stackpole, 2022). At its heart, program evaluation can be used to improve services and service delivery (Loesch, 2001). Recent trends in program evaluation have evolved to more closely examine the clinical significance of program evaluation results. As Lenz (2021) puts it: "the real-world meaningfulness that an intervention or program has on quality of life for clients or those with whom they interact." This enhanced focus on the real world impact of services represents an opportunity for professional counselors to enhance not only service quality, but also to present those results more clearly as evidence that our services are effective (Lenz, 2020a). Throughout this chapter, we'll look at some basics in program evaluation, such as sources of program evaluation information and the basic types of program evaluation. We'll also look at some best practices and basic steps in program evaluation, then we'll practice applying some of those best practices and basic steps to actual program examples. Finally, we'll take a look at two program evaluation models that lend themselves well to practitioners.

DOI: 10.4324/9781032706139-15

Down on the Farm: A Quick Look at Information Sources in Program Evaluation

Program evaluation is an essential tool for practitioners. Three types of feedback contribute to good program evaluation: External evaluation, internal evaluation, and stakeholder feedback. External evaluation means gathering feedback from an outside source. Internal evaluation comes from within (employees, program staff, etc.) and is often not obvious to outsiders. Stakeholder feedback is a more inclusive term. This type of feedback comes from anyone who may be benefiting from the program – clients, donors, staff, and so on. It is important to note that stakeholders may also be community members who benefit from the overall impact of your program. Good program evaluation is constant and contributes to everyday operations while helping to produce change based on the interests and input of multiple parties. In the following three sections, we'll use a story to examine the different sources of information in program evaluation: External evaluation, internal evaluation, and stakeholder feedback.

The Power of the External Evaluation

Let's say, for example, it is 1772 and you were working on your farm. Your task is to get water from the stream that runs through the valley to the carrot fields on the plateau. You, being a good farmer and the innovative type, might design a state-of-the-art bucket-carrying system that carries four buckets on a pole. You hump it down to the water, fill up your buckets, and start the long climb uphill. The hill is steep, and you are focused on the work of moving up the hill smoothly so that you keep spills to a minimum. Your eyes are constantly scanning the ground in front of you for rocks and slippery points so you can stay on track. All in all, the system works fairly well, and you find that you reach the top with most of the water. You're rocking right along!

One day, you run into your neighbor at the post office. (Post office? In 1772? I know, I know, work with me here, OK?) Your neighbor fills you in on what she sees when she watches you work. Your neighbor, watching you from across the valley as you work each day, notices that when you fill up the buckets on one side, you have to lean the pole down to fill the other side, causing some spillage. The buckets also jostle a bit as the pole bounces when you walk, causing slightly more spillage. You suspected this but have been so busy getting this vital job done that you haven't been able to take the time to think about fixing it. Your neighbor notes that, if you attached ropes to your buckets, then the buckets to the pole, it might solve this problem. You do, and it works! Remember the old saying: **"You don't know what you don't know."** External evaluation is helpful in helping us to figure out what we don't know by providing an extra pair of eyes from an outside perspective. You have improved your process as a result of the external feedback! This is the power of an **external evaluation**.

The Power of the Internal Evaluation

OK. You've gotten pretty good at this water-transporting business, and your farm has grown. You've hired some folks to carry some of the water and passed along your newly developed technology. Things are going fairly well.

One day, you notice that some workers are having more success than others. You gather your employees to discuss the differences. "I'm pretty short," one worker says, "and the ropes on the buckets are a bit too long. It slows me down." Another worker says, "I could carry more using a different setup. My legs are stronger than my shoulders."

You now have two new ideas that can improve your business, neither of which would have been obvious to an outsider. A Toltec saying applies here: **"Practice creates the master"** (Ruiz, 2001). The people that do the work are the masters. Getting their feedback into the program evaluation is a critical piece of any program evaluation process. This is the power of an **internal evaluation**.

The Power of Stakeholder Feedback

OK! Now you've got a thriving business, and you have incorporated some excellent feedback into the process of delivering your service. Life is good, right?

One day, after buying a batch of carrots from your field, a local merchant approaches you. "Your carrots are OK," he mentions, "but I've got to tell you, Lisa's carrots from the next valley over are just incredible. My local chefs have asked about switching over to her carrots in my market."

You are gobsmacked! You've just figured out a great way to do business, you've improved your overall program, crops are growing better than ever, and now the consumers want to buy different carrots!

"Wait," you say, "what do the chefs want in a carrot?"

The market owner thinks for a minute. "Ah, I think that I heard them say they want a softer flesh when cooked, but I'm not sure. I'm not a chef."

You think back to how your business has developed from other feedback.

"I've got an idea," you say. "Let's get all of the local chefs together and explore what they want and need in terms of produce. Maybe Lisa can produce the carrots and I can produce the leaf lettuce. That will play to both farms' strengths."

The chefs agree, the meeting takes place, and each farm makes the requested changes.

Bam! You've improved both the process of your business and its long-term prospects using feedback from stakeholders. As Helen Keller once said: **"Alone, we can do so little; together, we can do so much"** (Keller, 1996). That is the power of **stakeholder feedback**.

Terms Used in Program Evaluation: When Do We Use What?

Good program evaluation is a constant process of internal and external evaluation, along with client and stakeholder feedback. This process informs the everyday operation of the program, "feeds back" into the program design (why the farm exists), and changes are made based on what is in the best interests of all of the stakeholders.

In the helping professions, this can happen with a program that serves clients with depression or a program that serves people with severe mental illnesses, or it can happen in a counselor program that trains counselors. Good program evaluation is at home in any business.

There are as many potential program evaluation designs as there are types of programs. *The design and type of program evaluation depends on the questions we want to answer*. In our previous section, we explored different sources of program evaluation data. In the following section, we'll explore different types of program evaluation based on what we need to know about the outcomes of our program and/or the process of our program. Each type of program evaluation has its own format and its own goals.

Let's say we want to know about the impact of our program (outcomes) – specifically, whether our program is effective at helping clients with depression. This type of program evaluation is looking at **outcomes or the product** that we deliver. **Outcome-based** program evaluation is called **summative evaluation**. We're looking at the sum total, or the bottom line.

Does the program help people feel less depressed? (outcome/product). Other examples of summative evaluations may include program cost, program impact in the community, and program impact on clients.

Let's look at a graphic example of the summative evaluation design in Figure 15.1. We're wondering about whether our counseling program is effective in treating clients with depression. We'd look to our external feedback sources first: Hospitalization rates or opinions of any external reviewers (e.g., such as accreditation bodies). We'd then look at internal feedback sources (e.g., employees, staff members, staff psychiatrists). Finally, we'd look at stakeholder feedback sources (e.g., clients, clients' family members, community members). We'd use these three sources of data to form impressions of our overall program effectiveness, as demonstrated in Figure 15.2.

While an outcome of the program is a common goal of program evaluation, other program evaluation designs help to answer different questions. Let's say that we want to know about our program's process. Maybe we have questions about how effectively staff personnel are communicating with each other within the program. Since this question has to do with the **process** of how our program runs, it is a **process-based** or **formative evaluation**. In this evaluation, we're looking at how well staff communicate within the program as it is running. Does our staff communicate effectively (process)?

Let's look at Figure 15.3, a graphic example of this formative evaluation design. We'd utilize the same data sources: External feedback (e.g., reviewer opinions, reviewer's comments after speaking with program staff), internal feedback (e.g., employee comments, staff opinions on communication and efficiency), and stakeholder feedback (e.g., client's comments, client's family members feedback on the way that staff work together). This data, represented in Figure 15.4, would inform our conclusions on how well our program is functioning.

Other examples of formative evaluations include needs assessments, determining how clients define success, and examining how well a program operates in various phases.

While each of these designs can be used independently, in some settings, it may be important to understand both the process and outcomes of a program. We'll look at mixed-method designs as we move along.

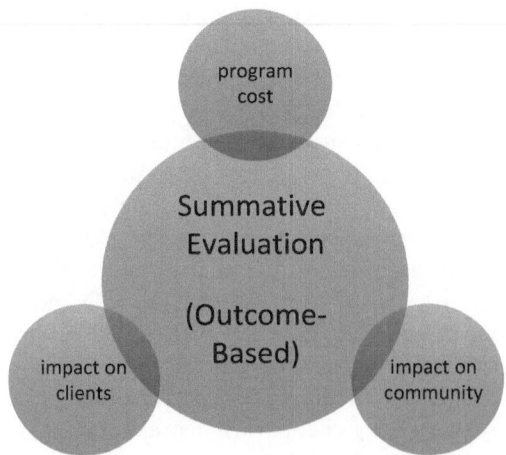

Figure 15.1 Summative (Outcome-Based) Evaluation.

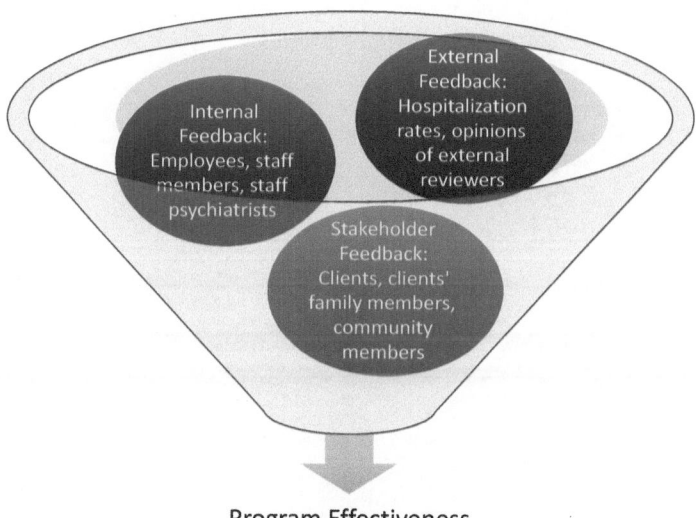

Figure 15.2 Feedback Types Informing the Summative Program Evaluation.

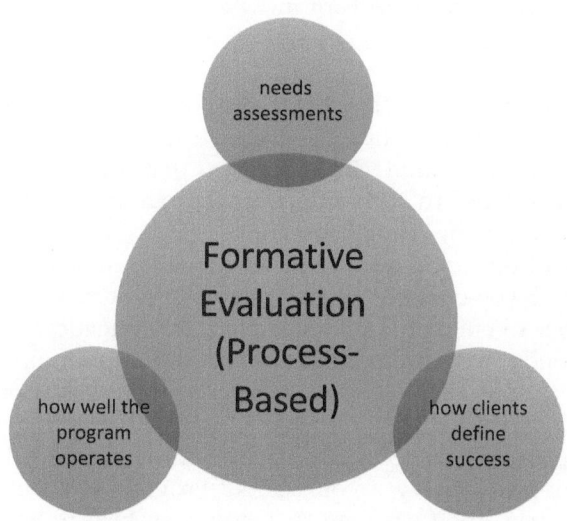

Figure 15.3 Formative (Process-Based) Evaluation.

Do We Really Need Program Evaluation? Who Can Afford That?

The term "program evaluation" gets thrown around a good bit in the larger nonprofit world. Donors often want to know whether the money that they donate is doing the good deeds it is supposed to be doing. Funders want to know that the grants they make are well placed or that the dollars they send to a program are being well spent. As a result, much of the information related to program evaluation has been developed for the larger world of big money and big systems (Kellaghan & Madaus, 2000) or has such discipline-specific language that it is difficult to apply it outside of its intended field (Astramovich & Coker, 2007).

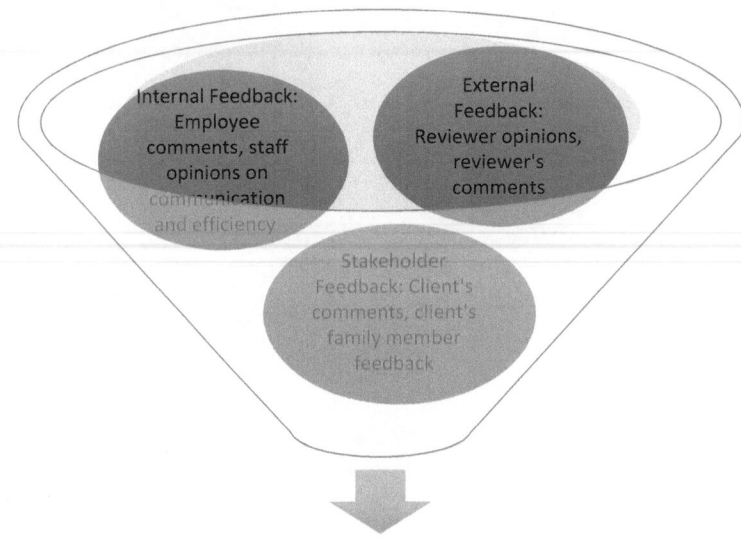

Program Functioning

Figure 15.4 Feedback Types Informing the Formative Program Evaluation.

As practitioners, we often need to scale these ideas down to fit our projects and programs. This involves financial as well as practical planning. As an example, the United States Office of Planning, Research and Evaluation (2010) suggests that the "rule of thumb" for planning program evaluation costs is 15% to 20% of the overall program budget. These are huge numbers, especially when considering a small operation.

Obviously, as a practitioner, you need to be able to scale these numbers to make them fit for the program in which you operate. When designing a program or budgeting for program needs, always remember to build in funding for program evaluation.

Further, as practitioners, we have an ethical obligation to make sure that the programs we deliver are effective. In the American Counseling Association's Code of Ethics (2014), Standard C.2.D states, "Counselors continually monitor their effectiveness as professionals and take steps to improve when necessary. Counselors take reasonable steps to seek peer supervision to evaluate their efficacy as counselors." Program evaluation is not a luxury, it is an obligation. Fortunately, good program evaluation can help to enhance a program. Just look what it did for our farm!

On another happy note, these ideas are very "scalable" to any size project. The secret is often in the program evaluation design. Specifically, many small programs, offices, or schools do not have large administrative staffs that can operate and monitor a complex program evaluation process. Many can be one- or two-person operations that work on a shoestring budget. If that is the case, it is important to *base your program evaluation in work you already do*. This will allow you the flexibility to respond to additional needs as they develop.

Finally, given the shift toward accountability in public policy, health care, and the helping fields in general, it is clear that a working knowledge of program evaluation (PE) and effective PE development is essential for helping professionals.

Trends in Program Evaluation: Clinical Significance and Quality of Life

The professional literature in health sciences has begun to call for the addition of clinical significance to the lexicon of good outcome research (Carpenter, Waldrop & Carter-Templeton, 2021). Concurrently, a recent trend in professional counseling program evaluation is the examination and intentional inclusion of clinical significance in program evaluation (Lenz, 2020b). Simply put: How much did our intervention contribute to the quality of life experienced by an individual or group? In other words, what was the practical impact of our program? That's a fundamentally important question! It prevents us from getting so focused on what we *think* about how our programs work that we ignore the ways in which they *actually impact* our clients or our students.

Why collect this data? It allows us to examine the practical significance of our interventions. It also allows us to challenge our assumptions. For example, we may examine the results of our program evaluation in Case Study #1 ahead and, sure enough, folks report a lower score on the Beck Anxiety Inventory. Our program is designed to reduce anxiety, and we've done that, yes? Well sure … but we are making an assumption here. Specifically, that a reduction in anxiety symptoms leads to a better quality of life for folks. So we add a quality of life measure into the medium effects category to get a measure of the ways in which the quality of life of the individual has been impacted. Problem solved, right? Maybe … but maybe not. There is some important information that could really improve our evaluation process. Curious as to what that may be? Let's look at the following program evaluation example (Case Study #1), and then we'll come back to the ways in which we can develop and use clinical significance data to enhance our program evaluation.

Sample Case Studies and Program Evaluation Questions

Program #1: Four-person private practice specializing in treating clients with anxiety disorders.

Problem: A funder wants program evaluation (outcomes) data, and the practice has no administrative staff available to compile data. The four partners in the practice also want to evaluate how successful they have been in treating clients for the past year. They also wonder if the practice is operating as efficiently as it could be (process).

Analysis: This program evaluation is looking for outcome (summative) data (are clients feeling less anxiety?) as well as process (formative) data, so this is likely to be a mixed-methods program evaluation.

Program #2: Mid-size counseling program in a university counseling center.

Problem: The trustees want a justification for spending the money on the counseling center. They simply want an answer to the question: Is this program helping our students?

Analysis: This program evaluation is looking solely for impact/outcome (summative) data.

Program # 3: Four-person private practice with a general caseload consisting of both adolescents and adults. These clients are mostly low income and utilize Medicaid to pay for services. The practice is enrolled as a Medicaid provider.

Problem: The state is now requiring the practice to be accredited. The practice must choose an accrediting body and begin the self-study process.

Analysis: This program evaluation will be driven, to a degree, by the standards called for by the accrediting body. The self-study and on-site reviews will examine both formative (process) data and summative (outcome/impact) data. Interestingly, most accrediting bodies deal more with process data than with outcomes. This makes sense when you think of the function of most accrediting bodies in the clinical world. They are primarily quality-improvement organizations designed to help organizations improve how they do things (process), which can lead to better outcomes. Their main focus is on helping organizations get better at doing what they do, which is mostly process.

Best Practices in Program Evaluation

As shown in Figure 15.5, The Centers for Disease Control (CDC, 2021) proposed six universal steps for effective program evaluation. In this section, we'll identify each of those six steps and apply each to our Program #3 as the case study.

Step One: Identify and Involve the Stakeholders

This means thinking about who benefits from the service. It also means thinking about program staff. Anyone who "has a horse in the race" is a stakeholder. That means clients, board members (if applicable), staff, and any interested vendors or third parties. It is very important to remember that while staff are also considered sources of internal evaluation data, staff are also stakeholders and, as such, can be an invaluable source of stakeholder data. Now, let's apply Step One to Case Study #3:

Case Study #3

In this case, clients are clearly stakeholders. As a part of the informed consent process, it is helpful to remind clients that, just like they are doing in their own lives, the practice always tries to improve and to grow. Asking permission up front to involve the client in the quality-improvement process is a best practice. Not only does this process model the growth and

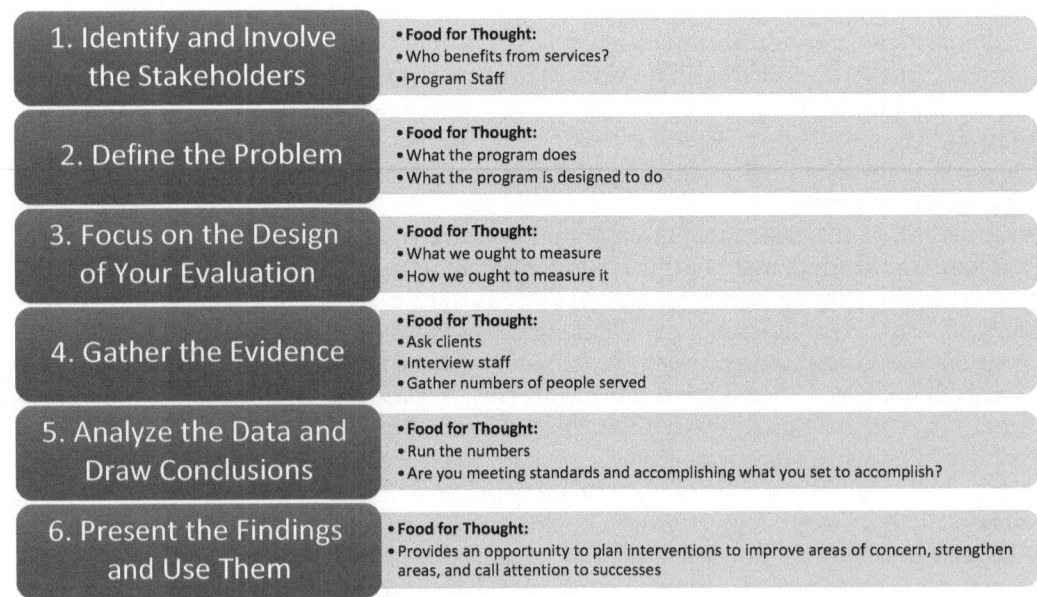

Figure 15.5 Best Practices in Program Evaluation According to the CDC.

development process for the client, it also allows the client to be at the heart of the program evaluation process. From an ethical standpoint, this makes sense, as we have a fiduciary duty to do what is in the best interests of those clients. Best of all, clients won't be surprised when you ask for feedback!

Staff are also stakeholders here. It is imperative that staff be involved in the program evaluation and quality-improvement process. This is a vital source of internal evaluation data!

The partners in the practice are also stakeholders in the process. It is their practice, after all! These folks are also great internal evaluation sources!

Third-party funders are stakeholders in this process. They have an interest, for example, in how well you are documenting your billing time and the services for which they are paying.

Interested third parties may be other organizations or agencies with whom you interact. Maybe you refer folks to the local vocational rehabilitation agency or the local mental health center. All of these "partner" agencies are stakeholders in how well your program functions. This feedback can be invaluable. Sometimes you get good ideas from these other organizations. Other times, they may provide a particularly valuable perspective. For example, they may say, "We've noticed that when you refer folks, they are sometimes confused as to exactly what it is we do." This provides you the opportunity to improve your process of educating those folks and thereby likely improving their ability to be successful with this additional service.

Finally, and not to be forgotten, there is the accrediting body itself. Examples may be: The Commission on Accreditation of Rehabilitation Facilities (CARF), the Joint Commission on Accreditation of Healthcare Organizations (JCAHO), or another accrediting body. These accrediting bodies are also known by another name: **Quality-improvement organizations (QIOs)**. They are designed to help organizations to improve and enhance their operations.

Now that we have identified the stakeholders, it is time to involve them. This may mean reaching out to clients and letting them know that, just like we discussed in our informed consent process, we need their input in our program evaluation process. A best practice here is never to burden a client with cumbersome tasks. Develop an estimate of how much time the feedback process will take and stick to it.

Step Two: Define the Program

This means thinking about exactly what the program does and what the program is designed to do. This allows you the opportunity to identify "program drift" or "mission creep." These are two things that commonly happen over time. A program that was designed to treat depression finds that it is dealing a good bit with anxiety, for example. The services then "drift" to cover the presented need. Soon, a program that was designed to treat just depression has "crept" into treating anxiety. No value judgment here. Again, this is very common. This step provides the program the opportunity to return to the mission statement of the organization and ask the questions: Are we still on target? Should the mission change? In short, you are asking the question: What is our program supposed to do?

Case Study #3: This Is a Counseling Private Practice With a Broad Mission to Meet the Complex Needs of Its Clients

Now that we have defined the program, we have a better sense of exactly what to measure. We now know that we are striving to meet the complex needs of our clients. That gives us some latitude, but it also offers us a very specific target. In our case, we also have a driving need to begin the accreditation process. That helps us in many ways. In an accreditation process, much of the evaluation design is dictated by the standards of the accrediting body, the self-study, and the on-site review processes. If we didn't have those standards and procedures as a road map, we'd just have to design our own PE plan. Fortunately, we now have a very clear definition of the process we need to follow as well as a very clear definition of our program. Without this critical step of clearly defining your program, you can't know what to measure!

Step Three: Focus the Design of Your Evaluation

This means thinking about what we ought to measure and how we ought to measure it. Do we want to know about outcomes? Do we want to know about process? Both?

It is now far more feasible to develop an evaluation plan on the basis of a clearly defined program. In this case, we have defined that our mission is to meet the complex needs of our clients. Now we can focus our design on exactly the area(s) in which we are most interested. Are we meeting those complex needs (summative)? and/or How are we doing that (formative)?

Case Study #3: Let's assume that we want to begin the self-study process for the Commission of the Accreditation of Rehabilitation Facilities (CARF). This will involve both formative and summative data gathering. The specific areas that we'll evaluate will be proscribed for us by CARF. We'll examine the 2024 Standards Manual for our type of accreditation to each standard. For example, in our setting, we would be using the behavioral health program standards. The self-study process would form the basis of the internal evaluation process. Once that self-study is complete and sent to CARF, an on-site evaluation (external evaluation) will be scheduled. It is at this meeting that the evidence gathered in the next phase will be presented. Evaluators will also speak with clients and stakeholders (stakeholder feedback) when they arrive.

This gives us the chance to triangulate our data a bit. Remember, we already spoke with staff as part of our internal evaluation process. When our external reviewers (on-site folks) also speak with staff, it provides us an opportunity to compare the answers that our staff and clients gave to us with those answers given to the reviewers. In this way, we have the opportunity to ensure that we are getting a complete and honest picture of our functioning that is free of undue influence. This concept of data triangulation is a critical one in assessment circles and is considered a best practice in evaluation. In this way, accreditation bodies help organizations to hit the key points (internal, external, and stakeholder-based) of the program evaluation process, and they also help us to ensure that our gathered data is accurate and well balanced.

In our example, for a CARF self-study, we are asked to examine each of the specific areas called for in the behavioral health standards. So, during the self-study, we'd utilize a variety of program evaluation tools, such as internal and external evaluation, stakeholder feedback, and evidence gathering. These program evaluation tools help us look at the following: Program structure and staffing, screening and access to services, individual treatment plans and progress notes, transition and recovery services, medication use policies and procedures, nonviolent practices (emergency procedures), and quality records review. We would look for evidence of how we are doing in each area and note any areas in which we come up short of the standards. We would then share the results of this self-study with the on-site reviewers (another example of a source of external evaluation data) and get their feedback on what they see as our strengths and areas for improvement.

That gives us an opportunity to leverage the experience and expertise of the on-site reviewers in the next step of the accreditation process. The important thing to remember here is that accrediting bodies are truly **QIOs**. The very best programs embrace this process and utilize it to enhance their programs.

Step Four: Gather the Evidence

This means actually gathering data. You may be asking questions of clients, gathering numbers of people served, or interviewing staff – whatever inquiries are appropriate for the information you need to gather.

Case Study #3: In this example, we would need the actual evidence that we have complied to a certain standard. While the self-study entails many different components as noted in Step Three, for the sake of an example, let's just look at standards related to transition and recovery services. In this evidence-gathering step, we'd be gathering examples of transition plans that our practice uses, whether that be the section of the treatment plan that addresses transition and discharge or whether we use a separate transition planning form. We would be gathering the actual examples that show the program meets that standard on an individual basis as well as on a systematic basis.

In other words, we will want to show evidence that we met the standard once and also show evidence that we have a system in place to meet that standard consistently. So, we may go to a specific client chart, pull out the section that deals with transition planning for that client, and use that example to show actual evidence that our program actively addressed that transition planning standard in that case. Further evidence may also be gathered, such as a copy of our blank treatment plan that contains a section entitled "transition plan." The first is evidence that we addressed the standard in a specific case. The second is evidence that the program addresses the standard systematically with each and every client.

It is never enough, in program evaluation, to say "Yep, we do that. I'm sure we do that somehow …". We always have to show actual evidence that it is being done in the form of a working example. In this way, we retain the integrity of the program evaluation process and can be certain that we are getting an accurate look at what we do and don't do and thus where we may need to change or alter our program to meet our stated mission/definition and become more effective and efficient. During our CARF on-site review, we would be presenting this evidence to the reviewers and brainstorming ways to strengthen any areas in which we came up a bit short.

Step Five: Analyze the Data and Draw Conclusions

In this step, you run the numbers. Are you meeting the standards? Are you accomplishing what your program set out to accomplish?

Case Study #3: In our example, this is the step in which we look at five transition plan records that we collected in Step Four and conclude: Yes! In five of five, we met the standard that insists we address transition and discharge in the treatment plan. That is 100% compliance with that particular standard. We'd do the same for other standards. Let's say that the standard calls for us to address the strengths, needs, abilities, and preferences (SNAP) for each client. Let's also say that, as we examine the evidence, we find that two of our clinicians always talk about the SNAP profile of each client, but the other two do it only occasionally. That's less than 60% compliance with that standard. We may then make a decision to add a SNAP section to our treatment planning document, thereby ensuring that we examine, in each treatment planning session, the strengths, needs, abilities, and preferences of each and every one of our clients.

Step Six: Present Your Findings and Use Them

Program evaluation is a waste of time and resources if you don't use the results. Presenting the results of program evaluations to the board, partners, staff, and other stakeholders is a critical step to beginning to use those results. This provides an opportunity to plan interventions designed to improve areas of concern, strengthen areas that need strengthening, and call attention to your successes. Program evaluation can and should be an opportunity to celebrate the good work that you do. Don't let that opportunity pass you by!

Our best practice steps applied to our Case Study #3 are shown in Figure 15.6.

Case Study #3 Wrap Up

In our example, we'd present the findings of our self-study, as well as the results of our on-site review, and look for ways to improve where needed. We'd also have the opportunity (and this is vital!) to go back to our mission statement and program design and look for opportunities to improve our overall design, mission, or functioning. In this way, effective program evaluation becomes a self-sustaining loop that helps the program to continually grow and improve (Box 15.1).

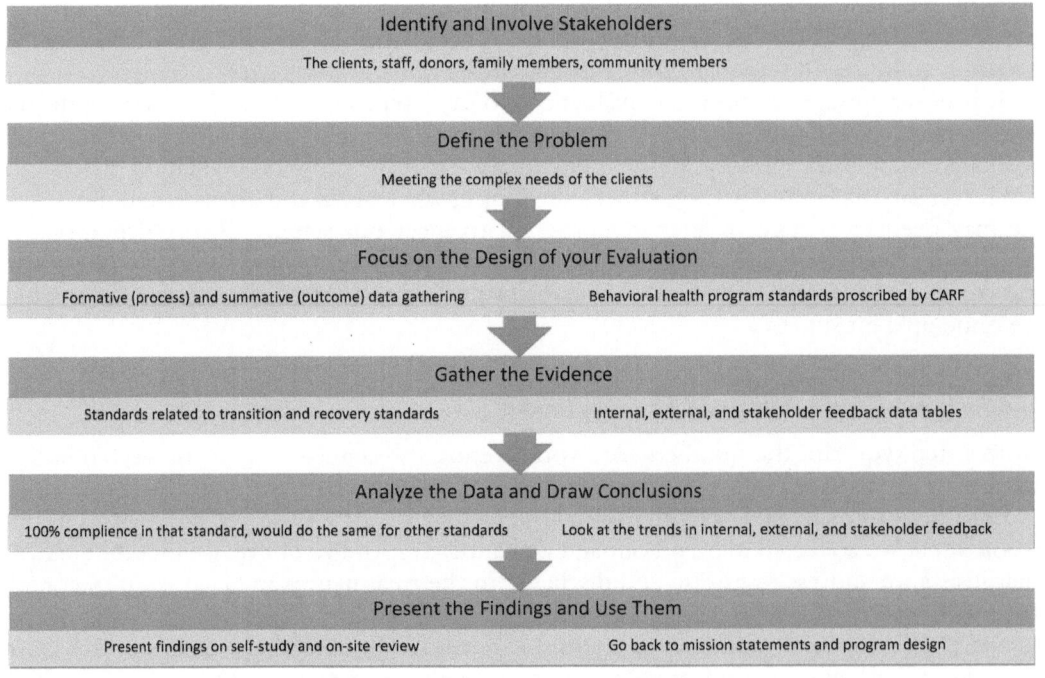

Figure 15.6 Best-Practice CDC Model Applied to Case Study #3.

Box 15.1   Practice Exercise

Apply the CDC Best Practice Steps to Case Studies #1 and #2

Look at the best practices steps in Figure 15.5. See if you can apply those steps to thinking about how you might go about designing a program evaluation plan for these two programs. Remember, these are case studies, so you may have to add some details (like a program focus and mission statement) to inform your process. Do the best you can. The more you can get into the habit of thinking like a program evaluator, the more naturally the PE process will flow for you. Pay particular attention to the Food for Thought sentences next to each step. These are the questions that will help you to plan and design the most effective program evaluation for any given program.

Models of Program Evaluation

Models of program evaluation combine the best practices mentioned earlier into a series of steps that help us to ensure we have considered all that we can in developing and designing our program evaluation plan. These models help us to visualize and conceptualize our overall program evaluation approach, and they help us to consider the many different program evaluation data sources. In this way, we have the chance to combine all of what we have learned about program evaluation into a cohesive approach that seeks to maximize our effectiveness in getting our questions answered. This section will look at two models of program evaluation that may lend themselves to adaptation in the helping professions field.

Logic Model

Joseph Wholey (1979) developed a model that breaks the program evaluation process down into workable "chunks" and then presents them in a graphic model designed to help the user understand the flow of the organization while also posing basic questions about the program's effectiveness. Logic models have been utilized in the counseling field; most recently, a logic model was developed in order to evaluate the ASCA national model in school counseling (Martin & Carey, 2014). Such work shows the applicability and adaptability of the logic model concept.

Wholey's logic model starts with a "situation statement" that is designed to sum up and present the need for the program, along with the circumstances surrounding it.

Taylor-Powell and Henert (2008) give us the basics of logic modeling:

* *baseline* – information about the situation or condition prior to intervention;
* *impact indicator* – evidence that an impact is being achieved;
* *inputs* – resources that go into programming such as staff time, materials, money, equipment, and so forth;
* *outputs* – the activities, products, and participation resulting from program activities;
* *outcomes* – results or changes from the program; the outcomes can range from immediate (short term) to intermediate (medium term) to final (long term).

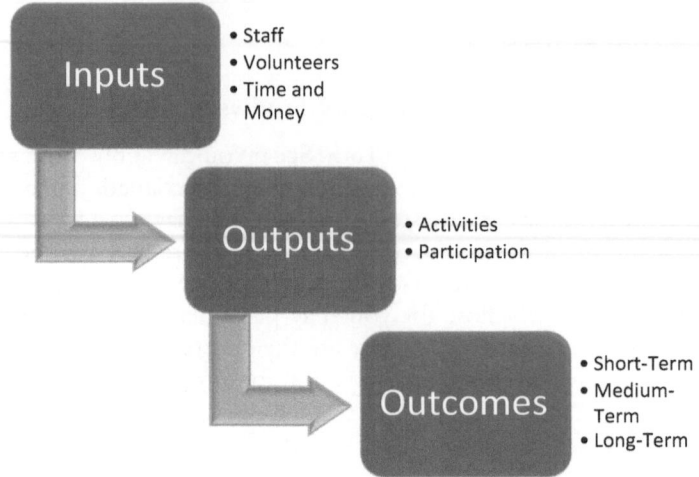

Figure 15.7 Generic Basic Steps of Logic Model.

Figure 15.7 shows an example of a basic logic model framework, which includes the components noted by Taylor-Powell and Henert (2008).

Logic Model in Action

Let's use Case Study #1 to illustrate the logic model concept in action:

Case Study #1 Situation: Four-person private practice specializing in treating clients with anxiety disorders.

Situation: A funder wants program evaluation (outcomes) data and the practice has no administrative staff available to compile data. The four partners in the practice also want to evaluate how successful they have been in treating clients for the past year. They also wonder if the practice is operating as efficiently as it could be.

Assumptions: Effective individual and group interventions can lead to better coping strategies. Better coping can lessen the symptoms of anxiety. Fewer anxiety symptoms may lead to better quality of life.

Inputs: Four counselors at $30/hour, rent at $1,000 per month, utilities at $10 per day, insurance and indirect costs at $85 per day.

Outputs: Client participation in one session per week, enrollment in a client support group for an additional hour per week, and client "homework" approximately a half hour each week. Client evaluation using Quality of Life Scale and Beck Anxiety Inventory (BAI).

Outcomes: Clients show a 22% reduction in week 2 of the BAI score (short term), clients report a 36% increase in the Quality of Life Scale by week 4 (medium term), followed by an overall 32% reduction in BAI score after week 6 (long term). This reduction stays stable for the measured timeframes.

First, we'll apply these basic steps and get a quick "down-and-dirty" look at inputs, outputs, and outcomes (see Figure 15.8). This is sometimes a helpful first step, as it allows us a quick peek at the "bottom line" features important to summative program evaluation designs.

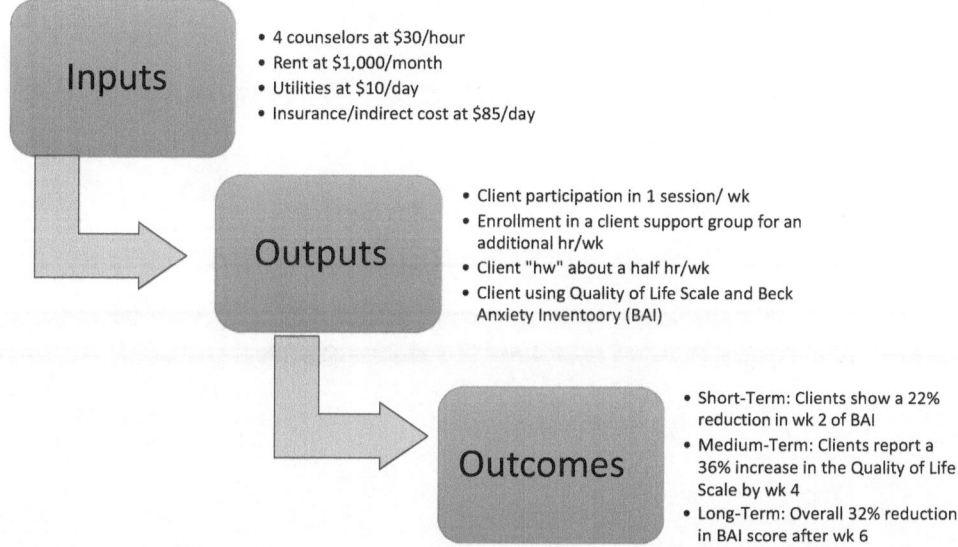

Figure 15.8 Logic Model Inputs, Output, and Outcomes Steps Applied to Case Study #1.

The Logic Model's Fundamental Program Evaluation Question

The fundamental program evaluation question for Case Study #1: Is the program, given its situation and assumptions, worth the input cost (staff time and resources devoted to operations) and output costs (client effort and participation) for the short-, medium-, and long-term returns on the investment? Now that we've gotten a quick look at the bottom line, we'll next plug our Case Study #1 into a full logic model and see how the logic model process may be helpful in examining our program in a good deal more depth (Box 15.2). But first …

Box 15.2   Pop Quiz Question

Is the example a summative evaluation or a formative evaluation?[1]

Keep in mind: Logic models can also be helpful in formative designs in that they help us to examine multiple facets of the program and present those facets in a graphic that is easy to follow. We are then better able to understand the ways in which different things connect and flow within our program, which helps us to better understand formative (process) questions. Let's take a look at Case Study #1 using a full logic model.

Case Study # 1 Logic Model Discussion

As you can see in Figure 15.9, this logic model allows us to see, at a glance, the effectiveness of our program (summative data) in the form of the 22% decrease in the BAI score in week 2, the 36% increase in the Quality of Life scores by week 4, and the 32% overall reduction in BAI scores after week 6. This model also gives us a graphic look at how our program "fits together." We can also see the assumptions under which we choose to operate, and we can check those

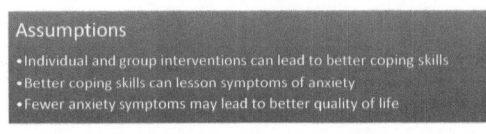

Figure 15.9 Full Logic Model Applied to Case Study #1.

* Note: Above graphic adapted from University of Wisconsin-Extension, Cooperative Extension, Program Development & Evaluation's Logic Model (Powell, Steele, & Douglah, 2013).

Credit: Adapted from University of Wisconsin-Extension, Cooperative Extension, Program Development & Evaluation's Logic Model

assumptions against the actual data (i.e., Do fewer anxiety symptoms lead to improved quality of life?). In our case, we can see that it seems that our assumptions are holding up against the actual data. If they were not, we would then have the opportunity to change our program, and we may be able to see exactly where the change would have the most impact.

As you may have noted, there is an external factors section that also influences our results. Let's say, for example, that we encountered a 40% reduction in service availability due to a funding source deciding to approve less of our services. We would then have the opportunity to see if that external factor made an impact. We could also use this same model to look for ways to offset that impact. We could, for example, note that we are only utilizing one half hour of "homework" per week. Given the service reduction, might we want to enhance our use of homework? Are there other opportunities to improve our outcomes or processes? What potential opportunities do you see?

Putting Clinical Significance to Work in Program Evaluation

Let's return to Case Study #1 and our program evaluation process. Clinical significance has to do with quality of life … and we have a quality of life measure. We're golden, right?!

See … we don't know what the quality of life score may have been was before our intervention! So … a better way to intentionally include quality of life data would be to use a pre and post methodology and include a quality of life measure prior to our intervention (baseline) and then employ that same measure after our intervention. Pre and post methodology has been indicated in past studies to be a best practice in the program evaluation process, while the addition of follow up/follow on data gathering may be even more robust (Roberts & Ilardi, 2003).

How might that work? We could utilize a complex statistical approach in which we weigh the various outcome data numbers using a structural equation modeling (SEM) approach. This idea was advanced by Alessandri, Zuffianò, and Perinelli (2017). In essence, this involves using the professional literature and our experience to develop a theory about the ways that our various program elements come together and using that theory to design an equation to "test" that theory. We then would load that equation and the outcomes scores into software that "models" the data and reports on the relationships between the variable that we measured (measured variables), as well as those variables that are harder to measure directly (latent variables). While a complete exploration of that approach is beyond the scope of this chapter, the aforementioned Alessandri, Zuffianò & Perinelli (2017) article is excellent. If you'd like to learn more about using SEM as a tool, please check out Kline (2016), *Principles and Practice of Structural Equation Modeling*, 4th Edition.

Another way of collecting quantitative data on Clinical Significance was advanced by Blanchard and Schwarz (1988) and is called the percent improvement measure. This is an approach that has been used in professional counseling (Balkin & Russo, 2021; Ikonomopoulos et al., 2021). Lenz (2020a) details this measure as follows:

"A proportion representing intervention gains with respect to pre-intervention severity/functioning." Here is how it is expressed/calculated:

$$\text{Percent Improvement} = 100 \times \frac{\text{Preintervention Scores} - \text{Postintervention Scores}}{\text{Preintervention Scores}}$$

In our Case Study #1, then, we would need the preintervention baseline Beck Anxiety Inventory average for our group, and the postintervention Beck Anxiety Inventory average for our group. Then, we'd divide that number by our preintervention average score and then multiply by 100. That would give us the percent improvement for our group and enable us to both evaluate and to tell the story of the clinical significance/impact of our intervention. This sort of straightforward and easy to understand approach benefits us by helping us to more clearly understand our program's practical impact. It can also help by providing us with an easy-to-understand way for outside stakeholders to appreciate the impact of our program. In the current environment of increased accountability and shrinking funding sources, this can be an invaluable asset.

Finally, we may even collect qualitative data (word-based data from interviews with participants) from our clients after our intervention inquiring as to their perception of what was most meaningful in the quality of life change. This could lead to insights on what worked as well as insights on things like ease of access to services, interactions with program staff, and so on. This way, we can gather good quantitative data about our program while also gathering good qualitative data about both outcome (**summative**) and process (**formative**).

Gathering this data allows us to represent the clinical significance of our data in a way that maximizes both efficiency and clarity. This allows us to use the program evaluation process to enhance the quality of the program, and also to better illustrate the practical impact of our programs to potential funders and community stakeholders (Box 15.3).

Box 15.3   Practice Exercise 2

Apply the logic model and Clinical Significance Assessment to a program with which you are familiar

Ask yourself: Does this logic model help me to better understand this program and the way it works (formative assessment)? What does the logic model indicate about the way the program works? Are there areas for improvement that are apparent after examining the logical structure? Is the program worth the input and output costs (summative assessment)? How can I/Do I have a better sense of the practical impact of my program? How can I use that data to enhance my program? To tell the program's story to stakeholders?

Accountability Bridge Model

As noted in Walsh and Stackpole (2022), the accountability bridge model (Astramovich & Coker, 2007) combines the clinical evaluation steps typical in the counseling field with modern and very important business and accountability concepts popular in the corporate world (Ernst & Hiebert, 2002). The resulting accountability bridge takes into account the unique context and needs of a program while supporting the need for interactive and ongoing efficiency evaluation (Astramovich & Coker, 2007). It is this attention to the unique context of the program as well as to the process of gathering data that makes the accountability bridge unique. Though the accountability bridge is a model designed from counseling program evaluation, it can be applied to other fields and specialties within the helping professions.

As you can see in Figure 15.10, the central hubs of the accountability bridge are the counseling program evaluation cycle and the counseling context evaluation cycle. This represents, according to Astramovich and Coker (2007), *"an ongoing refinement of services based on outcomes, stakeholder feedback, and needs of the population served."* In other words, the feedback of all stakeholders, including clients, is constantly being fed back into the program

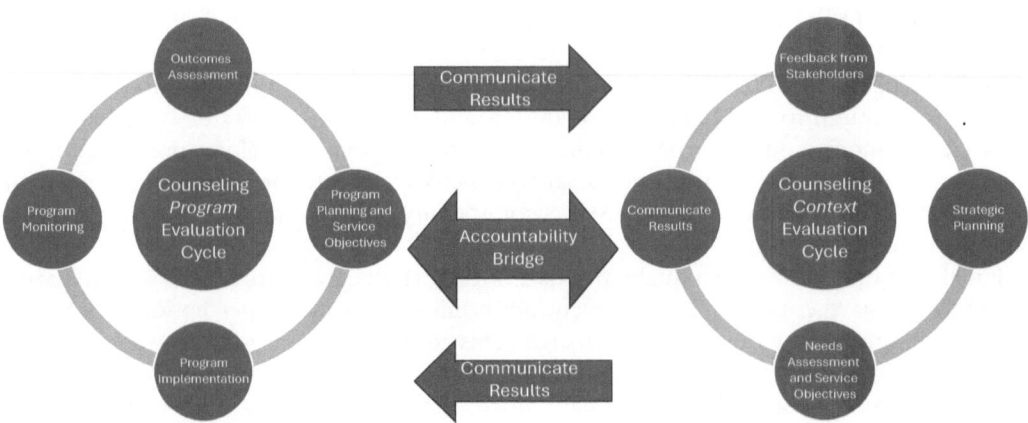

Figure 15.10 Accountability Bridge Model.

Source: Astramovich & Coker, 2007, used with permission.

design and evaluation process, allowing for the ongoing needs of the program to be accounted for, in addition to accounting for the ongoing environment and context of the program.

Consumer-driven service design is acknowledged as a best practice (Fenton, 2003; Fischer, 2006; Hamann et al., 2005). Using the accountability bridge, this consumer feedback is leveraged to its full potential while continuously being tested and refined, while the unique needs and context of the program are also considered. This allows for more culturally competent and community-driven program evaluation.

Accountability Bridge Applied

Let's apply Case Study #2 to the accountability bridge and see if it can help.

Case Study #2: Mid-size counseling program in a university counseling center.
Problem: The trustees want a justification for spending the money on the counseling center. They simply want an answer to the question: Is this program helping our students?
Analysis: This program evaluation is looking solely for impact/outcome (summative) data.

The hubs around which we'll build our accountability bridge are:

1. The counseling center's program evaluation cycle.
   The program's program evaluation cycle likely occurs periodically as accreditation visits happen, so we can start there. We can also assume that, because the trustees have asked questions, more program evaluation than normal is likely. That helps us to understand the type of data we'll be getting. We know, for example, since it is an accreditation-related process, we're likely to get lots of formative (process) data during the PE process. That's good, but it doesn't necessarily help us to answer the trustees' question, which seems to be much more summative (outcome-oriented) in nature. That's OK, though, because we know there will likely be more data than we need to answer the basic questions here.
2. The counseling program's unique evaluation context.
   We know that the trustees are looking for summative (outcome) data, and that is driving this particular round of PE. We also know (see earlier) that we will have accreditation data – see how one feeds the other? – so we'll be able to find formative data that backs up the summative data. That will likely help with the trustees. In this case, as we move through the process, we can see a wealth of opportunities to connect different pieces of the PE process.

Let's apply our universal steps and the accountability bridge:

First, we identify the stakeholders. In this case, clients are clearly stakeholders, but so are our trustees! This gives us the chance to involve them from the beginning. What are their concerns? Fears? Hopes? We now have an opportunity to work that feedback directly into our program evaluation process. This helps to bring the trustees aboard as allies, as opposed to "judge and jury," thus, possibly enhancing buy-in. It also allows a funder to have direct input into our evaluation process. That enhances both trust and the opportunity to design a program that is more efficient.

Second, we define the program. This is our second hub, so we can work to define exactly what the mission of the counseling center is. We involve our stakeholders and gain feedback from clients on this question (What would you want your counseling center to do?), trustees (What do you hope that we do?), and staff (What do you wish that we would do?) and feed the answers to all of these questions directly back into our program-design loop. In this way, we become a dynamic and growing organization that is responsive to stakeholder needs and desires as opposed to a static entity.

Third, we focus on our design. Using the feedback loop, what should we be looking at? Are we doing what we want to be doing? Where should we look? How might that help, given all of our stakeholder concerns and questions?

Fourth, we gather the evidence. This is great, because we are gathering the exact evidence that we need. Best of all, having involved our staff and internal stakeholders, we aren't burdening them with new and unexpected tasks. They are more likely to buy in and are very likely to have given us invaluable ideas on efficient ways to gather this data. These may even be ways we would have never come up with ourselves!

Fifth, we crunch the numbers. This gives us an incredible chance to look at our program critically but in full context. It gives us a chance to celebrate our successes and plan for improvement, knowing we have complete buy-in from stakeholders and partners.

Sixth, we present the findings and use them. Again, we have advance buy-in here. Trustees are informed by outcome data that solidifies their commitment. Additionally, we are able to back up the summative data we present to them with valuable formative data that helps them to understand our unique needs and contexts.

In short, the accountability bridge helps all stakeholders, program staff, and administrators to have ownership of the program evaluation process. Ownership leads to buy-in, and buy-in leads to better data. Better data, you guessed it … leads to better program evaluation! In this way, a good program evaluation design is as important a tool as good program staff (Box 15.4).

Box 15.4   Practice Exercise 3

Apply the Accountability Bridge Model to a Program with Which You Are Familiar

Ask yourself: Does this model help me to better understand this program and the way it works? What stakeholders need to be involved? How could we make that happen? How might it help? What does this model indicate about the way the program works? Are there areas for improvement that are apparent after examining the context of this model? How about opportunities to improve the program evaluation process itself?

How might *you* incorporate the concept of clinical significance be incorporated into this model? It might fit on the Context side of the wheel, right? In the Feedback from Stakeholders or the Needs Assessment piece. That's a great place to add data on practical impact and quality of life from clients and families, yes? And … might it not *also* fit on the Program side? Maybe in the Program Monitoring and Outcome Assessment areas? In other words, we can the *systematic collection of the data* to the Program side and the *actual data and use of the data* to the Context side. This way, we are systematically gathering, processing, and utilizing the clinical significance data to inform and enhance our program. And that's the name of the game: Program evaluation!

Chapter Summary

We first took a trip down to the old farm. I know ... 1772, right? At the farm, we took a look at the vital sources of information for effective program evaluation: Internal evaluation, external evaluation, and stakeholder feedback. Truly effective program evaluation involves all three of those sources.

We then examined the different types of program evaluation that are typically done: Summative (outcome-based) evaluations or formative (process-based) evaluations. We agreed that both could be required (mixed methods), and we looked at a variety of different cases across a range of clinical settings.

We took a look some recent trends in program evaluation like clinical significance and the use of various tools to assess and utilize that data.

We worked with the six universal steps for effective program evaluation design and applied those steps to a specific case study. We also utilized two additional case studies in different contexts. We examined a small private practice, a university counseling center, and a medium-sized private practice in the context of effective program evaluation design.

We also looked at two powerful tools in program evaluation, logic modeling and accountability bridge modeling, and then we applied case studies with these models. Throughout our exploration, we had practice sections with questions for reflection and review.

Practice-Based Application

Think about the client-presenting concern, symptom, or situation that you identified in Chapter 1, and use that to answer the following questions:

- If you were to design a program to address the presenting concern, symptom, or situation you identified in Chapter 1, how might you use the CDC recommendations to design a good way to evaluate whether that program was working?
- How might you go about about identifying and communicating with all of the stakeholders in your newly developed program?
- How might you incorporate both formative (process) and summative (outcome-including clinical significance) into your accountability bridge for your program?

Resources for More Information

Program Evaluation

The program manager's guide to program evaluation (Office of planning research and evaluation). (2010). Retrievedfromwww.acf.hhs.gov/opre/resource/the-program-managers-guide-to-evaluation-second-edition

Logic Modeling

Accountability bridge model. (Astramovich & Coker, 2007). Retrieved from www.counseling.org/knowledge-center/vistas/by-subject2/vistas-assessment/docs/default-source/vistas/introducing-the-accountability-bridge-model-a-program-evaluation-framework-for-school-counselors
Program evaluation: Logic Modeling-University of Wisconsin-Extension. (2013). Retrieved from http://fyi.uwex.edu/programdevelopment/logic-models/

Clinical Significance (Lenz, 2021). Retrieved from: https://www.tandfonline.com/doi/full/10.1080/21501378.2021.1877097

For an examination of the use of clinical significance in recent professional counseling literature, please see:Jessica M. Holm, Elizabeth A. Prosek, Justin R. Lockhart, Melanie S. Rawls & Jessica Gerthe. (2023) Program Evaluation of a Community-Engaged Partnership Between a Counselor Preparation Program and Adult Probation Services. *Counseling Outcome Research and Evaluation* 15, pages 1–17.

A. Stephen Lenz, Danielle A. Pester, Kami Tran, Karen Buckwalter, Kelly Green & Debbie Reed. (2023) A Non-Inferiority Evaluation of Standard and Abbreviated Developmental Trauma and Adjustment Programming for Adopted and Foster Youth in Residential Care. *Residential Treatment For Children & Youth* 41, pages 1–19.

Danielle A. Pester, A. Stephen Lenz, Karen Doyle Buckwalter, Kelly Green, Debbie Reed & Christin Dobbs. (2023) Evaluation of the Developmental Trauma and Attachment Program for Decreasing Disruptive Behavior Among Adolescents in a Residential Setting. *Counseling Outcome Research and Evaluation* 14:2, pages 108–121.

Javier Cavazos Vela, James Ikonomopoulos, Clarissa Salinas & Elizabeth Zamora. (2023) Using Quantitative Research Designs to Conduct Outcome-Based Research with Children and Adolescents. *Journal of Child and Adolescent Counseling* 9:2, pages 149–169.

For an exploration of Using Counseling Skills in Program Evaluation, please see:Coleman, M. L. (2022). The Use of Counseling Skills Within Evaluative Contexts. *Counseling Outcome Research & Evaluation*, *13*(1), 22–29. https://doi.org/10.1080/21501378.2022.2025771

A. Stephen Lenz. (2022) Counseling Program Evaluation: A Key Pathway Through Implementation, Improvement, and Social Change. *Counseling Outcome Research and Evaluation* 13:1, pages 1–2.

Carl John Sheperis & Bryan Bayles. (2022) Empowerment Evaluation: A Practical Strategy for Promoting Stakeholder Inclusion and Process Ownership. *Counseling Outcome Research and Evaluation* 13:1, pages 12–21.

Questions for Further Review and Application

(See Practice Exercises throughout the chapter).

A Word From the Authors

Our hope is that each of us now has a new program evaluation toolkit. Whether it is a fresh, new vocabulary surrounding program evaluation types, experience in using the six universal steps to program evaluation and design, new skill in developing logic models, or new skill in deploying the accountability bridge model of program evaluation, my invitation to each of you is to reach into that toolkit often. These conceptual tools (logic modeling, accountability bridges, clinical significance) only work efficiently when you become familiar enough with them that they become cognitive habits. Pull out these tools and practice exercises often, play with them, make them your own.

Having been active in the professional clinical world for almost 17 years, we can tell you that folks who are skilled in program evaluation are some of the most in-demand folks in the field. Perhaps this is because many are intimidated by program evaluation and all it entails; maybe they fear finding that a service isn't effective (Lusky & Hayes, 2001), or maybe they lack training in program evaluation (Whiston, 1996) or the skill to apply the results (Isaacs, 2003). Those that are not intimidated and those that have some skill with these concepts tend to thrive in the helping fields. They also tend to get their professional needs met more often because they have skills to make the case that their services are both vital and of value to organizations and communities. As Mike's grandfather used to say, the buffet is open. Feel free to make any of this your own. May your own buffet always be as full as you want it to be.

—Michael Walsh, PhD, LPC, CRC, and Amy Allison, MRC, CRC

Note

1   Answer: Summative! This is an outcome-based (summative) question – based on BAI and Quality of Life scores—and therefore a summative design. Did you get this one right?

References

Alessandri, G., Zuffianò, A., & Perinelli, E. (2017). Evaluating Intervention Programs with a Pretest-Posttest Design: A Structural Equation Modeling Approach. *Frontiers in psychology*, *8*, 223. https://doi.org/10.3389/fpsyg.2017.00223

American Counseling Association. (2014). *ACA code of ethics*. https://www.counseling.org/resources/aca-code-of-ethics.pdf

Astramovich, R. L., Coker, K. J. (2007). Program evaluation: The accountability bridge model for counselors. *Journal of Counseling & Development*, *85*(2), 162–172.

Balkin, R. S., & Russo, G. M. (2021). Evaluating perceptions of working alliance and crisis stabilization for adolescent males in residential treatment for substance abuse: A time-series analysis. *Counseling Outcome Research and Evaluation*, *12*(1), 4–15.

Blanchard, E. B., & Schwarz, S. P. (1988). Clinically significant changes in behavioral medicine. *Behavioral Assessment*, *10*(2), 171–188.

Carpenter, R., Waldrop, J.B., & Carter-Templeton, H.D. (2021). Statistical, practical and clinical significance and Doctor of Nursing Practice projects. *Nurse Author & Editor*, *31*(3–4): 50–53.

Centers for Disease Control. (2021). *Evaluation steps*. Retrieved from www.cdc.gov/eval/steps/index.htm

Coleman, M. L. (2022). The Use of Counseling Skills Within Evaluative Contexts. *Counseling Outcome Research & Evaluation*, *13*(1), 22–29. https://doi.org/10.1080/21501378.2022.2025771

Ernst, K., Hiebert, B. (2002). Toward the development of a program evaluation business model: Promoting the longevity of counselling in schools. *Canadian Journal of Counselling*, *36*, 73–84.

Fenton, W. S. (2003). Shared decision making: A model for the physician-patient relationship in the 21st century? *Acta Psychiatrica Scandinavica*, *107*, 401–402.

Fischer, E. P. (2006). Shared decision-making and evidence-based practice: A commentary. *Community Mental Health Journal*, *42*(1), 107–111.

Gargani, J. (2016, May). Message from the president – Why evaluation and design? AEA Newsletter. https://www.eval.org/Full-Article/aea-newsletter-may-2016

Hamann, J., Cohen, R., Leucht, S., Busch, R., Kissling, W. (2005). Do patients with schizophrenia wish to be involved in decisions about their medical treatment? *American Journal of Psychiatry*, *162*, 2382–2384.

Ikonomopoulos, J., Garza, K., Weiss, R., & Morales, A. (2021). Examination of treatment progress among college students in a university counseling program. *Counseling Outcome Research and Evaluation*, *12*(1), 30–42. https://doi.org/10.1080/21501378.2020.1850175

Isaacs, M. L. (2003). Data-driven decision making: The engine of accountability. *Professional School Counseling*, *6*, 288–295.

Kellaghan, T., and Madaus, G. F. (2000). Outcome evaluation. In D. L. Stufflebeam, G. F. Madaus, T. Kellaghan (Eds.), *Evaluation models: Viewpoints on educational and human services evaluation* (2nd ed., pp. 97–112). Boston, MA: Kluwer Academic.

Keller, H. (1996). *The story of my life*. Dover Publications.

Kline, R. B. (2016). *Principles and Practice of Structural Equation Modeling* (4th ed.) New York, NY: The Guilford Press.

Lenz, A. S. (2020a). Estimating and reporting clinical significance in counseling research: Inferences based on percent improvement. *Measurement and Evaluation in Counseling and Development*, *53*(4), 289–296. https://doi.org/10.1080/07481756.2020.1784758

Lenz, A. S. (2020b). The future of Counseling Outcome Research and Evaluation. *Counseling Outcome Research and Evaluation*, *11*(1), 1–3. https://doi.org/10.1080/21501378.2020.1712977

Lenz, A.S. (Editor) (2021) Clinical Significance in Counseling Outcome Research and Program Evaluation, *Counseling Outcome Research and Evaluation*, 12:1, 1–3, https://doi.org/10.1080/21501378.2021.1877097

Loesch, L. C. (2001). Counseling program evaluation: Inside and outside the box. In D. C. Locke, J. E. Myers, E. L. Herr (Eds.), *The handbook of counseling* (pp. 513–525). Thousand Oaks, CA: Sage Publications.

Lusky, M. B., Hayes, R. L. (2001). Collaborative consultation and program evaluation. *Journal of Counseling & Development*, *79*, 26–38.

Martin, I., Carey, J. C. (2014). Development of a logic model to guide evaluations of the ASCA National Model for School Counseling Programs. *The Professional Counselor*, *4*, 455–466.

Powell, E. T., Steele, S., Douglah, M. (2013). *Planning a program evaluation*. Madison, WI: Division of Cooperative Extension of the University of Wisconsin-Extension.

Taylor-Powell, E., Henert, E. (2008). *Developing a logic model: Teaching and training guide*. Madison, WI: University of Wisconsin-Extension, Cooperative Extension, Program Development and Evaluation. Retrieved from www.uwex.edu/ces/pdande

Roberts, M. C. & Ilardi, S. S. (2003*). Handbook of Research Methods in Clinical Psychology*. Oxford: Blackwell Publishing.

Ruiz, M. (2001). *The four agreements: A practical guide to personal freedom*. Amber-Allen Publishing.

United States Office of Planning, Research and Evaluation (2010) *The Program Manager's Guide to Evaluation* (2nd ed.). Washington, DC.: Office of Planning, Research and Evaluation Administration for Children and Families U.S. Department of Health and Human Services.

Walsh, M., Balkin, R. (2017). Program evaluation. In Balkin (Ed.), *Counseling research: A scholar-practitioner approach to research in the counseling profession*. Alexandria, Virginia: American Counseling Association.

Walsh, M., Stackpole, K. (2022). Program evaluation. In Balkin (Ed.), *Counseling research: A scholar-practitioner approach to research in the counseling profession*, (2nd ed.). Alexandria, Virginia: American Counseling Association.

Whiston, S. C. (1996). Accountability through action research: Research methods for practitioners. *Journal of Counseling & Development, 74,* 616–623.

Wholey, J. (1979). *Evaluation: Promise and performance*. Washington, DC: Urban Institute Press.

Index

Pages in **bold** refer to tables.